*For Churchill Livingstone:*

*Commissioning Editor:* Ninette Premdas
*Project Development Manager:* Mairi McCubbin
*Project Manager:* Andrew Palfreyman
*Designer:* Sarah Russell
*Illustrations Manager:* Bruce Hogarth
*Illustrator:* Graeme Chambers

# Surgical Nursing
# of Children

**Margaret A. Chambers** BSc(Hons) MSc PGDipEd
RGN RSCN DPSN RNT
*Senior Lecturer in Children's Nursing, University of Plymouth, Plymouth, UK*

**Sue Jones** BSc(Hons) MSc RGN RSCN
*Assistant Director of Nursing, Practice Development, Trust Headquarters,*
*United Bristol Healthcare NHS Trust, Bristol, UK*

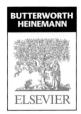

BUTTERWORTH
HEINEMANN

ELSEVIER

Edinburgh  London  New York  Oxford  Philadelphia  St Louis  Sydney  Toronto 2007

BUTTERWORTH
HEINEMANN
An imprint of Elsevier Limited

First published 2007

ISBN 10: 0 7506 4807 4
ISBN 13: 978 0 7506 4807 3

**British Library Cataloguing in Publication Data**
A catalogue record for this book is available from the British Library

**Library of Congress Cataloging in Publication Data**
A catalog record for this book is available from the Library of Congress

**Notice**
Medical knowledge is constantly changing. Standard safety precautions must be followed, but as new research and clinical experience broaden our knowledge, changes in treatment and drug therapy may become necessary or appropriate. Readers are advised to check the most current product information provided by the manufacturer of each drug to be administered to verify the recommended dose, the method and duration of administration, and contraindications. It is the responsibility of the practitioner, relying on experience and knowledge of the patient, to determine dosages and the best treatment for each individual patient. Neither the Publisher nor the editors and contributors assumes any liability for any injury and/or damage to persons or property arising from this publication.

**The Publisher**

 your source for books,
journals and multimedia
in the health sciences
**www.elsevierhealth.com**

The
Publisher's
policy is to use
**paper manufactured
from sustainable forests**

Printed in China

# Contents

# Contributors

**John Bastin** BSc FLS
*Senior Lecturer in Biology, Faculty of Health and Social Work in Cornwall, University of Plymouth, Truro, Cornwall, UK*

**Jilly Bradshaw** RGN RSCN
*Paediatric Nurse, Bournemouth Eye Unit, Royal Bournemouth Hospital, Bournemouth, UK*

**Margaret A. Chambers** BSc(Hons) MSc PGDipEd SRN RSCN DPSN RNT
*Senior Lecturer in Children's Nursing, University of Plymouth, Plymouth, UK*

**Judith Clegg** BSc(Hons) RGN RSCN DIPSN
*Advanced Neonatal Nurse Practitioner, Neonatal Unit, Royal Cornwall Hospital, Truro, Cornwall, UK*

**Annette K. Dearmun** BSc(Hons) PhD RGN RSCN DN DNE RNT
*Principal Lecturer and Senior Nurse, Oxford Brookes University, Oxford Radcliffe Hospital, Oxford, UK*

**Maggie J. Doman** BA(Hons) MSc RGN RSCN ONC
*Senior Lecturer in Nursing (Child), Exeter, University of Plymouth, UK*

**Orla Duncan** RGN RSCN
*Cleft Lip and Palate Clinical Nurse Specialist, Royal Hospital for Sick Children, Edinburgh, UK*

**Christine English** BSc(Hons) MSc PGDE RGN RSCN DPSN
*Senior Lecturer, Nursing and Midwifery, Children's Division, University of Newcastle and Northumbria, Newcastle upon Tyne, UK*

**Karen Evans** RGN RSCN
*Professional and Practice Development Nurse, Bristol Royal Hospital for Children, Bristol, UK*

**Caroline Haines** BN(Hons) MSc PGDE RNT RGN RSCN
*Nurse Consultant, Paediatric Intensive Care, Bristol Royal Hospital for Children, Bristol; Associate Senior Lecturer, University of the West of England, Bristol, UK*

**Sue Harris** RSCN
*Clinical Nurse Lead Paediatrics, Chelsea and Westminster Healthcare Trust, London, UK*

**Chris Holden** MSc PGDE MCGL RGN RSCN
*Head of Department and Clinical Nurse Specialist, Nutritional Care, Diana, Princess of Wales Children's Hospital, Birmingham, UK*

**Sue Jones** BSc(Hons) MSc RGN, RSCN
*Assistant Director of Nursing, Practice Development, Trust Headquarters, United Bristol Healthcare NHS Trust, Bristol, UK*

**Anthony Lander** PhD FRCS DCH
*Consultant Paediatric Surgeon, Institute of Child Health, Diana, Princess of Wales Children's Hospital, Birmingham, UK*

**Ann Macfadyen** BA(Hons) MSc PGCE BN RGN RSCN
*Senior Lecturer, Childhood and Family Studies, Northumbria University, Newcastle, UK*

**Lindy May** MSc Neuroscience; DipCouns RGN RSCN
*Nurse Consultant in Pediatric Neurosurgery, Great Ormond Street Hospital for Children, NHS Trust, London, UK*

**Alyson Methven** BSc RSCN RGN
*Senior Staff Nurse, Royal Hospital for Sick Children, Glasgow, UK*

**Tracy Morse** BA(Hons) BSc(Hons) CertEd DipHS RGN RSCN
*Lecturer Practitioner, Institute of Health Studies, University of Plymouth, Taunton, UK*

**Sarah Neill** BSc MSc PGDE RGN RSCN RNT
*Senior Lecturer in Children's Nursing School of Health, University of Northampton, Northampton, UK*

**Heather Newton** DipPSN CertEd RGN
*Nurse Consultant in Tissue Viability, Royal Cornwall Hospitals NHS Trust, Truro, UK*

**Carolyn Patchell** BSc SRD
*Head of Dietetic Services, Diana, Princess of Wales Children's Hospital, Birmingham, UK*

**Vanessa Unsworth (nee Peden)** RN(Child) Dip, BSc(Hons), MPhil
*Practitioner Health Lecturer, Derbyshire Children's Hospital Derby, UK/University of Nottingham, Nottingham, UK*

*Position, Astra Charnwood Research Nurse, Academic Division of Child Health, University of Nottingham, Derbyshire Children's Hospital, Derby, UK*

**Sandra Pedley** BA (Hons) PGDE RGN RSCN
*Education Sister, Paediatric Intensive Care Unit, Bristol Royal Hospital for Children; Bristol, UK*

**Elizabeth Thomas** RGN RSCN
*Paediatric Urology Nurse Specialist, Surgical Ward, Bristol Royal Hospital for Sick Children, Bristol, UK*

**Shelley Thomas** BSc (Hons) RN
*Senior Nurse, University of Bristol Dental Hospital, Bristol, UK*

**Alison Twycross** MSc DMS CertEd(HE) RGN RMN RSCN PhD
*Principal Lecturer in Children's Nursing, Faculty of Health and Social Care Sciences, Kingston University, Surrey*

**Jan A. Walmsley** BSc(Hons) RN RSCN
*Staff Nurse, Day Surgery Unit, Treliske Hospital, Truro, UK*

# Foreward

I am delighted to write the Foreword to this much-needed text, which brings together many different aspects of caring for a child prior to and following surgical intervention.

The care of children following surgery has changed considerably over the last 30 years, along with an expanding range of surgical procedures and less invasive techniques. Today there is an increasing emphasis on greater involvement of the family, child friendly environments, shorter hospital stays, more day surgery and a growing number of community children's nurses to enable early discharge and family support within the home environment. Advances in surgical techniques and sound research evidence have also led to changes in practice in areas such as pre- and post-operative care, as well as vastly changing professional preconceptions over required fasting periods.

Caring for a child is undoubtedly a team approach. Nowhere is this more evident than for a child undergoing surgery, with the team including parents and play specialists, porters, doctors and nurses. Nurses have a particular role in managing and pre-empting pain, yet all too often studies and audits highlight a lack of attention to this most-important aspect of care. The importance of ensuring adequate psychological support and preparation prior to interventions for children should not be underestimated. Children often have great difficulty understanding events, becoming overwhelmed by untoward and unexplained interventions resulting in potentially life-long adverse effects. Achieving a successful outcome for the child and family depends on early identification, adequate support, preparation and appropriate treatment and care from the entire multi-professional team.

Surgical nursing of children is undoubtedly a specialty in its own right, requiring the attainment of specific knowledge and skills. The text reflects the various changing patterns and challenges facing practitioners, outlining the knowledge and skills which must be acquired in order that children and their families receive a high standard of care. This quite rightly includes an emphasis upon meeting a child's psychological and social needs, as well as physiological considerations.

Congratulations to all the chapter authors, and the editors who have created a textbook that will, I am sure, be a standard reference for all child health nursing students, as well as those seeking to specialise in the field of children's surgical nursing.

Fiona Smith
Adviser in Children and Young People's Nursing
Royal College of Nursing

# Preface

The motivation for this book was many years in clinical practice undertaking various aspects of the nursing care of surgical infants and children with no recent text dedicated to the subject. This book will be of interest to all students of nursing on child branch programmes whether at degree or diploma level and all qualified nurses undertaking the care of children with surgical conditions.

The underpinning framework of this traditional text book is systems theory, with initial chapters which address common themes such as quality, pain and nutrition. There is a strong focus throughout on the concept of family-centred care. The chapters have all been written by respected UK children's nurses, all of whom are experienced in their field, and each chapter is supported with evidence in accordance with contemporary medical and nursing practice.

The children's nurse today practices against a background of continuing change, role development and boundary threat. There is increased emphasis on the role of the family in the care of sick children, on children's rights as citizens and users of the service, and on listening to the voices of children. In the centre of this maelstrom sit the child and family requiring care. The aspirations of children's nurses to meet the challenges of contemporary practice must not allow them to lose sight of the basic principles of nursing care that are clearly identified in this book.

We hope that children's nurses in every setting find this book useful and would encourage feedback via our publishers.

Plymouth, 2006                    Margaret Chambers
                                           Sue Jones

# Acknowledgements

We would like to acknowledge R Spicer, Consultant Paediatric Surgeon, Bristol Royal Hospital for Children, United Bristol Healthcare NHS Trust for his verification of the text, and the Hospital Play Specialists at Bristol Royal Children's Hospital for organising the cover photographs.

We would also like to acknowledge the patience of our authors who have waited along time for this book

The Surgical Nursing of Children
Margaret A Chambers and Sue Jones (Editors)

# Chapter 1

# The context of care in surgical nursing

Margaret A Chambers, Jan A Walmsley and Sarah Neill

## CHAPTER CONTENTS

## INTRODUCTION

The purpose of this chapter is to set the context within which the surgical nursing care of babies and children takes place. First, the concept of family-centred care, the philosophy that underpins all aspects of children's nursing, will be discussed in relation to surgical nursing care. The value of therapeutic play activity and its role in the psychosocial care of the surgical patient who is a child will be examined. This will be followed by a discussion of pre- and postoperative care, including fasting for surgery and discharge planning.

## FAMILY-CENTRED CARE

Family-centred care is the philosophy that underpins all aspects of contemporary children's nursing practice. For many years, the individual child was the primary focus of care for the children's nurse, but more recently the child and family have been placed at the centre of nursing care.

The history of family-centred care, from the exclusion of parents from hospital wards to the notion that the family has a pivotal role in relation to the care of its children, extends over more than half a century. Health and social policy are influential in the development of philosophical approaches to care, and in turn ideology influences the development of policy (Clayton 2000). Key principles of family-centred care, for example, are evident in the Platt Report (Ministry of Health 1959), *The Welfare of Children and Young People in Hospital* (Department of Health 1991a), *Children First* (Audit Commission

1993) and more recently *The Patient's Charter* (Department of Health 1996) and the *Children's National Service Framework* (Department of Health 2004). The principles of family-centred care are in congruence with those emphasised in the *Children Act* (1989) and consistent with contemporary thinking about the involvement and empowerment of the recipients of health-care services (Callery 1997a).

There have been attempts to define the term 'family-centred care', notably Wong & Wilson (1995): 'The term family-centred care defines the focus of pediatric care because nursing of children cannot be optimally performed unless each family member is designated the patient or client.' (p15)

The expression family-centred care is a misnomer if the family is not placed at the centre of care (Coyne 1996). However the terms parental involvement, parent participation, care by parents and family nursing are often used synonymously with the term family-centred care.

At the heart of the concept of family-centred care is the belief that the family is the one constant in the child's life (Wong & Wilson 1995). All healthcare services are directed towards enabling and empowering, supporting, developing and respecting the ability of the family to carry out its decision-making and care-giving roles. Care, therefore, is individualised to meet the needs of the whole family and not merely those of the individual child, and parents and professionals work in equal partnership towards the provision of optimal quality in care.

The fundamental elements of family-centred care include consideration of family structure and culture, the individual roles of family members and their need for information and support, negotiated parental involvement in care and the effects of the child's need for care on the whole family (Nethercott 1993). Just as important is the idea that in true family-centred nursing it is the family and not the nurse that is recognised as the expert carer of the child. This is in direct conflict with the medical model of care that promotes the nurse's role as the expert carer (Thorne & Robinson 1988) and may account for the perceived dichotomy between philosophy and practice (Bruce & Ritchie 1997).

There are two basic concepts that underpin the practice of family-centred care – enabling and empowering. Enabling allows family members to demonstrate their capabilities and offers opportunities for them to develop new competencies that may be needed to meet the healthcare needs of the child, whilst empowering allows families to gain or retain

a sense of control over their family lives (Wong & Wilson 1995).

Family-centred care, whilst accepted as best practice, nevertheless has implications for families and for the delivery of nursing care. Parental demands for nursing support and time may present nurses with problems in managing their work (Callery 1997b) and parents are users of resources (Coyne 1996). There are subsequent implications for nursing numbers, skill mix and budgets. Involvement in care can be challenging for parents. In undertaking nursing procedures they may experience role conflict and disruption to the normal protective parental role (Callery 1997b), and parents sometimes find it tedious to be with their child continuously (Sainsbury et al 1986). Since an essential tenet of family-centred care is the recognition of the diversity of what constitutes a family, nurses need to understand the difficulties faced by some families in caring for their hospitalised child. It may be difficult, for example, for single parents to stay in hospital with a sick child when there are other children to be cared for at home. The importance of a holistic and individual assessment of each family member, and collaboration between the nurse and the family about what can or cannot be managed by the family, cannot, therefore, be over-emphasised.

## FAMILY-CENTRED CARE AND THE SURGICAL EXPERIENCE

The principles of family-centred care have relevance for the child undergoing ambulatory, planned or emergency surgery. Parents need support if they are to be able to nurture and care for their children at such times, as anxiety associated with helping children to cope with painful procedures or accompanying them to the operating theatre has been reported (Callery 1997a).

Parents can be empowered to care for their children throughout the surgical experience. For ambulatory and planned surgical experiences, pre-admission clinics (see Ch. 8) can and should involve the child's family as well as the child. Parents cannot be enabled or empowered to care if they do not have the information they need to answer any questions their child may have, and the pre-admission clinic is the ideal place for the transfer of information from professional to parent to take place. In an emergency the parent should be party to all the information given to the child, and opportunities must be offered for parents to ask questions and to be actively involved in all aspects of the preparation of their child for surgery. Many hospitals operate a system of preoperative visiting by operating theatre staff (see Ch. 5). This is an ideal opportunity for parents to make contact and begin a therapeutic relationship with the staff who will be caring for their child through the surgical episode. Familiarity with the theatre staff will help to allay anxiety in both the parent and the child.

Family-centred philosophy requires professionals to empower parents to care for their children but also to respect their right to decline to undertake aspects of care delivery as they choose. In recent times it has become accepted practice for parents to accompany their children to the anaesthetic room and to stay with them during the induction of anaesthesia. The presence of a parent during induction reduces the effects of separation anxiety in young children and the fear and anxiety associated with anaesthesia in older children (La Rosa Nash & Murphy 1997), as well as reinforcing the caring parental role. However Callery (1997a) has reported that some parents find watching their child go to sleep in this way to be especially distressing. If parents are properly prepared and supported by the family's named nurse throughout the experience, they will be better able to develop the coping skills they need. Parents who opt out of accompanying their children to the anaesthetic room are likely to cite their own anxiety as the reason for the decision (La Rosa Nash & Murphy 1997). If parents decide not to accompany their child, their right to exclude themselves from the anaesthetic room must be respected.

There is a similar increasing trend towards encouraging parents to be with their child in the recovery room during the immediate postoperative recovery period (Edwards 1998). Innovative concepts such as the provision of bleepers to call the family to the recovery room as soon as the child arrives from the operating theatre are becoming embedded in practice and demonstrate a high commitment on the part of professionals to the principles of family-centred care. Callery's study (1997b), however, also suggests that the recovery period may be another major stress point for the family. Parents may be distressed by seeing their children in a high dependency environment with airways, drains and infusions in situ and their child potentially in pain. Adequate preparation for and encouragement and support during this experience are essential if parents are to be able to cope effectively.

Other aspects of the surgical experience may be challenging for parents involved in their children's care. For example, holding children during potentially painful procedures such as dressing changing and cannula insertion, or cooperating with staff in withholding diet and fluids can be particularly difficult for them and may be seen as a threat to their nurturing parental role. Sharing knowledge with parents about the child's developing cognitive ability can help parents to understand and cope with their child's reactions to events such as these, and this may be especially important if the child's anger is directed towards the caring parent.

Pain management is discussed in detail in Chapter 6. However it is important to note here that a family-centred approach to pain management in the pre- and postoperative period helps to restore parental control and empowers families in the management of their child's pain after discharge – another period of high anxiety for parents.

Whilst the challenge of sharing care with parents is rewarding for children's nurses, family-centred care means more than just inviting parents to participate in the care of their child. Furthermore it is not enough to espouse the principles of family-centred care, it is the role of the children's nurse to ensure that these principles are put into practice. This means that children's nurses must recognise the family as the constant in the life of each child and that the concept of family must be properly understood. Because the presence and active involvement of parents in the care of their children affects the work roles of nurses (Casey 1995), it means that children's nurses must accept new roles as educators and facilitators in order to enable and empower parents who are the most appropriate people to care for their child.

## THERAPEUTIC PLAY

Play is any activity that is undertaken for intrinsic pleasure not extrinsic purposes, and is the natural activity of childhood. Therapeutic play is the use of play as therapy to help distressed or potentially distressed children come to terms with their fears and to master their experiences (Chambers 1993). Children's nurses can use therapeutic play techniques to communicate with children, to facilitate understanding and to correct misconceptions about nursing and medical experiences. Through therapeutic play techniques children can rehearse or relive their anxiety-provoking experiences in order to develop the skills they need to cope. Providing opportunities for therapeutic play activity is therefore essential for the emotional wellbeing of the child in hospital. Since emotional wellbeing is at least as important as physical wellbeing and contributes to the child's recovery, it is important that children's nurses incorporate therapeutic play techniques into their everyday nursing practice.

Delpo & Frick (1988) described two important types of therapeutic play: directed play, in which the adult directs the play activity and determines its objectives; and non-directed play, in which the child controls all aspects of the play activity, although the adult may select the environment and materials in order to stimulate specific play activity. Examples of directed play are preparation for medical procedures and surgery, whilst non-directed play includes free medical play that allows the child to access medical equipment whilst being supervised but not controlled by the adult.

## PLAY AND THE SURGICAL PATIENT

Children's reactions to a surgical event are not related to the seriousness of the surgery but to the fantasies aroused by it (Freud 1952). Such fantasies may include the idea that hospitalisation and surgery are a punishment for wrong doing, or that castration and mutilation will take place, and are clearly related to the child's cognition and understanding of illness causation and body concepts. Therapeutic play techniques can assist children's nurses to dispel myths and promote understanding. They are therefore powerful tools that can help children's nurses to support children undergoing ambulatory, planned and emergency surgery.

## PREOPERATIVE THERAPEUTIC PLAY PREPARATION

Preparation for medical procedures, and especially for a surgical event, reduces associated stress and promotes recovery. As a result of this many hospitals now have well established pre-admission preparation programmes for children undergoing ambulatory or planned surgery and their families. Similarly, children undergoing emergency surgery receive as much preoperative information as their medical condition permits. Before undertaking play preparation, it is important to establish what the child already knows and understands so that play

activity can be geared towards meeting the needs of the individual child and family, and the child's fantasies and misconceptions can be addressed during the preparation procedure. Play preparation programmes must take account of the individual child's age and, more importantly, cognitive ability, which may be affected by stress.

Play activity can continue during transfer to the operating theatre and the induction of anaesthesia. This usually takes the form of transportation on theatre trolleys that have been disguised as trains, rockets and sleighs, or in toy cars instead of trolleys, and diversionary techniques for those children who find it difficult to cope in the anaesthetic room.

## POSTOPERATIVE THERAPEUTIC PLAY

Postprocedural play is less well developed as a therapeutic tool but therapeutic play is just as valuable in the postoperative recovery period. Some children may need to play out their anxiety by reliving the whole event through their play. Others communicate their fears, anxiety and even pain through play. Therapeutic play techniques can help children avoid complications during the recovery period: for example, blowing bubbles is one way in which to persuade the reluctant child to undertake breathing exercises following surgery. Postoperative therapeutic play is especially important for those children whose medical condition dictated speedy removal to the operating theatre and who may not have been well prepared as a result.

Whilst they are in hospital children are exposed to numerous threats to their wellbeing, not the least of which is the surgical event. These require children to develop the skills to cope and therapeutic play activity is one way in which children's nurses can reduce threats to personal growth and bolster children's feelings of control.

## PREOPERATIVE CARE

The role of the children's surgical nurse has developed dramatically since its emergence and continues to evolve in response to attitudinal theories and health and social policy reforms. Developments in technology and advancements in surgical procedures has led to an increase in day surgery admissions and shorter stays for inpatients, which subsequently results in the need for strategies to prepare children and their families for rapid through-put and early discharge. Day surgery for children is one of the fastest developing branches of health care in Western society. It is proving to be cost-effective and beneficial to children and their families by maximising the use of healthcare resources, cutting waiting lists and maintaining family integrity (Glasper & Lowson 1998) (see Ch. 8). Consequently, the philosophy of family-centred care, now an integral aspect of children's nursing, has become a fundamental concept that helps to facilitate the current trend towards shorter pre- and postoperative admission periods and early discharge.

## ASSESSMENT

The role of the surgical nurse commences with assessment prior to surgery; it takes place either in outpatient clinic following consultation with the surgeon, one or two weeks prior to admission during a pre-admission visit to the ward or, particularly in the case of an emergency, shortly before surgery takes place. Government reports and others acknowledge the need for adequate preparation of children and their families prior to surgery (Department of Health 1991a, Thornes 1991), although currently there are no clear guidelines to determine the content of such visits, which can result in disparity. Since the introduction of clinical governance (Department of Health 1998), children's nurses are challenged to scrutinise their practice and develop strategies to address the barriers that may impinge on the quality of care purposed to meet the changing needs of children and their families. The detrimental impact of hospitalisation has been well documented over the past half century (Bowlby 1951, Committee on Child Health Services 1976, Robertson 1958); however, many strategies are now being implemented to ensure that an episode in hospital no longer carries the lasting psychological damage it once threatened. The value of psychological preparation for the child and family and the exchange of information the child, family and named nurse (Department of Health 1991b) alliance affords has long been recognised and this has been implemented for over a decade. However, an optimum time frame for pre-admission assessment and subsequent preparation strategies has not yet been defined, although the cognitive developmental stage of each individual child is fundamental to the equation. Frequently, pre-assessment takes

place 7–10 days prior to admission for practical purposes. This permits time to arrange medical or clinical investigations and implement therapeutic strategies in a holistic approach to optimising the child's health prior to elective surgery; or to find a replacement for the list following any necessary cancellation or deferment.

Assessment, whenever it takes place, is the key to identifying potential or actual problems and establishing deficits in knowledge, information or resources. Assessment, the first stage of the nursing process, enables the nurse, in partnership with the child and family, to formulate an individualised plan of care to meet the family's holistic care needs based on specified time frames and environmental options available. Assessment of suitability for day-case or inpatient status is frequently based on a nurse-led assessment encompassing physical, social and psychological considerations.

## CARE PLANNING

The process of care can be structured around a nursing model, for example the 'Activities of Daily Living' model (Roper et al 1996) with its straightforward vocabulary that is readily understood by each participant of the partnership, and which helps to promote the concept of equal autonomy and avoids disempowerment through ineffective communication. Communication is one of the most effective tools the children's surgical nurse can employ. Effective communication helps to ensure that children and their families are well informed and psychologically prepared to safely undergo the surgical episode, whilst establishing the boundaries of responsibility and defining expectations and limitations. Care planning can be time consuming, but the essence of redressing the balance of shared responsibility is via the vehicle of negotiation and through investment in family education to meet deficits in knowledge.

Regardless of the nursing system used, several nurses may be involved in implementing care, therefore a written care plan is a relevant communication tool that avoids fragmentation and provides documentary evidence of family-centred goals and actions selected to facilitate them. Quality care plans include acknowledgement of the child and family's own preferences where choices can be offered. The depth of information included is dependent to some extent on the length of stay expected. Care planning is an ongoing activity, which is revised in response to evaluation. Evaluation of response to actions identifies when goals have been reached and aspects of care can be discontinued or adapted.

Effective communication and well developed organisational skills ensure the accurate timing of preparatory measures and promote the preemption of postoperative interventions, ensuring the child is safely prepared and smoothly transferred throughout the theatre episode. Coordination of care frequently falls upon the named nurse, therefore it is helpful to establish good working relationships with the medical, anaesthetic and theatre personnel, promoting the efficient management of the theatre list which inevitably benefits the patient.

## IMPLEMENTATION OF THE CARE PLAN

One of the main tasks of the children's surgical nurse is to ensure the safety of the child and family pre- and postoperatively by providing a safe environment and adhering to local and national policy, protocols and guidelines. The ward manager is responsible for providing the right skill mix of personnel to cope with the workload and for the provision of safely maintained equipment.

On admission, a child and family's first impressions can be predictive of the whole theatre episode. It would, therefore, be pertinent for the nurse to ensure a positive reception with a friendly welcome and orientation to the ward. This brief encounter can allow an experienced nurse to discern and allay particular anxieties and select the best approach to suit the individual family's needs. Young or unprepared children may be reluctant to comply with investigations and interventions, particularly if they are in pain or are fearful. Children's surgical nurses should use their specialist knowledge of child development and cognition to formulate strategies that encourage the child to comply. However, most Health Authorities now employ hospital play specialists who are adept at intervening in this situation and can be utilised to assist in obtaining baseline observations to determine fitness for surgery and height and weight, which are particularly important to determine correct anaesthetic drug dosages. Children can usually be encouraged to wear an identification band, which could be decorated with coloured stickers, and are frequently allowed to wear their own clean pyjamas or shorts and T-shirt for the theatre episode rather than an unfamiliar the-

atre gown that can cause unnecessary distress. It is recognised that many children in hospital have a major fear of needles. To address this problem, a local anaesthetic gel is routinely applied to the proposed cannulation site as an effective method of reducing anxiety and painful cannulation. Its skin numbing properties should first be explained and successful cannulation may be demonstrated with the aid of a specially designed doll.

## PREOPERATIVE FASTING

Whilst much has been written in the nursing literature about the need for psychological pre-procedure preparation, much less attention has been focused on the physical preparation of the child for a general anaesthesia. Crucial to the child's perioperative safety, the main concern is to avoid the occurrence of aspiration pneumonitis, with its potentially life-threatening consequences (Pandit & Pandit 1997). Box 1.1 lists the risk factors for pulmonary aspiration.

A review of the literature around perioperative fasting times (Neill 1995) found that guidelines suggest fasting times of 4 hours for fluids and 6 hours for food with, in some examples, consideration given to the age of the child and

---

**Box 1.1  Risk factors for pulmonary aspiration (Schreiner 1994, Dowling 1995, Schreiner & Nicolson 1995, Hata 1997, Splinter & Schreiner 1999)**

- Emergency surgery (therefore including those who have had a recent full meal)
- Trauma or severe illness (including systemic infection and sepsis)
- Depressed consciousness from drugs or injury
- Increased intracranial pressure
- Impaired cough – decreased consciousness and bulbar palsy
- Difficult airway
- History of vomiting during anaesthetic induction
- Factors leading to increased gastric volumes or pressure
  - obesity,
  - ascites,
  - gastrointestinal motility problems or obstruction,
  - autonomic neuropathy (diabetes mellitus),
  - pregnancy

consequent reduced fasting times for younger children (Bates 1994). However, even where protocols for optimal fasting times exist, there is evidence to suggest that children are often fasted for as much as 12–24 hours (While & Crawford 1992, Maclean & Renwick 1993, Bates 1994, Stack & Stokes 1995).

There are a number of adverse consequences associated with prolonged fasting. These include increased irritability, hypoglycaemia, hypotension, dehydration, headache and unhappiness, sometimes leading to the cancellation of surgery if the child becomes uncooperative. The discomfort of a thirsty child has the potential to increase anxiety at induction with consequent increased distress on waking (Zuckerberg 1994). Prolonged fasting, together with the effects of some anaesthetics, may predispose the child to postoperative nausea and vomiting, increasing the likelihood of an overnight stay. Dehydration alone will increase the time interval to micturition and could potentially delay discharge (While & Crawford 1992).

Fluids leave the stomach faster than solids and different solids also empty at different rates. The type of fluid also influences emptying rates, with clear fluids of neutral pH, iso-osmolarity and calorie free emptying at the fastest rate. Amongst food types, lipids or fats are the slowest to leave the stomach, carbohydrate-rich foods have an intermediate emptying time, whilst protein-rich foods leave the stomach at the fastest rate for solids (Splinter & Schreiner 1999). Solids are defined as those foods that are in the solid state in the stomach. There are important clinical implications for children's nurses here as milk is digested into liquid whey and solid curds in the stomach, which means milk needs to be treated like a solid for fasting purposes, whilst gelatine may be solid on ingestion but liquefies in the stomach, making jellies permissible as clear fluids preoperatively, which may facilitate more effective fluid management of children who have difficulties swallowing liquids.

Breast milk is known to leave the stomach more quickly than formula milk due to the high proportion of casein in formula milks (Thomas 1994), therefore breastfed babies can potentially normally feed for longer than those on formula prior to general anaesthesia, and some of the recent guidelines now incorporate differential fasting time for breast and formula milk feeding.

Current evidence suggests that clear fluids can be safely given to healthy children with no known risk factors for pulmonary aspiration up to 2–3 hours prior to the induction of anaesthesia (Splinter & Schreiner 1999), whilst the recommendation for fasting after ingestion of solid food continues to be 6 hours following a light meal. However, it should be noted that gastric emptying following a heavy meal may be as much as 9 hours. Further research is needed to clarify the minimum safe fasting times for breastfed infants and current guidelines take a cautious approach, opting for a 4 hour fast. Fluid fasting guidelines are given in Box 1.2.

The benefits of clear fluid ingestion up to 2 hours before surgery include increased child and parent satisfaction, increased gastric pH, ingestion of calories, decreased risk of hypoglycaemia, decreased lipolysis and ketosis, and improved fluid homeostasis (Splinter & Schreiner 1999). Enabling parents to provide a drink 2 or 3 hours before the operation would fit more easily with the family's normal daily activity and remove the misery of excessive thirst. However, this needs to be supported by verbal and written information explaining the rationale for this approach. Giving this information to parents will have the effect of improving their sense of personal control and as a result may enhance their ability to deal with their child's hospital admission and the necessary care after discharge. Furthermore, nausea and vomiting and the risk of hypoglycaemia and dehydration would be reduced, resulting in fewer postoperative complications and lessening the chance of delayed discharge or an overnight stay in hospital.

Premedications are seldom used in day surgery; however, if a premedication is prescribed for an inpatient, parents need to be aware of the effect and be encouraged to help their child to relax or sleep in a safe environment. Prior to administering a premed, the nurse is responsible for ensuring that valid informed consent has been obtained (see Ch. 3) fasting guidelines have been adhered to, and all other preoperative safety considerations have been addressed in accordance with the theatre checklist (see Fig. 1.1). Preoperative checklists vary

---

**Box 1.2 Fasting guidelines (Association of Anaesthetists of Great Britain and Ireland 2001)**

2 hours clear non-particulate and uncarbonated fluids
4 hours breast milk
6 hours solid food, infant formula or other milk

| PATIENT LABEL | YES | NO | N/A | COMMENTS |
|---|---|---|---|---|
| Fasting – time of last diet.......... time of last drink... | | | | |
| Name band | | | | |
| Details correct | | | | |
| Consent signed | | | | |
| Medical case notes | | | | |
| X-rays | | | | |
| Site marked | | | | |
| Jewellery removed | | | | |
| Dentures removed / in situ | | | | |
| Caps / Crowns / Loose teeth | | | | |
| Prosthesis removed / in situ | | | | |
| Hair clips | | | | |
| Glasses / Hearing aid | | | | |
| Premedication | | | | |
| Prescription chart | | | | |
| Make-up/Nail varnish removed | | | | |
| Allergies | | | | |
| Bladder emptied | | | | |

**Additional Information:**

**Nurse Signature**.....................................

Figure 1.1  Theatre checklist.

in format but are all designed to ensure that the child is safely prepared to undertake the planned anaesthetic and surgical procedure. Any potential problems or significant additional information should be highlighted when the patient is handed over to the anaesthetic/theatre personnel.

The benefits of having parents accompany their children to the anaesthetic room are now well established; however, parents need careful preparation and support to enable them to undertake this role effectively (see Ch. 5). During the perioperative period, parents may welcome a period away from the ward or may prefer to stay close by. The family may require support, refreshment or further information during this time. It is imperative to keep parents fully informed throughout the procedure of any delays and to know where to find parents if they leave the area.

Parents can be very distressed to see their child emerging from anaesthetic and may assume the child is in pain, therefore they need to be prepared for what to expect with explanations of any specialist equipment that may be present. If the child is expected to go to intensive care or high dependency following surgery, a visit prior to theatre should be arranged for the benefit of all the family.

## EMERGENCY PREOPERATIVE CARE

When a child is admitted to the ward for surgery as an emergency, the urgent demand for psychological and physical care presents the children's surgical nurse with the challenge of minimising the impact. The nature of an emergency admission exacerbates levels of fear and anxiety for the child and family who may feel out of control because of the speed at which events occur.

Children undergo emergency surgery for many reasons, ranging from serious accidents and acute exacerbation of common childhood conditions, e.g. hernia, torsion of testes, or appendicitis, to minor procedures involving manipulation or examination for foreign bodies under anaesthetic.

On admission, in addition to routine surgical preparation, it may be necessary to undertake medical investigations, for example blood tests, X-rays or scans, to assist or confirm a diagnosis. The child's condition may also warrant immediate medical intervention, for example fluid replacement or intravenous analgesia and antibiotics to stabilise or optimise the child's condition prior to surgery.

On a child's admission, the surgeon, anaesthetist and named nurse will each make an initial assessment of the child and family's needs. The surgical and anaesthetic examination allows the physical risks to be assessed and a time for surgery to proceed may then be calculated. The physical care of the child will always take priority over the psychological care when a child presents in a poorly condition; however, a period of observation, for example in suspected appendicitis, may precede surgery, allowing time for psychological preparation. Usually nil by mouth will be ordered and intravenous fluids will be commenced to maintain fluid balance. Unless the child's condition is imminently life threatening, the normal physical and psychological preparation routine may be followed; however, some aspects, for example fasting guidelines, may be omitted or modified depending on the urgency of the surgery.

Children arriving for emergency surgery may well present with severe pain, bleeding, vomiting or may be lethargic or gravely ill. Parents may also be burdened with feelings of guilt, particularly following any type of accident; it is therefore particularly important to be sensitive to parental anxiety and to maintain the principles of family-centred care whilst preparing a child for emergency surgery.

## POSTOPERATIVE CARE

Following surgery under a general anaesthetic, children will usually be transferred to a recovery area where continuous monitoring is undertaken until they are able to maintain their own airway, pain is adequately controlled and observations have returned to normal limits (see Ch. 5). If this is not achieved, for example following major surgery, the anaesthetist may transfer the child to high dependency or intensive care for a further period of recovery. Recovery practitioners need to ensure that all criteria for discharge from recovery have been achieved and documented prior to transferring the child to the ward staff and parent. Whilst the value of a parent's presence in the anaesthetic room has long been recognised, the concept of parents in recovery attending their children as they emerge from the effects of surgery and anaesthetic is currently being explored (see Ch. 5).

Pain assessment is deemed to be most effective if pain assessment tools are introduced prior to surgery. Several analogue scales are available to help children describe their pain level (see Ch. 6). Pain should be assessed and adequately controlled prior to transfer, and intravenous infusions, patient controlled analgesia, epidurals and so on should be set up so the anaesthetist can make any necessary adjustments. Pain management can be an onerous task for the children's nurse; however, nurses can harness valuable information if they recognise parents as the most effective judges of pain by interpreting their child's general demeanor and behaviour. Pain relief measures include analgesia, but comfort, massage, reassurance and distraction strategies delivered by perceptive parents can also provide much alleviation.

Liaison with the ward staff prior to transfer allows the nurse to ensure that all preparations for maintaining a safe environment are in place and that parents are made aware of what to expect, for example the attachment of intravenous infusions, drains, monitors and so on.

Hand-over frequently takes place in recovery, often with a parent present. A comprehensive verbal hand-over accompanied by clearly written documentation ensures all aspects of the perioperative episode are addressed and helps the nurse and family to formulate a postoperative care plan based on the changing care needs of the child.

Hand-over should include:

- An account of the anaesthetic episode including drugs administered
- The surgical procedure and any complications
- Method of wound closure and type of dressing
- Postoperative prescription and any postoperative instructions
- A résumé of the child's recovery episode.

Using the child's bed for transfer avoids a further manoeuvre, which may be distressing or painful. To maintain safety, portable oxygen, suction, monitoring or resuscitation equipment may be necessary to accompany the child throughout the transfer. The family should be reunited with their child as soon as possible and kept informed of the child's condition. Monitoring of the child should continue as appropriate, keeping a record of observations, pain assessment and interventions implemented throughout the recovery period. Any restrictions or instructions ordered by the surgeon should be made clear to the child and family to enable them to resume care appropriately. Cot sides may be in place whilst the child is recovering; however, parents should be shown how to lower them to access their child, so that they do not pose a barrier.

A postoperative care plan may have been negotiated with the child and family prior to surgery; however, an ongoing review and evaluation optimises its efficacy. The care plan should incorporate realistic postoperative goals, which include a safe recovery from anaesthetic, early detection and prompt treatment of postoperative complications, maintenance of dietary and fluid requirements and a return to normal mobility. As the child's condition allows, the level of monitoring may be reduced and the parents encouraged to resume their parental role to minimise discontinuity and prepare them for coping after discharge. Initially, a safe, suitable environment may be needed to promote sleep and rest, but following minor surgery strategies may be utilised to keep children occupied until they are discharged. Following surgery, various members of the multidisciplinary team may be employed to aid recovery. The play specialist provides appropriate activities to suit the child's individual needs; however, if a prolonged hospital stay is necessary the hospital school service may also be employed for school-aged children. Surgery can impose restricted mobility resulting in complications, therefore physiotherapy may be necessary to promote recovery, maintain skin integrity and facilitate rehabilitation.

Sometimes an intravenous cannula will be in place following surgery. With young children it needs to be safely secured with tape, splint and bandage to prevent accidental premature removal, bleeding and loss of venous access. However, following minor elective surgery, the cannula may be removed more hastily when fluids are tolerated and oral pain relief is adequate. The presence of an intravenous device can be more distressing for a young child than the surgery itself. Accurate recording of fluid balance is important following surgery, to ensure urinary retention is quickly recognised and dehydration is avoided or effectively managed (see Ch. 7). The surgical wound site should be inspected on arrival on the ward and at appropriate intervals to ensure any dressing remains intact and any bleeding, bruising, inflammation or infection is reported. The wound or dressing should also be inspected prior to discharge and any instructions regarding wound care should

DISCHARGE PLAN – DAY SURGERY | PATIENT DETAILS

| CHECKLIST | YES | NO | N/A | COMMENTS |
|---|---|---|---|---|
| VITAL SIGNS WITHIN NORMAL LIMITS | | | | |
| PAIN SCORE (0-10) | | | | SCORE ......... |
| DRESSING / WOUND CHECKED | | | | |
| STEADY GAIT / ORIENTATED | | | | |
| FLUIDS / DIET TOLERATED | | | | |
| HAS PASSED URINE | | | | |
| CANNULA REMOVED | | | | |
| WRITTEN INFORMATION LEAFLET | | | | |
| VERBAL INFORMATION AS STATED | | | | |
| T.T.O'S / INSTRUCTIONS | | | | |
| DRESSING / EQUIPMENT SUPPLIED | | | | |
| DENTURES / VALUABLES RETURNED | | | | |
| DISCHARGE SUMMARY TO GP | | | | |
| FOLLOW UP APPOINTMENT | | | | |
| PATIENT FEELS READY FOR DISCHARGE | | | | |
| DISCHARGED WITH ESCORT | | | | |
| CARER FOR 24 HOURS | | | | |
| PRIMARY CARE TEAM INFORMED | | | | |
| TIME OF DISCHARGE ............................ | | | | |

PATIENT ADMITTED TO WARD
WARD .........................................
NOTES TRACED   YES / NO
X-RAYS TRACED   YES / NO /N/A
RELATIVES INFORMED   YES / NO
PATIENT PROPERTY TO WARD   YES / NO

NURSE SIGNATURE

Figure 1.2 Discharge plan.

be given verbally and clearly written (see Ch. 4). Prior to discharge, the nurse is responsible for ensuring all discharge criteria have been met and that the child and family are successfully discharged from hospital back to the primary care team. This may simply involve sending a surgical discharge summary to the general practitioner (GP) but liaison with a health visitor, district or practice nurse or children's community nurse may be necessary to ensure a seamless web of care.

## DISCHARGE PLANNING

Discharge can be a daunting experience for parents who may experience a sense of abandonment; therefore, a discharge plan is best commenced at pre-assessment to allow parents to prepare for the period after discharge. It can be used as a risk assessment tool of the patient's readiness for discharge and it prompts the nurse to identify which interventions need to be employed. As the recovery period progresses the discharge plan will be activated to ensure the coordination of care. Parents need to be aware of what support mechanisms are available and informed of how to access them. Some hospital trusts employ a discharge liaison officer to coordinate care at the acute and primary interface, or a hospital liaison health visitor may be engaged to assess and negotiate the community care needs of the child and family prior to discharge.

A discharge plan (see Fig. 1.2) may comprise of a document that prompts the nurse to consider each aspect of care according to local discharge policy and provides documentary evidence of interventions employed. Clinical observations should be satisfactory and any bleeding minimal and in relation to the individual surgical procedure. Pain should be controlled with oral analgesia, which should be provided according to local policy. Dressings should be supplied as necessary to ensure the parent or district nurse is equipped to undertake any dressing changes. Parents may be willing to change dressings themselves; however, they need to be prepared to undertake the procedure satisfactorily with careful instructions or by demonstration, including how to observe for signs of healing or infection.

Prior to discharge a child should be able to tolerate fluids and diet. Passing urine prior to discharge following a day surgery procedure may result in a lengthy unnecessary delay, therefore if the surgery is not of a urological nature, advice may be given with instruction to report any problems. Parents need to be adequately equipped to continue the care of their child at home, therefore information and instructions need to be clearly written and unambiguous. A copy of any instructions may also be sent to the district or practice nurse to enable continued planned care to take place after discharge. A follow-up appointment may be made prior to discharge and points of contact where parents can seek help or advice need to be clearly documented.

Before discharge, the nurse must assess the parents' willingness and capability to continue care safely at home. Nurses may assume parents want to be involved in the nursing care of their child; however, some parents may find clinical intervention, e.g. changing dressings, distressing as it may present a challenge to their role as protectors (Neill 1996). Early discharge from hospital places a heavy burden of responsibility upon the family; therefore support in the community is fundamental to success. Accountability does not end when a child leaves the hospital ward unless responsibility has been transferred back to the parent and colleagues in the community, thus enabling the nurse to relinquish her duty of care.

## References

Association of Anaesthetists of Great Britain and Ireland (AAGBI) 2001 Pre-operative assessment – the role of the anaesthetist. AAGBI, London

Audit Commission 1993 Children first: a study of hospital services. HMSO, London

Bates J 1994 Reducing fast times in paediatric day surgery. Nursing Times 90(48): 38–39

Bowlby J 1951 Maternal care and mental health. World Health Organisation, Geneva

Bruce B, Ritchie J 1997 Nurses' practices and perceptions of family-centred care. Journal of Pediatric Nursing: Nursing Care of Children and Families 12(4): 214–222

Callery P 1997a Paying to participate: financial, personal and social costs to parents of involvement in their children's care in hospital. Journal of Advanced Nursing 25(4): 746–752

Callery P 1997b Caring for parents of hospitalised children: a hidden area of nursing work. Journal of Advanced Nursing 26(5): 992–998

Casey A 1995 Partnership nursing: influences on the involvement of informal carers. Journal of Advanced Nursing 22(6): 1058–1062

Chambers MA 1993 Play as therapy for hospitalised children. Journal of Clinical Nursing 2: 349–354

Children Act 1989 HMSO, London

Clayton M 2000 Health and social policy: influences on family-centred care. Paediatric Nursing 12(8): 31–33

Committee on Child Health Services 1976 Fit for the future: report of the committee on child health services. (Chairman Professor SDM Court) HMSO, London

Coyne IT 1996 Parent participation: a concept analysis. Journal of Advanced Nursing 23(4): 733–740

Delpo EG, Frick SB 1988 Directed and non-directed play as therapeutic modalities. Children's Health Care 16(4): 261–267

Department of Health 1991a Welfare of children and young people in hospital. HMSO, London

Department of Health 1991b The patient's charter – raising the standard. London

Department of Health 1996 The patient's charter: services for children and young people. HMSO, London

Department of Health 1998 A first class service: quality in the new NHS. Department of Health, London

Department of Health (2004) National service framework for children, young people and maternity services. Department of Health, London

Dowling JL 1995 'Nulla per os [NPO] after midnight' reassessed. Rhode Island Medicine 78(12): 339–341

Edwards J 1998 Parents in recovery: a paediatric recovery nurse's view. British Journal of Theatre Nursing 8(6): 5–6

Emerson BM, Wrigley SR, Newton M 1998 Pre-operative fasting for paediatric anaesthesia. A survey of current practice. Anaesthesia 53(4): 326–330

Glasper EA, Lowson S 1998 Innovations in paediatric ambulatory care: a nursing perspective. Macmillan, London

Hata T 1997 Preparation and intraoperative management of the pediatric patient. Pediatric Annals 26(8): 471–503

La Rosa Nash PA, Murphy JM 1997 An approach to pediatric perioperative care: parent-present induction. Nursing Clinics of North America 32(1): 183–199

Maclean AR, Renwick C 1993 Audit of pre-operative starvation. Anaesthesia 48(2): 164–166

Ministry of Health 1959 The welfare of children in hospital. (Chairman H Platt) HMSO, London

National Association for the Welfare of Children in Hospital 1990 Needs and services: children in surgery. Nursing Standard (special supplement) 4(24):14

Neill S 1995 Fasting for day surgery: the parental role. Paediatric Nursing 7(2): 20–23

Neill S 1996 Parent participation 2: findings and their implication for practice. British Journal of Nursing 5(2): 110–117

Nethercott S 1993 A concept for all the family: family centred care: a concept analysis. Professional Nurse 8(12): 794–797

Pandit UA, Pandit SK 1997 Fasting before and after ambulatory surgery. Journal of Perianesthesia Nursing 12(3): 181–187

Robertson J 1958 Young children in hospital. Tavistock, London

Roper N, Logan WW, Tierney AL 1996 The Elements of nursing, 4th edn. Churchill Livingstone, Edinburgh

Sainsbury CPQ, Gray OP, Cleary J 1986 Care by parents of their children in hospital. Archives of Disease in Childhood 61(6): 612–615

Schreiner MS 1994 Preoperative and postoperative fasting in children. Pediatric Clinics of North America 41(1): 111–120

Schreiner MS, Nicolson SC 1995 Pediatric ambulatory anesthesia: NPO – before or after surgery? Journal of Clinical Anesthesia 7(7): 589–596

Splinter WM, Schreiner MS 1999 Preoperative fasting in children. Anesthesia and Analgesia 89(1): 80–89

Stack CG, Stokes MA 1995 Preoperative fasting for paediatric anaesthesia. British Journal of Anaesthesia 75(3): 375

Thomas B 1994 Manual of dietetic practice, 2nd edn. Blackwell Scientific, Oxford

Thorne C, Robinson SE 1988 Health care relationships: the chronic illness perspective. Research in Nursing and Health 11(5): 293–300

Thornes R 1991 All in a day's work. Paediatric Nursing 3(1): 7–8

Walmsley JA 2000 Discharge plan – day surgery. Royal Cornwall Hospital Trust, Treliske, Truro, Cornwall

While AE, Crawford J 1992 Paediatric day surgery. Nursing Times 88(39): 43–45

Wong D, Wilson D 1995 Whaley and Wong's nursing care of infants and children, 5th edn. Mosby, St Louis

Zuckerberg AL 1994 Perioperative approach to children. Pediatric Clinics of North America 41(1): 15–29

# Chapter 2

# Quality in children's surgical services

## Dr Annette K Dearmun

## INTRODUCTION

This chapter will explore some of the overall quality issues in relation to children undergoing surgery. The chapter highlights the importance of ensuring that care meets agreed standards and introduces the reader to the origins of standards for children undergoing surgery. This is followed by an exploration of seminal reports that have identified best practice for this client group. Finally, some of the ways in which quality of care may be monitored will be discussed. It is not intended to describe in detail the ways in which standards, guidelines and protocols can be developed and the reader is referred to other texts on these topics.

## CLINICAL GOVERNANCE

The introduction of clinical governance (Department of Health 1997, Department of Health 1998), reinforced in *The NHS Plan* (Department of Health 2000), has provided a framework for the development of strategic quality initiatives and given prominence to quality improvement within the National Health Service agenda. Accountability, effectiveness and continual improvement in quality are hallmarks of clinical governance. In this way professionals are expected to strive to provide clinical care of a consistently high quality. In order to meet these demands for clinical excellence it is the responsibility of all professionals to ensure that their practice is effective and based upon recognised best practice (accepted standards) underpinned, wherever possible, by research evidence from systematic reviews, rather than by custom and ritual (Callery 1997, Glasper & Ireland 2000). This acknowledges the symbiotic relationship between effective practice, evidence-based practice and the resultant quality of care. The consequences of not accepting this responsibility may be twofold: first, being liable to investigation or inquiry, such as the Bristol Royal Infirmary Inquiry (Kennedy 2001), and having to respond to complaints from the consumers of health care, that is parents and children, acquiring a poor reputation and being unsuccessful in accreditation; secondly, an increase in reported adverse incidents or even increased mortality rates and the possibility of litigation. The latter has particularly distressing consequences for all those individuals involved and potential financial penalties for the Trusts implicated.

## THE HISTORICAL CONTEXT

Surgery on infants and children is still a relatively new and emerging science. The earliest reported surgical procedures were generally palliative, for example drainage of cerebral spinal fluid for babies with hydrocephalus and Ramstedt's procedure performed on babies with pyloric stenosis. From a technical point of view, in the absence of sophisticated and safe anaesthesia, surgery on children was often inhumane and carried significant risk. There was little understanding and appreciation of asepsis and therefore postprocedural infection was commonplace. Furthermore, beliefs prevailed that infants and children did not feel pain in the same way as adults and thus they were given minimal analgesia. It is suggested that within this historical context the measurements of quality of care were based more upon morbidity or mortality data and in terms of outcome – the ultimate success was the survival of the patient.

The advent of refined anaesthetic agents and antibiotics heralded an increase in the range of surgical procedures and techniques that could be perfected for use on children and this in turn increased the effectiveness of surgical interventions. It became possible to focus upon the processes as well as the outcomes of care, the former involving contextual, psychological and social as well as physiological considerations.

## EARLY QUALITY INITIATIVES

Action for Sick Children (http://www.actionforsick-children.org/), formerly the National Association for the Welfare of Children in Hospital (NAWCH), pioneered the setting up of multiprofessional and multiagency project groups, to include consumers and to explore and disseminate best practice in relation to these processes of care. It may be interesting to note that the original impetus for this arose in the 1960s from concerns of mothers of children experiencing surgery. At that time they complained that they were not allowed to stay with their children in hospital or accompany them to theatre.

In the last 15 years two seminal reports have been published – *Just for the Day* (Thornes 1991) and *Meeting the Needs of Children and Young People Undergoing Surgery* (2004). The ideas in these reports are discussed later in the chapter.

It could be argued that as the range and complexity of surgical techniques expanded the number of children with conditions for whom surgery could be the first line treatment of choice increased. However, traditionally, and for largely pragmatic reasons, very few surgeons were specifically allocated and trained to operate on children. As a consequence, a number of surgeons from different adult specialities were drawn in to perform surgery on children. Thus most surgeons had a caseload that extended throughout the age range from infants to older persons. It was not uncommon for patients to be nursed on wards according to clinical speciality rather than age. Therefore, children and adults admitted to hospital for surgery were often nursed in close proximity to one another and little attention was given to the quality of the environment for either client group. Gradually the far-reaching physiological and psychological implications of nursing children alongside adults were recognised. Although in some places this situation still prevails, it is now appreciated that under such circumstances quality of care for both the adult and child client group is compromised, and the need to define quality charter marks to ensure equity of care for children requiring surgery has been highlighted. Overall, the professional consensus is that specific health and safety issues will receive greater consideration and quality will be enhanced when the environment is specifically designed with children in mind and equipped for their care.

In 1996 a comprehensive review of children's surgery was undertaken in preparation for the House of Commons Select Committee (Health Committee 1997). This involved a thorough appraisal of all the reports relating to services for children requiring surgery, the accumulation of research, where available, and the collection of expert witness evidence of best practice and cited examples of inadequate practice. Accordingly, the medical and nursing perspectives were presented to government via the committee. As a direct result of this work the Royal College of Surgeons Children's Forum was set up to explore the findings, to develop strategies for implementing the government's recommendations, and to ensure there were mechanisms for ongoing monitoring. One of the outcomes was the publication of *Children's Surgery: A First Class Service* (Royal College of Surgeons of England 2000, due for revision in 2005). The Royal College of Nursing Children's Surgical Nursing Forum, set up in 1990, played a significant part in this work. One of the most exciting aspects of this initiative was the way in which the expertise of surgeons, representing their respective specialities and colleges, and the perspective of children's nursing, were combined, universally endorsing the previous published guidelines (Dearmun 2000). Thus professionals with potentially different value systems, approaches and contributions reached a consensus about the centrality of the needs of the child and family, putting aside professional self-interest. From this premise recommendations about minimal acceptable standards of care were detailed, acknowledging previous published guidance, including recommendations from the Clinical Standards Advisory Group (CSAG) and National Confidential Enquiry into Peri-operative Deaths (NCEPD) reports and the two main seminal reports about children's surgery.

## DEFINING QUALITY IN CHILDREN'S SURGICAL SERVICES

This section explores the quality standards pertaining to children undergoing surgery. Many of the recognised standards of care are the outcomes of reviews of practice and the identification of limitation and deficits in the services for children. Several reports have made credible attempts to define standards of care for children within acute and community settings. Such generic standards pertaining to services for children have relevance for the nursing of children undergoing surgery (e.g. Department of Health 1991, Department of Health 1996, Smith 2003, Department of Health 2003a, Department of Health 2003b) and these are acknowledged.

However, there are two specific documents in relation to children's surgery worthy of further attention because arguably they form the foundations for subsequent work:

- *Just for the Day* (Thornes 1991), which has the primary focus on day surgery, and
- *Setting standards for Children Undergoing Surgery* (Hogg 1994), which superseded the above and concentrated on the needs of children admitted as inpatients for surgery.

## JUST FOR THE DAY: CHILDREN AND DAY SURGERY

On the surface day surgery for children appears to have been a recent innovation although some of the earliest day surgery procedures were undertaken in children in outpatient settings at the turn of the century. Concurrent with a growth in inpatient services was an apparent decline in popularity of day surgery. This was also attributed to increasing concerns about safety and mediocre quality, in other words risk management and quality issues. In the 1980s there was a revival, underpinned by government initiatives, in particular the drive within the National Health Service (NHS), to increase throughput, to reduce waiting times and to use resources more efficiently. By the early 1990s 30% of all surgical interventions were undertaken as day cases (Moores 1995) and this rising trend towards day surgery and ambulatory care has continued.

On one level children were seen as ideal candidates for day surgery and this was a persuasive rationale for developing ambulatory approaches to health care. The endeavour was to minimise the disruption to the child and family of admission to hospital. The many advantages associated with reducing the amount of time children spend in hospital, thus minimising separation disruption and stress, have been well documented (Dearmun 1994).

Until 1991, guidance on day surgery in children was inconclusive and incomplete. The *Just for the Day* report (Thornes 1991) has been considered a milestone in providing a blueprint for the development of day surgical services for children. It was primarily designed as a tool for use by managers to identify minimal standards and enhance quality of care.

The premise of *Just for the Day* was the overall conviction that reducing length of stay in hospital for children through the expansion of day surgery was positive, but 'Day admissions have to be carefully planned if they are not to cause unnecessary stress to children and families.' (Thornes 1991, p. 1) Research and audits have shown the limitations of this ambulatory approach to organising care, in particular inadequate information, poor discharge planning and the pressure on carers, who often have to take on additional responsibility at home (While & Crawford 1992, Lane & Baker 2000). To this end the report offers twelve quality standards that can be used as performance indicators, including criteria regarding the selection of children who are suitable for day surgery so that social as well as 'condition related' considerations are taken into account. There are also recommendations about the advice given to carers regarding aftercare and guidance about the referral and support from community nursing services, especially the need for input from community children's nurses.

## STANDARDS FOR CHILDREN UNDERGOING SURGERY AS INPATIENTS

In 1994 Hogg produced a report that complemented the work started by Thornes (Hogg 1994). This set of recommendations, infused by examples of good practice, has as its primary focus children admitted for surgery as inpatients and is also valuable as a managerial tool for monitoring standards. The themes address all aspects of the experience of the child and family, from pre-admission through to discharge home, providing a wealth of information. The overall standards are identified in Box 2.1.

## DEFICITS IN CURRENT PROVISION

Overall, many of the deficits in the provision of services for children experiencing surgery identified in all the reports mentioned so far were attributed to two main aspects:

- the environment in which the children are nursed, and
- the aptitude, competence and technical expertise of healthcare professionals, in particular their appreciation of children and adolescents as distinct groups with specific developmental needs.

## ENVIRONMENTAL ASPECTS OF SURGERY

As suggested earlier in this chapter, the environment or context within which care is delivered can

---

### Box 2.1  Setting standards for children undergoing surgery (Hogg 1994)

- **The decision to operate:** including the provision of information, informed consent and confidentiality
- **Admission to hospital:** including criteria for admission, the experience and training required of surgeons and anaesthetists
- **Preparation for the operation:** including the preparation of parents, the preparation of children using a range of media, the utilisation of pre-admission programmes that draw on contributions from all members of the multidisciplinary team
- **Ward procedures:** including strategies to minimise anxiety, starvation regimes, clothing worn to theatre
- **Going to the theatre:** including imaginative modes of transport to theatre and communication to minimise waiting times
- **Anaesthetic room:** including the environment and procedures and the support to be given to parents to enable them to reassure and comfort their child during induction of anaesthesia
- **Recovery room:** including the environment and procedures and the provision for parents to be available when their child wakes up
- **After the operation:** including pain management policies
- **Home again:** including preparation prior to discharge and liaison between the acute and community services
- **Contracting for quality – purchasers:** this includes a checklist in terms of overall strategy, placing contracts, contract specifications and monitoring
- **Quality services for children – providers:** this uses the above themes and offers a checklist or audit tool for managers in the form of questions about the services provided

---

have a profound influence and sometimes a detrimental effect on the approaches to care and especially the extent to which children's specific developmental needs are recognised and met. The diversity and number of surgeons operating meant that children could often be found within an environment that was more equipped to provide care to adults. In relation to children admitted for day surgery, those admitted and discharged within 12 hours, there seemed to be a particular variability in the quality of care provided and this was dependent to a large extent upon where they were located. The *Just for the Day* report (Thornes 1991) offered an evaluation of several options in order to identify the relative strengths and limitations of each and the resultant quality issues.

## The creation of ambulatory care specifically for children

The expert panel suggested that the optimal approach to serving this population was the creation of an ambulatory care facility or day unit specifically designed for children. However, in reality this is not always considered feasible for two main reasons:

- First, managers often maintain that there are insufficient numbers of children admitted for day surgery to warrant special attention. Whilst this may be supported by the statistical evidence available, it is argued that the total numbers of children fulfilling this category are concealed because of lack of robust data and poor data collection techniques. These do not take into account that a large number of children experiencing day and inpatient surgery are under the care of adult surgical teams and are therefore inappropriately coded to adult, rather than children's services.
- Secondly, it is considered that additional resources are required to redesign the current provisions to provide facilities specifically for children and this is not seen as a viable option.

Recognising that these are particular challenges in day surgery, commonly a compromise is sought and children may be admitted to an inpatient children's ward instead. Although this may be more appropriate than admission to an adult facility, it may be seen that there is still a need to exercise caution. There is a likely expectation that the philosophy of care operating within a children's inpatient ward will acknowledge the developmental needs of children and other important aspects of care, such as working in partnership with their families. Whilst this may be true in such settings, priority is generally given to caring for the children with longer term and high dependency needs, thus the specific needs of the child having day surgery may still be neglected.

Two other alternatives have been put forward:

- to create a designated area within an adult day surgery unit, or
- to devote a particular day to children's surgery within the adult day surgery unit.

Both these options are considered to be poor practice. The *Just for the Day* report (Thornes 1991) held the view that the admission of children to an adult day care facility is undesirable, not least because if they have postoperative complications and need to stay overnight there may not be inpatient children's services within the same geographical location. Hence, it is probable that children will be admitted to the adjacent adult ward or they may have to be transported some distance to a children's centre and this transfer may involve an inherent risk to their safety.

A comparative study undertaken by While & Crawford (1992) found that when children were admitted to an adult facility the quality of care was compromised and the prudence of using occasional sessions in such an environment was questioned. They concluded that care was considered inadequate on at least three counts.

- First, there was evidence that children were sent the pre-admission information that had been designed for adults. The consequence of this was it was neither appropriate nor child friendly.
- Secondly, there was little consideration of the psychological preparation required for a child and family's admission to hospital and surgery.
- Finally, frequently the approaches to care did not demonstrate an affinity to children's specific needs because staff did not always possess the knowledge and skills to work with children and their families, especially in terms of giving appropriate information and the assessment and management of pain.

When allocating a designated day within an adult facility for children's surgery, forethought is required with regard to the careful planning of the operating lists so that the children can be admitted on the same day, and to ensure the safety and aesthetic aspects of the environment in the adult unit are suitable on the day designated for children, not least ensuring that paediatric resuscitation equipment is available.

Maintaining a consistent quality of care for children receiving treatment outside a designated children's unit may be a challenge. To this end, in some Trusts registered children's nurses have been employed to coordinate care for the children admitted to other departments, for example Accident and Emergency, X-ray and adult wards. There is some anecdotal evidence to suggest that access to the expertise of registered children's nurses has served to educate nursing staff and raise awareness of the needs of children (Stower 1998, Valentine & Smith 2000).

However, in the final analysis, despite such strategies to ensure quality care in this way, the main recommendations encapsulated in all the reports were that all services for children should be affiliated to comprehensive children's centres and share their philosophy of care.

## THE APTITUDE, COMPETENCE AND TECHNICAL EXPERTISE OF HEALTHCARE PROFESSIONALS

A conjecture is put forward that healthcare professionals who are not regularly involved in caring for children will not necessarily have the aptitude, competence and experience to care for children. Thus they may not subscribe to the values inherent in family-centred approaches to care; but perhaps more importantly, they will not have the knowledge base to practise competently and safely and to support children and families through the total experience of admission to hospital and surgical interventions. In contrast, nurses who consistently work with children having surgery develop particular expertise, which includes being able to assess the child's physiological status and be proactive in identifying and minimising complications, providing psychological preparation for events in hospital, assessing and managing postoperative pain, and offering appropriate aftercare advice.

In addition to the aptitude and competence of nursing staff, the technical expertise of surgeons and anaesthetists has also been scrutinised. This was the focus of a Royal College of Surgeons Paediatric Forum publication *Children's Surgery: A First Class Service* (2000) and the *Paediatric and Congenital Cardiac Services Review Report* (Department of Health 2003a). Here the main emphasis was upon the surgeon's competence to perform surgery on children and the Trust's responsibility to develop strategies to ensure that specific surgeons are allocated to operate on children with the expectation that these individuals would have chosen to gain expertise in the paediatric surgical speciality. It was also deemed important that the designated surgeons have a workload of adequate volume to

maintain their level of surgical competence with this age group.

The above aspects of environment of care and aptitude and technical expertise of personnel could be classified as the overarching contextual quality issues for children experiencing admission for the day or as inpatients.

Managers may be more ready to accept that specific technical expertise is required in order to anaesthetise and operate on children. However, when it comes to convincing them of the need for children to be cared for in a child-oriented environment by children's nurses, as embodied in reports and recommendations, the systematic research and evidence base to support these arguments needs to be more robust.

In the following section other quality aspects permeating the reports will be discussed.

## INFORMATION GIVING

Lack of information and poor communication is one of the most common complaints made by consumers of health care. The importance of providing adequate information is stressed within the quality standards. The purpose of effective communication and information giving is identified in Box 2.2.

> **Box 2.2 The purpose of effective communication and information giving**
>
> - To help to prepare children and families for events prior to admission, during their hospital stay and after they return home
> - To facilitate effective decision making and informed consent by ensuring that the parent and child understand the procedures to be undertaken and have the opportunity to discuss fully the implications of the surgery and anaesthetic, including the risk and benefits
> - To enhance the parents' understanding of their role in relation to caring for their child in hospital, encouraging them to negotiate their contribution to care alongside other healthcare professionals
> - To provide guidance on aftercare including the community resources, the management of their child's pain, incisions and dressings, and recuperation or readjustment to usual recreational activities and patterns of daily living.

In respect of Box 2.2, the information should be tailored to the individual, taking into account the child or adolescent's age and stage of development.

The value of providing information for children and families prior to day surgery has been the subject of many research studies (for example, Jonas et al 2000). There are numerous recommendations about the accessibility of information in order to make informed decisions and the association between the giving of information and the reduction of anxiety. Information giving can take several forms. For children having elective surgery, initially it is given verbally during early visits to the GP or at outpatient consultations and through pre-admission visits. Sometimes nurses are appointed to undertake pre-admission clerking or provide a link between the inpatient and outpatient departments (Dearmun & Gordon 1999), and such individuals are in a prime position to provide information prior to admission. Written material (Stone 2000) or other media such as audiocassettes, slides and videos can support verbal information. It is anticipated that in the future information will also be provided via CD-ROM or Internet sources. For those children admitted in an emergency this is more difficult, and the timing and reinforcement of the information given is crucial.

## FAMILY-CENTRED CARE

The shift over the last 50 years towards making family-centred care pivotal to the nursing of children is very well documented (Savage & Callery 2000). It is widely accepted that parents or carers should be involved in all decisions affecting their child's treatment and care and in the actual physical and psychological support of their child. In all quality standards emphasis is placed upon healthcare professionals playing a facilitation role in enabling this to happen. It is interesting to note that some of the first studies in this area were undertaken on children having tonsillectomy (Visintainer & Wolfer 1975). It was found that children accompanied by their parents experienced fewer postoperative complications.

In terms of children's surgery there are a number of other specific considerations. First of these is the recognition of children or young people's need to be involved in their own care and to contribute to decisions of differing magnitude according to their understanding and competence. In obtaining con-

sent it does not follow that gaining consent from the parents is synonymous with procuring consent from the child (Bijsterveld 2000). Secondly, two reports (Thornes 1991, Hogg 1994) have maintained that a planned and shared approach to parental participation in the care of the child offers a positive experience for parents, and Hogg (1994) stated that: 'A parent should be enabled to be with the child and help with care when ever the child is conscious and should be given timely on-going information and support.' (p. 8) This gives support for parental presence in the anaesthetic and recovery rooms, a contentious issue that has traditionally been criticised, largely by anaesthetists and anaesthetic nurses. Some of the barriers have now been overcome and there are some examples of effective practice in this area.

## PROVISION OF COMMUNITY REFERRAL

The paucity and inequity of community children's nursing services has been recognised (Hunt & Whiting 1999) but the value of such services in providing essential aftercare advice to children and families following discharge should not be underestimated. Audits of day surgery have shown that parents would appreciate support and advice when they are first discharged home, but they are reluctant to contact healthcare professionals with what they perceive to be trivial concerns and thus this remains an unrecognised and unmet need.

## WAYS OF MONITORING QUALITY

This section looks at some of the ways in which standards of care may be monitored. Several approaches to quality measurement are identified. These include:

- professional self regulation, including benchmarking and clinical audit and integrated care pathways
- consumer surveys or user satisfaction.

The former involves an audit tool or checklist to monitor the implementation of predefined standards (as available in Hogg 1996) and can be used when commissioning services. The consumer survey or user satisfaction comprises the distribution of survey questionnaires, rating scales or interviews to parents and/or children to ascertain whether they are satisfied with the service received in relation to particular aspects of care (e.g. Higson & Bolland 2000, Higson & Hawkins 2001).

## PROFESSIONAL SELF-REGULATION

Some of the principles for the monitoring and auditing of standards specified in the reports already discussed are identified in Box 2.3.

## BENCHMARKING

Another way of monitoring the quality of the service is through benchmarking. This has been undertaken informally for a number of years in industry but Ellis (1999) offered a more structured process that has gained some popularity in the National Health Service. Expert practitioners construct benchmarks of standards by amassing evidence from a number of literature and intelligence sources, for example systematic reviews of research, examination of national guidelines and standards, identification of local guidelines and protocols; these are synthesised with the perspectives of carers, parents and other professionals. It could be argued that this multi-source approach improves the authenticity of the benchmark. The benchmark is then presented as the standard against which to compare services and practices (Ellis 1995). A peer review approach is used with a standardised system to score practice against the benchmark. One of the first benchmarking groups to be established in 1996 was the paediatric neurosurgery group and benchmarking of elective surgery has also taken place. The rigour of benchmarking has been questioned and work is currently underway to evaluate this process.

---

**Box 2.3  Principles when monitoring and auditing standards**

- There should be an audit which separates the provision for children
- Inpatient and day case data should be separated
- In terms of day surgery, there should be a review of the transfer to inpatient care and readmission rates
- There should be evidence of seamless care between acute and community care
- There should be evidence of the consumer perspectives of patient satisfaction.

---

## CLINICAL AUDIT

Audit has been defined as the degree to which actual care delivered conforms to preset criteria for good care (Donabedian 1966).

The features of clinical audit have been identified by Harvey (1996). Central to these are the systematic analysis and evaluation of current practice to improve patient care. On the surface there are similarities between research and audit but their distinctiveness lies in distinguishing between seeking new knowledge, which may be seen as research, and implementing espoused knowledge in the form of accepted quality criteria, which is classified as audit. Commonly, audits are undertaken to highlight deficits and improve practice or to look at the effectiveness of a particular intervention.

Initially, audit was exclusively related to morbidity and mortality and the systematic and critical analysis of the quality of medical care. This emphasised the outcome and quality of life for the patient. Arguably this reaffirmed the pre-eminence of the medical profession, but this uniprofessional perspective is now estranged from contemporary policy. The current drive is for clinical governance and the notion of multiprofessional audit programmes that are led by a variety of professional groups and examine a wide range of topics, for example a telephone service for children following day surgery (Feasey 2000, Higson & Bolland 2000), or adherence to advice on starving times or the incidence of pain, nausea or vomiting (Keeton 1999).

## PATHWAYS OF CARE

It is suggested that pathways of care are tools that provide another approach to auditing care. There are many synonymous terms, including: integrated care pathways (ICPs), anticipated recovery pathways, multidisciplinary pathways of care, care protocols, critical pathways and care maps. The idea, originating in the United States of America (USA), was introduced into the United Kingdom (UK) in the early 1990s. Within the context of American health care these tools were driven by the heath insurance-based system, whereas in the UK they have been seen in terms of monitoring clinical effectiveness and the focus has been on their use as a quality improvement tool (Johnson 1997), hence their relevance to this chapter.

Johnson (1997) has offered a definition of pathways of care that embraces three main features:

- An amalgamation of all the anticipated elements of care and treatment given by all members of the multiprofessional team
- An agreed time frame, action plan and outcomes of care
- A system for documenting the variance from the agreed outcomes.

It is the latter feature that provides the data with which to review current practice.

In essence pathways of care are similar to standardised or core care plans. However, it could be argued that their distinctiveness lies in the multiprofessional approach to their development and the way in which they encourage practitioners to review and coordinate current processes, practice and the care delivered by all health professionals coming into contact with the child and family. Best practice is acknowledged and discussed and, where possible, the care is based upon quality standards, available evidence and research (Currie & Harvey 1998). In the absence of systematic research, the benefits of using pathways of care remain conjecture but anecdotal evidence suggests that they can lead to improved teamwork, and enhance the consistency and equity of care received by children and families, and this is an area for future research. Johnson (1997) offers a further explanation and examples of pathways of care.

## THE USER'S PERSPECTIVE

There is an increasing trend towards recognising and valuing the user's contribution when evaluating and commissioning care (Woodfield 2001, Carney et al 2003). This recognises the government agenda within *The NHS Plan* (Department of Health 2000) and the premise inherent in the *United Nations Convention on the Rights of the Child* Article 12: 'Children have a right to express an opinion about their hospital experiences and have these taken into account for future service provision.' (United Nations 1989)

Eliciting users' views is sometimes fraught with methodological and ethical challenges, as identified by Callery & Luker (1996) and Woodfield (2001). In relation to children's services there may be a tension between child and parents in terms of who is the direct recipient of care and thus whose opinions have most significance. Traditionally, the priorities have been set by the professionals and address areas they consider to be important (McIver 1991).

Moreover, reaching a consensus view about the constituents of quality is a challenge because parents, children, nurses and medical staff may all have differing views as to what constitutes quality care, and this is still an area that deserves more attention (Lindsay 1995). Lindsay's work (1995) and that of Cunliff & English (1998) have begun to address the ways in which children and families could be more involved in the origin of standards. For example, Cunliff & English recognised that the mechanisms for gaining feedback from children in relation to their views of quality were inadequate. They described a project that elicited the ingredients of quality as seen by children by using questionnaires, answer phones, suggestion boxes and children and young people's panels. This is a good example of innovation in this area.

## CONTRACTING FOR QUALITY: COMMISSIONING CHILDREN'S SURGERY

The commissioning process often entails identification and monitoring of standards. For example, *Health Services for Children and Young People: A Guide for Commissioners and Providers* (Hogg 1996) identifies the principles for commissioning for and providing services, and attention is drawn to three main areas (see Table 2.1).

Most of the aspects of the audit tool in this document are concerned with overall quality issues for

**Table 2.1** Principles for commissioning and providing services

| Principle | Key actions |
|---|---|
| The rights of the child | - Practice is such a way as to respect children<br>- Recognise their rights as identified by the *UN Convention on the Rights of the Child* (United Nations 1989)<br>- Develop strategies to gain their views when developing services |
| Partnership with parents and children | - Respect the skills of parents and carers<br>- Provide appropriate information and support |
| An integrated and comprehensive service | - Develop a service plan for children that integrates all the services for children and families |

children cared for in a variety of settings with a range of health problems. There is a section comprised of audit checklists and two pages with a specific focus on surgery (Hogg 1996, pp. 15–16). These attend to aspects such as the use of designated surgeons and anaesthetists, transfer of children less than 3 years of age requiring emergency surgery, involvement of parents and child in decisions, and preparation of child and family for events. The British Association of Paediatric Surgeons (1995) has also produced a *Guide for Purchasers and Providers of Surgical Services.*

## CONCLUSION

This chapter has explored some of the overall quality issues in relation to children undergoing surgery and has introduced the reader to the origins of standards for children undergoing surgery. The recognised standards of care have been identified and ways in which they may be monitored were discussed. In terms of the standards currently available, there is growing consensus regarding the quality charter marks for children's surgical services. However, the evidence from systematic review to support these standards is limited. English & Bond (1998) have identified that the psychological care of hospitalised children is not a priority in the NHS Research and Development agenda, and whilst there is some evidence to guide practice there is a lack of systematic testing or hypotheses. This situation may need to change in order to move forward.

At the moment the view of the professionals tends to hold sway in terms of setting standards that reflect their agenda. However, there is a lobby to increase children's and parents' contribution to setting standards, as advocated by Hogg (1994): 'standards developed with children, young people and their families are often the best indicators of quality' (p. 29).

If this trend increases, practitioners will need to further develop creative approaches to involving children in the audit process and may need to consider some of the ethical issues associated with this.

It is appreciated that standards are not set in stone and will need to be reviewed in the light of new and emerging evidence and services, but familiarity with the available standards will reduce the need for replication of effort. Instead, increasingly practitioners working in the children's surgical care arena will be tasked with sharing good practice and ensuring that care provided for this client group is equitable and consistent. Traditionally there has been a failure to implement the standards that have been well documented. It could be argued that successful implementation relies on robust monitoring processes. It is anticipated that the Commission for Health Improvement Agency, the National Institute for Clinical Effectiveness guidelines and the implementation of the National Service Framework (Department of Health 2004) for children and young people will assist in ensuring the effectiveness of this quality programme and that practitioners will continue to make a positive contribution to these initiatives.

## References

Bijsterveld P 2000 Competent to refuse. Paediatric Nursing 12(6): 33–35

British Association of Paediatric Surgeons 1995 A guide for purchasers and providers of surgical services. British Association of Paediatric Surgeons, London

Callery P 1997 Using evidence in children's nursing. Paediatric Nursing 9(6): 13–17

Callery P, Luker K 1996 The use of qualitative methods in the study of parents' experiences of care on a children's surgical ward. Journal of Advanced Nursing 23: 338–345

Carney T, Murphy S, McClure J et al 2003 Children's views of hospitalisation: an exploratory study of data collection. Journal of Child Health Care 7(1): 27–40

Cunliff L, English C 1998 Kids count: a children's rights project. Paediatric Nursing 10(4): 16–19

Currie L, Harvey G 1998 Care pathways development and implementation. Nursing Standard 12(30): 35–38

Dearmun AK 1994 Defining differences: children's day surgery. Surgical Nurse 7(6): 7–11

Dearmun AK 2000 Children's surgery: a first class service. Paediatric Nursing 12(7): 8

Dearmun AK, Gordon K 1999 The nurse practitioner in children's ambulatory care. Paediatric Nursing 11(1): 18–21

Department of Health 1991 Welfare of children and young people in hospital. HMSO, London

Department of Health 1996 The patient's charter: services for children and young people. HMSO, London

Department of Health 1997 The new NHS, modern, dependable. HMSO, London

Department of Health 1998 First class service: quality in the new NHS. HMSO, London

Department of Health 2000 The NHS plan: a plan for investment, a plan for reform. HMSO, London

Department of Health 2003a Paediatric and Congenital Cardiac Services review report. HMSO, London. Online.

Available: http://www.doh.gov.uk/childcardiac/review-nov20. htm

Department of Health 2003b Getting the right start: the national service framework for children, young people and maternity services – Standards for Hospital Services. HMSO, London. Online. Available: http://www.doh.gov.uk/nsf/children/gettingtherightstart.htm

Department of Health 2004 National service framework for children, young people and maternity services. Department of Health, London

Donabedian A 1966 Institutional and professional responsibilities in quality assurance. Quality Assurance in Health Care 1(1): 3–11

Donabedian A 1980 Explorations in quality assessment and monitoring. Volume 1: The definition of quality and approaches to its assessment. MI Health administration, Ann Arbor

Ellis J 1995 Using benchmarks to improve practice. Nursing Standard 9(35): 25–28

Ellis J 1999 Benchmarking our stamp and its effects. Journal of Child Health 3(2): 33–35

English C, Bond S 1998 Easier said than done. Paediatric Nursing 10(5): 7–11

Feasey S 2000 Quality counts: auditing day surgery services. Journal of Child Health Care 4(2): 73–77

Glasper EA, Ireland L 2000 Evidence based child health care: challenges for practice. Macmillan, London

Harvey G 1996 Relating quality assessment and audit to the research process in nursing. Nurse Researcher 3(3): 35–46

Health Committee 1997 Hospital services for children and young people, session 1996–7, fifth report. HMSO, London

Higson J, Bolland R 2000 Telephone survey after paediatric surgery. Paediatric Nursing 12(10): 30–32

Higson J, Hawkins G 2001 Measuring quality in a paediatric day care unit. Nursing Times 97(10): 32–34

Hogg C 1994 Setting standards for children undergoing surgery: caring for children in the health service. Action for Sick Children, London

Hogg C 1996 Health services for children and young people: a guide for commissioners and providers. Action for Sick Children, London

Hogg C, Cooper C 2004 Meeting the needs of children and young people undergoing surgery. Action for Sick Children (Scotland), Edinburgh

Hunt J, Whiting M 1999 A re-examination of the history of children's community nursing. Paediatric Nursing 11(4): 33–36

Johnson S 1997 Pathways of care. Blackwell Science, London

Jonas D, Worsley J, Cox K 2000 Information giving can be painless. Journal of Child Health Care 4(2): 55–58

Keeton D 1999 Pain, nausea and vomiting: a day surgery audit. Paediatric Nursing 11(5): 28–30

Kennedy I 2001 Learning from Bristol: the report of the public inquiry into children's heart surgery at the Bristol Royal Infirmary 1984–1995. HMSO, London. Online. Available: http://www.bristol-inquiry.org.uk/index.htm

Lane M, Baker S 2000 Home sweet home – examining the interface between hospital and community. In: Glasper EA, Ireland L 2000 Evidence based child health care: challenges for practice. Macmillan, London

Lindsay B 1995 A matter of opinion. Perceptions of care in child health. Journal of Child Health 3(2): 33–35

McIver S 1991 An introduction to obtaining the views of users of health services. Kings Fund Centre, London

Moores Y 1995 The challenge ahead. Child Health 3(4): 131–135

Royal College of Surgeons of England 2000 Children's surgery: a first class service. Royal College of Surgeons of England, London

Royal College of Surgeons Paediatric Forum 2000 Children's surgery: a first class service. Royal College of Surgeons Paediatric Forum, England

Savage E, Callery P 2000 Parental participation in the care of hospitalised children: a review of the research evidence. In: Glasper A, Ireland L 2000 Evidence based child health care: challenges for practice. Macmillan, London

Stone KJ 2000 Can information leaflets assist parents in preparing their children for hospital admission? In: Glasper A, Ireland L 2000 Evidence based child health care: challenges for practice. Macmillan, London

Stower S 1998 A role in smooth transition. Paediatric Nursing 10(5): 6

Smith F 2003 Getting the right start: the children's national service framework. Paediatric Nursing 15(4): 20

Thornes R 1991 Just for the day: caring for children in the Health Service. NAWHC, London

United Nations 1989 United Nations convention on the rights of the child. United Nations, Geneva

Valentine F, Smith F 2000 Clinical governance in acute children's services. Paediatric Nursing 12(8): 6–8

Visintainer MA, Wolfer JA 1975 Psychological preparation for surgical paediatric patients: the effects on children's and parents' stress responses and adjustment. Paediatrics 56(2): 187–202

While A, Crawford J 1992 Day surgery: expediency or quality care. Paediatric Nursing 4: 18–20

Woodfield T 2001 Involving children in clinical audit. Paediatric Nursing 13(3): 12–16

# Chapter 3

# Ethics and consent

## Sue Jones

## INTRODUCTION AND CONTEXT IN CONTEMPORARY HEALTH CARE

Children's nurses have always been required and indeed seen it as their duty to act as advocates for the child, putting the best interests of the child forward and promoting what is in the child's interests to the medical team and the child's family. It is the role of the children's nurse to encourage children to express their views, help children to reach a better understanding of their surgery, understand the reasons for the surgery, and comply with their subsequent care. Much of this role is undertaken in partnership with the child's parents or person with parental responsibility. The nursing role in the consent process is paramount and is usually complementary to the medical practitioner's role.

However, the Nursing and Midwifery Council (NMC) (2002), in the new code of professional conduct, requires all registered nurses to obtain consent as a core skill across the healthcare professions. This new statement in the code of conduct makes explicit the nursing requirement to be the professional that obtains the consent where the nurse is the professional that conducts the procedure.

Gill Brook (2000) describes consent in children as a process whereby a greater understanding is gradually achieved. Children and their families need information and support from someone highly skilled in working with children; usually the children's nurse meets these criteria. For Gill Brook, a specialist children's nurse working with children having liver or bowel transplants, a full level of understanding of Frazer (or Gillick) competence (see below, 'Test cases in law') can be achieved for children as young as 6 or 7 years. The British Medical Association (BMA) (2001, p. 2) consent rights and choices steering group acknowledge that adults: '… often underestimate the abilities of children as young as 5 to understand what is at stake and with support take a significant part in decisions about their healthcare.'

For the sick child used to hospital, a far greater understanding develops over time. Decision making is an integral part of all children's development; it is also much more a part of the way children are viewed in society today, being encouraged to make choices from a very early age. Positive parenting hinges on allowing children to make choices. We also have to acknowledge that as adults we naturally shield children from difficult decisions, preferring to maintain the authority of parents to make difficult decisions, therefore underestimating the abilities of children. The privacy of family life is deep rooted and protected by politicians; the Prime Minister Tony Blair's reluctance to discuss his son Leo's measles, mumps and rubella (MMR) vaccination status is one such example.

*The NHS Plan* (2000) attaches very great importance to the needs and interests of patients, and the development of patient advice and liaison services (PALS) and partnerships with patients that are meaningful and that fully acknowledge and work with patients will be key elements in the NHS of the future. In children's nursing the philosophy of partnership working with the child and family has developed practice in such a way that the needs and wishes of the child and family are integral to the care that is given. Children's rights, on the other hand, have had a lesser emphasis, and any practice development initiatives that address consent to treatment for children must embrace the Human Rights Act (1998) and the *United Nations Convention on the Rights of the Child* (1989), ratified in the UK in 1991.

Recent public inquiries such as the Bristol Royal Infirmary Inquiry (Kennedy 2001) and the inquiry into organ retention at Alder Hey Hospital in Liverpool (Royal Liverpool Children's Inquiry 2001) prompted the biggest overhaul of consent to treatment ever in the UK. The Department of Health website now has very useful resources on consent for children and parents as well as health professionals, and is available at http://www.doh.gov.uk/consent. A national consent form for children has been developed and is now in use. The overriding message is the need for honesty and explanation, however difficult that honesty may be.

For the vast majority of children and young people, time will allow for their involvement in decision making and their parents will serve their best interests. The purpose of this chapter is to provide guidance on the nursing role in the consent process.

## AGE OF CONSENT

In England, Wales and Northern Ireland the age of adulthood is 18 years; in Scotland the age of majority is also 18 years, but at 16 years many decisions can be made legally by the young person, including consent to treatment. Adults at the age of 18 years not only have the vote, but can consent to treatment and refuse treatment without having to be assessed as competent. If decisions to refuse treatment are dubious, as long as adults are not mentally incapacitated their right to refuse treatment is respected. The provision of information and the requirements for informed consent remain paramount, and very often professional accountability hinges on whether or not the patient has had the opportunity to give a fully informed consent.

At 16–18 years of age young people are at a transitional stage, old enough to leave school, start work, be convicted of a criminal offence, pay for an adult ticket etc, but still dependent on parents to support many aspects of decision making. Children under 16 are often referred to as minors in the legal system.

> Adolescence is a period of progressive transition from childhood to adulthood and as experience of life is acquired and intelligence and understanding grow, so will the scope of the decision-making which should be left to the minor, for it is only by making decisions and experiencing the consequences that decision making skills will be acquired … good parenting involves giving minors as much rope as they can handle without unacceptable risk so that they will hang themselves!
>
> Lord Donaldson, Former Master of Rolls
> (BMA 2001, p. 6)

## WHO CAN PROVIDE CONSENT?

The following can provide consent:

- Adults who have reached the age of consent (18 years of age in England and Wales and 16 years of age in Scotland)

- The child's parents if married
- The child's mother if the parents are unmarried
- Any child assessed as Frazer/Gillick competent
- The local authority for looked after children (children in the care of the local authority).

## UNMARRIED FATHERS

Unmarried fathers do not automatically have parental responsibility and cannot automatically give consent for treatment of their children. They can apply for parental responsibility through courts that can formalise a parental responsibility agreement with the mother. The government are seeking to change this, so that in the future parents who are not married but who have signed the birth certificate will have joint parental responsibility.

## IMPORTANCE OF FAMILY ASSESSMENT ON ADMISSION

When admitting children to hospital it is extremely important not to make assumptions about parental responsibility, and there are ways of sensitively asking questions so that the team is clear about who can/cannot consent to treatment for the child. It is quite possible that an unmarried father is unaware that he does not have automatic parental responsibility and this assessment may require the children's nurse to liaise quickly with the medical social worker, particularly if the mother is unable to sign the consent.

Either on admission or at pre-assessment the children's nurse should also be ascertaining the child's wishes. Where children have already decided they want to sign their own consent, the nurse will then need to advocate on behalf of each child, assessing Frazer/Gillick competence and recommending to the surgeon that the children be given the time to give consent themselves. In a time pressured service this is by no means the easy option.

For planned surgery, the consent process should be part of the child's general preoperative preparation; whether children are giving their own informed consent or simply complying with a general anaesthetic and operation, they need information and preparation in a manner to suit their cognitive abilities. There should be absolutely no reason for a child to be restrained for a planned

surgical intervention. Parents should be encouraged to support their child's involvement in decision making about treatment. As a first step it may be appropriate for both the parent and the child to sign the consent.

## ETHICAL PRINCIPLES

Ethics is a form of moral philosophy '...designed to illuminate what we ought to do by asking us to consider and reconsider our ordinary actions, judgements and justifications'. The surgical care of infants and children can result in some very difficult ethical dilemmas. The nurse's role is as an equal partner in the surgical team, supporting decision making together with the child and family.

Beneficence and nonmaleficence are the most basic of ethical principles. They mean essentially that our actions should be of benefit to the child and family and ultimately do the child no harm (Brykczynska 1989). These principles form the basis of the United Kingdom Central Council (UKCC) Code of Professional Conduct (1992) and the newly updated NMC Code of Conduct (2002), and we uphold them through professional accountability. It is not always that easy, however, to know what is good or bad for a child. Informed decision making is what all children and their families should expect based on the child's cognitive ability and the nurse's skill in helping the child reach a greater level of understanding.

A third basic ethical principle is the principle of justice. Justice in ethical terms includes equal opportunities or fairness, an underlying principle of the NHS, with *The NHS Plan* (2001) seeking to end the 'postcode lottery' in NHS funding. Fairness for children and young people may mean having their rights respected.

The Royal College of Nursing (RCN) (2000) suggest using ethical principles to analyse a problem, looking at motives and consequences and seeking a balanced position. Thiroux's principles are suggested as a framework for their useful application in health care (Richardson & Webber 1995):

- The value of life
- Goodness and rightness
- Justice or fairness
- Truth telling and honesty
- Individual freedom.

Ethical decisions should not be made in isolation and should be discussed in teams with the involvement of the child and family.

Conflict between ethical principles can occur and choices will need to be made. For example, valuing life may be at the cost of quality of life and telling the truth may be honest but cause psychological harm. In one case where a patient with a progressive condition wanted to have her ventilator switched off the court ruled that she had the capacity to make the decision (Ms B v An NHS Trust 2002). Dame Elizabeth Butler Sloss, the judge in this case, was quoted in the press as saying that the 'doctor knows best' attitude must change, and that the rights of the competent adult were paramount. For children and young people under the age of 18 years in England and Wales and 16 years in Scotland, their rights are not as overriding as those of the competent adult. However, the importance of this ruling is the challenge to paternalistic decision making, and this case will have an impact on ethical decision making in the future.

Dearmun & McKinnon (2001) describe the role of the British Association of Paediatric Surgeons (BAPS) ethics group, where ethical problems can be raised and discussed by the profession at national level. A children's nurse nominated by the RCN has a seat on this committee and the committee welcome issues being raised by nurses. Ethical dilemmas can be forwarded to this forum by contacting Dr Annette Dearmun, Chair of the RCN Children's Surgical Nursing Forum.

The BMA medical ethics department (see Useful addresses, below) can also be contacted for information about developments since the publication of *Consent, Rights and Choices* (2001); alternatively the website contains further information.

## THE LAW

Consent to treatment has three dimensions: clinical needs, ethical issues and the law. The law relating to consent is common law and not specific legislation, and test cases in law are referred to in deciding cases.

The law relating to children and young people is briefly explained under each of the relevant acts and test cases. There are differences between the 4 UK countries, most notably in Scotland.

## FAMILY LAW REFORM ACT 1969

The Family Law Reform Act (1969) makes provision for 16 year olds to give a valid consent, whilst also stating that the right to provide consent by others, i.e. the parents, is not diminished.

## TEST CASES IN LAW

In civil law, test cases act to set a precedent and subsequent cases are measured against them. The Bolam test (1957) is particularly significant and is used by the NMC in deciding cases of misconduct. For nursing it essentially means care that could be expected of the average ordinary nurse. The most significant legal case for children was that of Gillick v West Norfolk and Wisbech Health Authority (1986). Mrs Gillick's case against the health authority centred upon her allegation that her daughter was too young to consent to take the oral contraceptive pill. Lord Frazer in the House of Lords ruled against her, commenting that it was: 'verging on the absurd that a boy or girl of 15 could not effectively consent for example to have a medical examination of some trivial injury to his body, or even to have his broken arm set'. Lord Frazer's ruling is known as 'Frazer competence' although many still refer to it as 'Gillick competence'.

## CHILDREN ACT 1989

The Children Act (1989) was regarded as a major piece of reforming legislation for children (Department of Health 2001). It was implemented in 1991, the same year in which the UN Convention on the Rights of the Child (1989) was ratified in the UK. The key message for practice from the Children Act is safeguarding and promoting children's welfare by:

- Working with parents
- Listening to children
- Strengthening interagency planning and provision of services
- Providing effective services.

## DIFFERENCES IN SCOTLAND

In Scotland, as in England, Wales and Northern Ireland, the age of majority is 18 years, but there are differences for young people aged 16–18 in that they can make many legally binding decisions, including consent to treatment.

## CHILDREN'S RIGHTS

The UN convention (1989), ratified in the UK in 1991, contains a series of articles about children's rights. It is a very useful tool for any children's nurse wishing to challenge accepted practice. It is not legally binding, but powerful if used with both the Children Act (1989) and the Human Rights Act (1998). The UN convention contains certain basic rights, such as a right to shelter and rights to information, and for children to have their wishes listened to and taken into account. The Human Rights Act applies equally to children and adults, it ensures that no public body can interfere in a person's private life without legal authority or a legitimate aim, and it affords legally competent children the same rights to confidentiality as adults (British Medical Association 2001).

## ADVOCACY AND CONFIDENTIALITY

The children's nurse is first and foremost an advocate for the rights and wishes of the child. This is done in the context of the whole family. Care needs to be taken to ensure that the voice of the child is always heard. Family friendly policies are all-embracing in contemporary UK health care, and opportunities for the children to have confidential conversations with their named nurses are few and far between. The children's nurse needs to be aware of non-verbal cues, and should always remember to communicate directly with the child as well as the family. Conflicts of interests with parents are unusual; parents rarely want something different to the child. There are, however, circumstances where a child or young person will not want parents to know something. When listening to children in confidence, the only circumstance where their confidentiality can be breached is in the case of child protection. The nurse listening to a disclosure of abuse should explain fully to the child what she will do with the information the child has given, acting to maintain the child's trust and confidence.

Confidentiality is also specifically mentioned in the new code of conduct for nurses and midwives (Nursing and Midwifery Council 2002). Children not wishing their parents to be informed about a treatment or condition should have their wishes respected while the health professional should seek to persuade them to tell their parents or offer to do this for them or with them.

## ASSESSING COMPETENCE

Assessing competence is one of the most difficult aspects of care, for which there is no easy answer. Children's nurses have a distinct advantage over other health professionals due to the extent of preparation they have at pre-registration about cognitive ability and the spectrum of development. There is no universal statement of competence. The context, type of decision, and particular circumstances all have to be taken into account.

Recommendations of competence by the BMA and the Law Society (British Medical Association 2001) indicate that assessment should consider a young person's:

- Ability to understand there are choices and that choices have consequences
- Willingness and ability to make a choice (including the option of choosing that someone else makes the treatment decisions)
- Understanding the nature and purpose of the procedure
- Understanding the procedure's risks and side effects
- Understanding of the alternatives to the procedure and the risks attached to them, and the consequences of no treatment
- Freedom from pressure.

Children's nurses must in particular utilise their communication and listening skills as well as their knowledge regarding cognitive development and ability.

## REFUSAL OF TREATMENT

The competent child may be able to consent to treatment, but as yet has no legal right to refuse treatment. Where refusal becomes an issue, the advice of the courts should be sought. In dealing with difficult circumstances, clinically the children's nurse's role will be that of communicator and lead negotiator with the child and family.

## WHEN LEGAL ADVICE IS REQUIRED

Clinicians can and should obtain legal advice where there are uncertainties about consent or refusal, or ethical issues that require an impartial view and a clear way forward.

## ORGAN DONATION

Organ donation is often a difficult subject to raise when a death is expected. Paediatric intensive care units should have local guidelines in place that support health professionals to broach the subject in a sensitive manner. The supply of organs for active treatment or for research has decreased dramatically since the Alder Hey Inquiry (Royal Liverpool Children's Inquiry 2001), and yet there is no drop in the number of organs required or the scope for successful transplant. Children's nurses should know where they can obtain advice on organ donation should they need it, and be aware of the need for parents to understand exactly what will happen if the coroner requests a post mortem or the parents consent to one. Parents need to be left under no illusion about what, if any, organs will be retained, and when they will be returned.

## ABORTION

While teenage pregnancy figures continue to rise, one option available to the young person is abortion. Abortions are unlikely to take place in an environment conducive to the care of young people. The children's nurse has a role in explaining procedures, maintaining confidentiality and advising areas of adult care that may be treating young people. Assessment of competence is extremely important, and a record of the assessment is vital. Young girls having abortions need to have a full understanding of the risks and immediate aftercare. The longer term psychological effects may emerge later on and young people should be encouraged to talk to their school nurses.

## CONCLUSION

- The law in relation to children and the age of majority varies across the UK.
- Parents usually want what is in the best interests of their children; where there are conflicts between the medical team and the child and family, legal advice will be needed and the courts may have to decide.
- Children as young as 5 years of age can be assessed as Gillick/Frazer competent.
- There is no single simple test for assessing competence.
- The Children Act (1989) was the last major piece of legislation to affect children and it concentrated on welfare.
- The Human Rights Act (1998) applies to children as well as to adults.
- The UN Convention on the Rights of the Child (1989) can be used to good effect to promote patient involvement and improve clinical practice.

## References

British Medical Association 2001 Consent, rights and choices in health care for children and young people. BMJ Books, London

Brook G 2000 Children's competence to consent: a framework for practice. Paediatric Nursing 12(5): 31–35

Brykczynska G 1989 Ethics in paediatric nursing. Chapman and Hall, London

Children Act 1989 HMSO, London

Dearmun A, MacKinnon E 2001 The surgical care of children: ethical dimensions. Paediatric Nursing 13(8): 29–30

Department of Health 2000 The NHS plan: a plan for investment, a plan for reform. Department of Health, London

Department of Health 2001 The Children Act now: messages from research. HMSO, London

Family Law Reform Act 1969 HMSO, London

Gillick v West Norfolk and Wisbech Health Authority [1985] 3 All ER 402

Human Rights Act 1998 HMSO, London

Kennedy I 2001 Learning from Bristol: The report of the public inquiry into children's heart surgery at the Bristol Royal Infirmary 1984–1995. HMSO, London. Online. Available: http://www.bristol-inquiry.org.uk

MsB v An NHS Trust 2002 EWHC 429

Nursing and Midwifery Council 2002 Code of professional conduct. NMC, London

Richardson J, Webber I 1995 Ethical issues in child health care. Mosby, London, p 3

Royal College of Nursing 2000 Ethical dilemmas: issues in nursing and health, 2nd edn. RCN, London

Royal Liverpool Children's Inquiry 2001 (the Redfern Report). Online. Available: http://www.ricinquiry.org.uk

United Kingdom Central Council 1992 Code of professional conduct. UKCC, London

United Nations 1989 United Nations convention on the rights of the child. United Nations, Geneva

## Useful Addresses

Medical Ethics Department
British Medical Association
BMA House
Tavistock Square
London
WC1H 9JP
Email: Ethics@bma.org.uk
Website: http://www.bma.org.uk

# Chapter 4

# Wound care

## John Bastin and Heather Newton

## INTRODUCTION

Over the last 30 years the science and art of wound care has evolved into a complex and demanding area of practice. This chapter will demonstrate an evidence-based approach to the surgical wound healing of babies and children, attempting to demystify the existing subject complexity and return to the fundamental principles to ensure clinically effective practice.

## WOUND HEALING PROCESS – AN OVERVIEW

Moy (1993) defines acute wounds as 'a destruction in the integrity of the skin including the epidermis and dermis'. A wound to the skin has implications for the whole homeostatic base of the body and therefore the importance of wound management should not be underestimated.

Surgical wounds can be classified as intentional acute wounds, which heal either by primary or secondary intention (Dealey 1999). Primary intention is a rapid healing process, which occurs in a wound where there is a clean incision and the wound edges are in apposition (see Figs 4.1, 4.2, 4.3), whilst secondary intention is a more protracted process and occurs where there has been tissue loss and the wound edges are further apart (see Fig. 4.4). Because of the nature of these wounds, healing occurs both from the edges and the bottom of the cavity. This method of healing surgical wounds is common when the wounds are infected or contaminated (Marks et al 1985). Occasionally, the surgeon

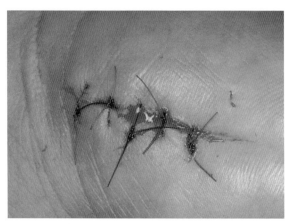

Figure 4.1 Sutured wound.

may consider closing a wound with sutures at a later stage of healing once any infection or contamination risks are minimised. The wound then continues to heal as a primary wound.

Once a wound has occurred, a process is set in motion to bring about repair in as rapid a time as possible (see Fig. 4.5).

Box 4.1 summarises the timescale and processes of wound healing.

Healing starts with the activation of the inflammatory response and the resulting redness and swelling are not only normal but also vital for this

process to move forward. Following tissue damage, a blood clot forms at the site of the damage. This can be initially delayed by the release of heparin from mast cells. This is a 'design feature' allowing flushing of bacteria and other debris to occur. The process is aided by the inflammation resulting from the release of histamine from other mast cells that occurs at the same time. Vasodilation also occurs at this stage. By the end of this phase the tissues are clean and able to move onto the next stage of the healing process (see Fig. 4.5a).

Neutrophils and macrophages move in and destroy damaged cells and cellular protein (including the blood clot) so that the injured site can now be rebuilt. The macrophages stimulate the development

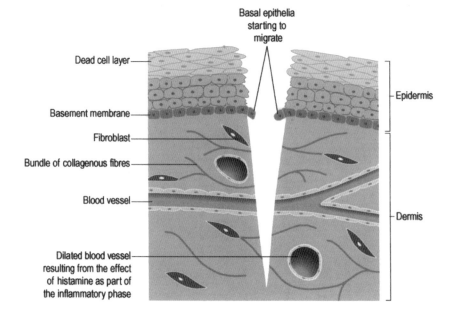

Figure 4.2  Surgical wound before healing.

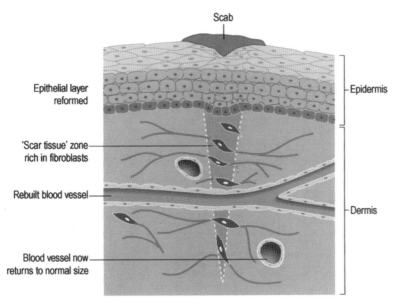

Scab

Epithelial layer
reformed

Epidermis

'Scar tissue' zone
rich in fibroblasts

Rebuilt blood vessel

Dermis

Blood vessel now
returns to normal size

**Figure 4.3** Surgical wound after healing.

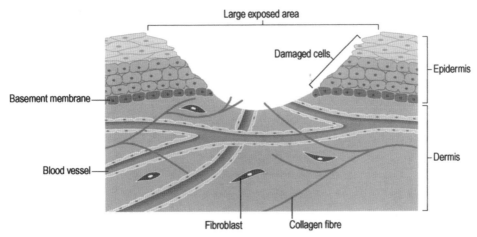

Large exposed area

Damaged cells

Epidermis

Basement membrane

Dermis

Blood vessel

Fibroblast          Collagen fibre

**Figure 4.4** Wound with tissue loss.

of fibroblasts from the surrounding tissue and start to secrete collagen, which will ultimately bridge the damaged tissue and form a matrix on which to 'hang' the new tissue cells of the skin. As this process ends the damaged area will have been filled with both collagen and a newly formed blood vessel and capillary network referred to as granulation tissue (see Fig. 4.5b). In wounds healing by primary intention this process is unseen.

Epidermal cells start to regenerate from the wound edges and grow across the bridge of granulation tissue in a process known as epithelialisation.

The maturation stage can take from 24 days to 2 years to complete. When this process is complete, any protective surface tissue will disappear following enzyme activity and over the next few months reinforcement of the area will take place. Depending on the amount of collagen produced, the wound site will blend into the surrounding tissue. Forester et al (1969) found that at 10 days an apparently well healed surgical wound has little strength and by 3 months the tensile strength is 50% that of normal tissue. Experimental studies have shown that a surgical wound is completely sealed

Figure 4.5 The wound healing process.

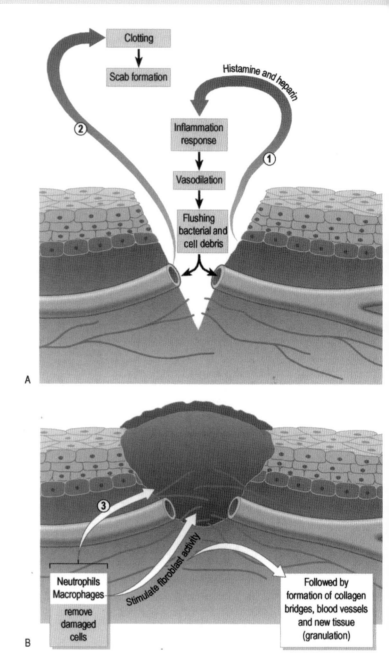

with fibrin within a few hours (Lindsay & Birch 1964, Heifetz et al 1952). However, wound healing by secondary intention will take longer than primary intention wounds because of the volume of tissue that needs to be generated and the potential to be damaged by dressing materials or by mechanical interventions. Because of the density of the collagen involved, the chances of scarring are increased.

It is interesting to note that scar tissue is historically a result of our evolutionary development. It was important to seal wounds quickly in the early days of man's existence to prevent both blood loss and infection. Mechanisms therefore evolved to repair wounds quickly by building rapid collagen bridges. If this legacy could have been prevented then scarring would not occur but healing would be a slower process (Graham-Rowe 2003). Current practice reflects the need to maintain a moist healing environment in order to promote epithelialisation and suppress this collagen bridging. Fetal wound healing has demonstrated that full thickness wounds can heal without scarring and this is dependent on factors associated with interuterine development (Adzick et al 1985). The skin is functionally mature at 33 weeks gestation yet all of the layers are very thin. The skin, however, will mature within 2–3 weeks of birth whatever the gestation period.

Children have a more vigorous healing rate than adults. In children aged from 1–3 years the dermis increases in thickness and from 4–7 years the dermis doubles in thickness, enhancing the rate of healing (Morison et al 1997).

## FACTORS WHICH INFLUENCE WOUND HEALING

The vast majority of wounds in children heal quickly with few or no problems (Rossiter 1997); however, there are factors that may influence the rate of wound healing which need to be considered. The following variables will influence the ability of the wound to heal and should be considered as part of the wound assessment process:

**1. Infection**: The very nature of the micro environment on the skin means that bacteria enter at the moment of damage, therefore a wound will always have some degree of invasion by the body's own bacterial flora. Minimising this invasion and that of potentially harmful bacteria is of prime importance in preoperative management. However, there is still much debate and many practice variations around this subject (Partridge 1998).

**2. Poor apposition of wound edges and tissue loss**: As with any repair process, the better aligned the areas then the stronger and more permanent the eventual repair will be. A well-aligned wound will have mechanical stress reduced to a minimum. If, however, there has been considerable tissue loss it may be difficult to align tissues therefore the wound would be better left to heal by secondary intention.

**3. Foreign bodies**: These could be from the incident itself, for example bone chips or environmental factors such as glass or gravel which have entered the wound prior to surgery. Secondary foreign bodies, in the form of dressing debris or sutures, could also give rise to sufficient irritation to prevent the cascading of the healing process by prolonging the inflammatory response.

**4. Characteristics of the wound**: The rate of wound healing could be influenced by the degree of necrotic material, the amount of slough and debris present in the wound, and the level of exudate.

**5. Repeated wound trauma and inappropriate dressings:** If a wound is continually reopened, either by design or accident, the normal progression of healing will eventually cease and the wound will become inactive. Some dressings can cause trauma by adhering to the wound interface and some delay healing if they do not fulfil the specific requirements of the wound, such as maintaining a moist environment.

**6. Poor blood supply**: Wound healing depends on a good supply of not only building materials but also control and stimulatory factors. If these cannot get to the damaged area because of poor blood supply then the rebuild process either fails to start or happens very slowly. Hypoxia of the tissues may result from a general anaesthetic and it must be remembered that parameters used to assess systemic perfusion, such as cardiac and urinary output, may not necessarily reflect peripheral perfusion.

**7. Underlying disease**: This could result in a child presenting in a compromised circulatory state as described above or in a poor nutritional state, both of which affect wound healing. A diabetic patient may have an increased potential to develop wound infection and tensile strength of wounds may be reduced (Partridge 1998).

**8. Nutritional status**: For many children the short period without food during the operative process will not be detrimental to wound healing; however, if there is a long period of preoperative fasting, together with a poor nutritional intake postoperatively, tissue breakdown may occur. A diet rich in protein, carbohydrates, vitamins and minerals (especially zinc) all promote good wound healing.

**9. Immunosuppression**: If a child is immunocompromised e.g. because of Cushing's disease or steroid therapy, the inflammatory process is suppressed and therefore the wound healing process is delayed or does not trigger the appropriate response. Physiological and psychological stress will raise corticosteroid levels, which not only suppress cell division but also the inflammatory process. Catecholamine levels are also elevated by stress and these will impair healing due to their vasoconstrictory action.

**10. Malignancy**: If a child presents with a tumour, early treatment may have included radiotherapy or chemotherapy prior to surgical intervention. This would not only affect the immune system but also influences the control mechanisms for cellular activity and division.

11. **Dry wound environment**: In order for the processes of granulation and epithelialisation to take place, the wound environment must be moist (Winter 1962). New cells not only require nutrients but also need the influence of cytokines to start the process of mitosis. Plasma fluids 'leaking' into the wound area would supply both of these. If this process did not occur, the cells would not be able to initiate new growth or physically migrate into the damaged area. Collagen fibres would also not be in a position to migrate if the interface was dry.

12. **pH**: Normal tissue pH is 7.3 and any factor which influences this will be detrimental to enzyme activity and molecular interaction. Protein structure is extremely complex and relies on hydrogen bonding for its molecular shape. Any change in hydrogen levels in the tissues will cause either depletion or addition of hydrogen bonds to the molecules, thus altering the shape of the protein, perhaps to the point where it becomes non-functional. In the case of control proteins and enzymes, this would prevent any forward movement of the healing cycle. It is vital that any solutions, creams or dressings that have direct contact with the wound area do not compromise the pH status of the wound.

13. **Temperature**: The ideal wound temperature is 37 degrees centigrade, however, the wound area is under the potential influence of ambient temperature and also thermal shock from irrigation at the time of dressing changes or cleansing. A reduction in temperature may inhibit the activity of the cells involved in the healing process. Lock (1980) found that after a wound was redressed it took 40 minutes for the temperature to return to normal and 3 hours for mitotic activity to return to normal.

14. **Existing scar tissue**: Repeated surgery in the same area would eventually lead to the tissue in that area becoming desensitised to the biochemical 'heal' commands. The increased amount of collagen would make it difficult for epithelialisation to progress.

15. **Position of the wound**: Consideration should be given to the position of the wound. This will influence the ability of wound dressings to stay in place, ensuring effectiveness of the product in relation to wound healing, e.g. across joints.

## WOUND ASSESSMENT

Wound assessment should be undertaken as part of a holistic approach and not in isolation. Benbow (1995) points out that wound care is not just about choosing dressings but is about managing local symptoms by accurate assessment of need and matching appropriate dressings. Consideration needs to be given to the physical and psychological needs of both the child and family and the effect of the wound on their lifestyle.

Factors that will be influential in the rate of healing, as previously described, will need to be assessed to ensure the maximum healing potential is realised. Once the child's clinical condition has been assessed, specific wound assessment can be undertaken. The characteristics of the wound (see Table 4.1) should determine the type of dressings selected. A baseline assessment will enable progress to be monitored and ensures that an appropriate dressing product is selected (Dealey 1999).

## PAIN ASSESSMENT

Pain has been described as a subjective experience arising from activity within the brain in response to damage to body tissues (Bond 1979). Surgical techniques have greatly improved over time and this strongly influences the degree of pain following surgery. Many operations are now undertaken through small incisions, reducing pain and tissue trauma. It is well known that vertical abdominal incisions hurt more than transverse incisions because of the nerve endings affected, therefore the implications of pain following surgery can be reduced if careful planning takes place in the operating theatre (Wall & Melzack 1995).

When removing or applying wound dressing products, the amount of pain should be minimal; however, if pain does occur it may well be due to poor technique or inappropriate dressing selection. Factors that also influence pain, e.g. exposure to the air, pressure on the tissues, excessive movement, irritant products, amount of dressing changes and clinical infection, should be acknowledged. The child's perception of pain should be assessed and documented. The use of a visual analogue scale especially devised for children (see Ch. 6) can assist in the accurate interpretation of both the level and frequency of the pain.

If the assessment process is comprehensive, it will enable a plan of care to be written which accurately reflects the individual child's needs.

Table 4.1  Wound assessment (after Dealey 1999)

| Wound assessment criteria | Rationale |
| --- | --- |
| Wound site | 1. The position may influence the risk of potential problems, e.g contamination, mobilisation<br>2. Influences dressing selection, especially awkward areas |
| Size and depth | 1. Needed to measure the effectiveness of treatments. It should be noted that necrotic wounds could increase in size during the debriding process<br>2. To aid dressing selection |
| Appearance: necrotic, sloughy, infected, granulating or epithelialising | 1. Indicates stage of healing<br>2. Enables effectiveness of treatment regime to be monitored<br>3. Indicates whether additional interventions are required |
| Level of exudate | 1. Influences dressing selection<br>2. Identifies the need for peri-wound protection<br>3. A sudden increase may be an early indication of wound infection |
| Condition of surrounding skin | 1. Influences dressing selection<br>2. Identifies if skin protection is required |
| Degree/cause of pain | 1. May affect the child/nurse relationship<br>2. Influences dressing selection and times of dressing changes |
| Effect of the wound on the child | 1. Influences dressing selection and compliance<br>2. Enables the nurse to plan individualised care to manage the holistic situation |
| The care environment | 1. May affect the psychological needs of the child<br>2. May require a family member to be involved in the dressing regime |

## WOUND MEASUREMENT

To monitor the effectiveness of the dressing regime it is advisable to record accurately the measurements of the wound. The simplest way is to measure the wound at its greatest length and breadth, although the accuracy of the measurement could be questioned. Another method is to trace the wound and there are special charts available which help to determine the surface area. Acetates or double sided plastic bags can also be effective; however, care is required to ensure the wound contact side is cleaned to prevent cross infection. Photographs provide a visual image of the wound; however, cameras may not be readily available in the clinical setting. Measuring depth is a more complex issue. Probes can be used with caution; however, again the accuracy is questionable. Computerised systems are available but are costly unless used on a regular basis.

It must be remembered that some wounds, especially if they contain necrotic material, may initially become larger as they are debrided and areas of inflammation should be carefully monitored in case the underlying tissues have been damaged.

## WOUND CLEANSING

Wound cleansing is still the subject of debate, with a lack of research supporting the technique and the type of solutions to use (Williams 1999). First, it must be determined whether the wound requires cleansing and what will be gained. Ritualistic cleansing of wounds is unnecessary and cleansing should only be undertaken to remove debris from the wound. It should not interfere with the normal conditions on the wound bed. The irrigation technique is the method currently favoured as it prevents the shredding of product fibres into the wound and reduces discomfort caused by the application of pressure when wounds are wiped (Williams 1999). Recommended solutions are sterile water, normal saline or tap water, all of which should be at room temperature to avoid cooling of the wound surface. If antiseptics are used to cleanse wounds the degree of damage to healthy tissues must be balanced against the bactericidal or bacteriostatic effect of the solution (Lawrence 1997). Children in particular may enjoy a bath or shower postoperatively; however, staff need to be aware of the infection control and wound management policies available within their own Trusts.

Some primary wounds will be sealed as early as 4–6 hours after closure, whilst others may take 24–48 hours or longer. This is dependent upon the child's natural response to healing and the type of closure used. Film dressings can provide a suitable protection when bathing or showering. There is little evidence to suggest an increase in wound infection following baths or showers; however, Gilchrist (1990) recommends showers as there is less likelihood of cross infection.

## WOUND INFECTION

Wound infection has been recognised as a factor responsible for delaying wound healing as it extends the inflammatory phase of healing, causing distress and discomfort (Flanagan 2000). The presence of bacteria in a wound does not necessarily mean that it is clinically infected. When bacteria are present in a wound but producing no host reaction this is known as colonisation. However, when the multiplying bacteria produce clinical signs and symptoms or a 'host reaction', clinical infection is indicated. The presence of pus, increased heat, redness, pain and exudate are all indications of infection together with an increase in temperature and a general feeling of malaise. Each individual responds differently to the presence of bacteria and children who have a reduced immune system, are malnourished, or are in a generally poor state of physical health prior to surgery may have an increased risk of developing wound infection. Length of preoperative hospital stay and the time on the operating table may also influence the risk of infection.

Wound swabbing is an unreliable and ritualistic method of detecting wound infection, therefore a thorough assessment should also be undertaken. A swab should only be taken if there are clinical signs to indicate a 'host reaction'. The presence of slough in a wound bed does not necessarily indicate that the wound is infected. If a wound is clinically infected the child should be treated with systemic antibiotics. There are no controlled trials to support the use of topical antibiotics in wound management (Flanagan 2000).

There is still much debate about skin cleansing prior to surgery, with some clinicians requesting preoperative baths whilst others prefer to cleanse the skin in theatre. Cruse & Foord (1980) claim that sepsis is more likely to occur during surgery, as tissue exposure to contamination reduces after this time by suturing and application of dressings.

## WOUND DRESSINGS

The wound management process should be seen as a continuum and dressing selection is integral to this. Dressings can greatly affect wound healing and can either inhibit or enhance the stages of the healing process. Winter (1962) undertook research that influenced the development of modern day wound dressings. He compared dry wound healing to moist wound healing and discovered that moist wounds granulated up to 40% faster than dry wounds. To ensure this process is promoted, dressing performance is often measured against the criteria in Box 4.2.

When selecting a dressing product there are other factors that need to be considered, especially when applying them to children. Dressing products should therefore:

- Allow normal activity and be acceptable to the child wherever possible. Bulky dressings should be avoided.
- Reduce the levels of pain. Some dressings have the ability to reduce pain through ensuring the nerve endings remain moist whilst other dressings require specific techniques to ensure a pain free removal.
- Be able to conform around awkward areas and be available in small sizes. This is especially important for children where surface areas are small and appropriate sized dressings are chosen to ensure maximum effect and fit.

---

**Box 4.2 Dressing performance (after Turner 1985)**

- Maintain high humidity at the wound surface/interface
- Remove excess exudate and toxic components
- Allow gaseous exchange
- Provide thermal insulation
- Protect from secondary infection
- Be free from particulate or toxic contaminants
- Allow removal without trauma at dressing change

• Be safe and easy to use. Only dressings which are licensed should be used. Many Trusts will have recognised formularies which guide practitioners on the most appropriate dressings to use. These are produced using the best available evidence to ensure safe, effective practice. If a dressing product is easy to use, the child's family members may be able to participate in the care if they so wish.

• Be cost effective. Nurses should be aware of the types of products available and their actions and indications to ensure that the right dressing is used for the right wound, on the right patient and in the right environment. Inappropriate use of dressings leads to increased cost both in the product itself and in healing time.

• Be available. Consideration needs to be given to the availability of dressing products across primary and secondary care settings to ensure continuity of care. The volume of dressings now available on FP10 has increased; however, it is important for nurses to be aware of availability and accessibility when choosing products.

## RECOMMENDED GOOD PRACTICE IN WOUND CARE

All healthcare professionals should have a fundamental level of knowledge and skill when undertaking wound care. An understanding of the principles of wound healing and factors that delay healing, and the ability to assess the wound characteristics and select the appropriate dressing regime are essential to achieve effective wound healing outcomes. The volume of dressing products now available provides an element of confusion for clinical staff and make this area of practice more complex. Access to education and training is vital and should reflect the needs of individual clinical specialities.

The emotional needs of the child must be considered when choosing dressings and it is important that staff build a relationship with the child and family to ensure that dressing changes are not seen as a traumatic experience. The level of involvement desired by the parents should be assessed. It may be appropriate to use 'explorative play' where the child experiences the sensation of the dressing first before it is applied to the wound. This may help to alleviate fear of the unknown and promote compliance with the treatment regime (see Ch. 1). The use of a play specialist may be considered to support treatment application.

## DRESSINGS FOR PRIMARY SUTURED WOUNDS

These types of wounds should heal rapidly with minimal cost attached to dressing products. Immediately postoperatively, wounds are covered by a simple adhesive dressing pad which protects the wound from external abrasion and absorbs any ooze from the wound edges. Examples include Mepore and Opsite Post Op. Occasionally when a limb swells following surgery, the adhesive dressing can cause friction at the epidermal/dermal junction and produce a blistering effect (see Fig. 4.6). Studies have shown that a simple wound dressing can be removed 24–48 hours after operation (Chrintz et al 1989). Where leakage or 'strike-through' occurs in dressings there is an increased risk of wound infection and dressings should be observed frequently and changed when indicated to reduce this risk.

## DRESSINGS TO PROMOTE HEALING BY SECONDARY INTENTION

In order for these type of wounds to heal effectively, healing must be encouraged from the base of the wound upwards and dressing selection should enable this to occur without the danger of leaving a hidden cavity beneath the epithelialised tissue. Wound dressings should promote a natural healing response by providing a moist, warm, non-toxic environment. The cosmetic appearance of the wound site is of fundamental importance, especially

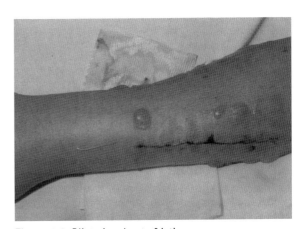

Figure 4.6 Blistering due to friction.

in children, with the aim being to minimise the degree of scar tissue. This can be promoted by maintaining the correct environment throughout all of the phases of wound healing to allow the wound to contract naturally.

The dressing selected should ensure a pain free application and removal and should not inhibit the normal activities of the child whenever possible. Attention should be paid to the condition of the surrounding skin, especially where it is fragile, dry, macerated or inflamed. Caution is required when removing film dressings and adhesive dressings to ensure the skin is not damaged in the process. Reactions to dressings can occur and usually present as irritation or erythema around the dressing site. A full assessment is then required to identify if there is a true allergic reaction or whether there is an irritant reaction caused by an inappropriate dressing selection or insufficient dressing changes.

## DRESSING SELECTION

The following dressing products are suitable for wounds healing by secondary intention, and technical information, indications for use and the contraindications will be discussed briefly. Local formularies for dressing selection may be restrictive in choice; however, many offer cost-effective solutions to wound management.

### HYDROCOLLOIDS

Hydrocolloids are interactive dressings that are made up of cellulose, gelatins and pectins which form a hydrocolloid base secured onto a backing of polyurethane film or foam. On contact with wound exudate the hydrocolloid material dissolves into a gel. No secondary dressing is required and they have been used successfully on awkward areas of the body. They are indicated for wounds which have low to moderate exudate and they have the ability to absorb, promote debridement, reduce pain by moistening exposed nerve endings, promote angiogenesis and provide an optimum healing environment.

The advantages are that the dressing can be left in situ for 5–6 days depending on the levels of exudate, and children can be bathed or showered without the need to remove the dressing. Hydrocolloid dressings can produce an odour from the gelling process. This is normal and patients

should be informed to avoid unnecessary concern. Occasionally the surrounding skin can become macerated if the level of exudate is too high and the dressing changes are infrequent. It is advisable to overlap the wound with the dressing by at least 5 cm.

Hydrocolloids are available as wafers of various absorbencies, granules, powders, gels and pastes. Examples include Granuflex, Comfeel plus, Tegasorb, Replicare ultra, Cutinova Hydro and Hydrocoll.

### ALGINATES

Alginate dressings contain calcium or sodium alginate that is derived from seaweed. In the presence of wound exudate a hydrophilic-like gel is formed. The calcium content in the dressing encourages clotting, therefore is promoted for its haemostatic properties. Alginates are indicated for use on moderate to heavily exuding wounds and can cause adherence to the wound surface if allowed to dry out. They require a secondary dressing to keep the alginate in position and to ensure a moist environment is maintained. They are available as flat sheets, rope or ribbon, extra absorbent pads or with an adhesive backing. Examples include Sorbsan, Kaltostat, Seasorb, Algisite M, Algosteril and Melgisorb.

### HYDROFIBRE DRESSINGS

Hydrofibre dressings contain sodium carboxymethylcellulose in which the sodium is formed into textile fibres. It forms a gel instantly on contact with moisture and can be used on wounds with moderate to heavy amounts of exudate. Because of the vertical spread of fluid through the dressing, the potential for skin maceration is very low and therefore it will not adhere to the wound bed. Dressings can be left in situ for up to 3 days but this is dependent on the volume of exudate. They require a secondary dressing to hold them in position. Aquacell is an example.

### HYDROGELS

Hydrogel dressings consist of insoluble polymers with a high water content. They provide a moist wound environment and have the ability to donate water to facilitate autolysis in necrotic and sloughy wounds. They can be used on flat wounds and cavities and require a secondary dressing. The type of secondary dressing will be dependent on the characteristics of the wound. Where a wound is dry a film dressing placed on top of a hydrogel will speed up the desloughing process; however, when a wound has softened a foam dressing may be more appropriate to absorb the exudate. Hydrogels should be avoided in wet wounds as the increased moisture may affect the peri-wound area and increase the frequency of dressing changes. Hydrogels are available in tubes or applicators in a variety of sizes or as flat sheets. Examples include Intrasite gel, Aquaform, Granugel, Purilon, Nugel and Sterigel, with Hydrosorb, Novogel and Geliperm being examples of sheet hydrogels.

## FOAM DRESSINGS

Foam dressings can be made from polyurethane or silicone and therefore can handle large volumes of exudate due to their absorbency. They have a non-adherent surface, although some adhesive foam dressings have an adhesive wound surface layer to facilitate the dressing staying in place. They can be used as a secondary dressing when used in conjunction with a desloughing agent next to the wound. Some foam dressings are made purposely for cavity wounds and form a foam stent for easy application and removal. Foam dressings are suitable for exuding wounds that are granulating or epithelialising. They are available as non-adhesive flat sheets with various degrees of absorbency, adhesive flat sheets, and cavity dressings. Examples include Allevyn, Lyofoam, Tielle, Biotain and Spyrosorb. Combiderm is a self-adhesive dressing which absorbs exudate by using cellulose granules in the core. It will not adhere to the wound bed and maintains a moist environment.

## CHARCOAL DRESSINGS

Charcoal dressings consist of activated charcoal that has been found to be effective in absorbing the chemicals released from malodorous wounds. Some dressings also contain silver, which is an antibacterial agent. These are recommended for wounds that are infected, necrotic or fungating, all of which may have an unpleasant odour. Some are advocated as a primary dressing whereas some are indicated as secondary dressings because of their ability to absorb exudate as well. They are available as charcoal pads or as a combination of charcoal and a dressing pad. Examples include Actisorb Plus, Carboflex, Clinisorb and Lyofoam C.

## ENZYMATIC PREPARATIONS

Streptokinase and Streptodornase are enzymes that when reconstituted facilitate the debridement of necrotic wounds. Streptokinase is a thrombolytic agent that acts directly on the substate of fibrin to break up thrombi. Streptodornase liquefies the nucleoprotein of dead cells or pus. Together they rehydrate hard necrotic material. The enzymes are activated when reconstituted with normal saline to form a liquid or can be made up with a combination of saline and a lubricating gel. The moist dressing can cause peri-wound maceration, and if the liquid version is applied using gauze this could dry out and cause adherence to the wound if not covered by a film dressing to maintain moisture. Varidase is an example which is licensed for use in children.

## IODINE PREPARATIONS

Iodine preparations are used in chronic wound management in adults; however, iodine may be absorbed through the unbroken skin of the neonate and the young child. Monitoring serum iodine levels and thyroid function are advisable in these patients.

## SEMI-PERMEABLE FILM

Film dressings are made up of a clear polyurethane-type film coated with an adhesive. They are semi-permeable and due to their extensibility and elastomeric properties they are conformable and are resistant to shearing forces. They do not absorb exudate but can be of value as a secondary dressing to create an optimum environment for healing. They can be used to protect vulnerable pressure areas, especially heels and elbows. Care is required when applying and removing these dressings as vulnerable skin may tear and cause further trauma. Examples include Tegaderm, Opsite, Mefilm, Bioclusive, Cutifilm and Epi View.

## LIQUID FILM

Liquid film is used to protect peri-wound areas, excoriated and macerated skin and stoma sites and can be used on the edges of surgical wounds. It is applied directly to the skin with either an applicator or as drops. It is a non-painful application and can protect the skin for up to 72 hours. Examples include Cavilon no sting barrier film and Superskin.

## TULLES

Tulle dressings consist of sheets of gauze impregnated with paraffin, antiseptics or other agents. They can be used on superficial wounds but do not have any absorbent capacity. They can adhere to the wound bed and cause pain and trauma on removal if allowed to dry out. Recent guidelines from the National Institute for Clinical Excellence (NICE) no longer recommend adhesive dressings for routine use (NICE 2001). Topical tulles need to be used with caution as they can lead to sensitivity and can occasionally produce bacterial resistance. Examples include Jelonet, Bactigras, Fucidin and Sofra-Tulle.

## RECORD KEEPING

In order to ensure effective communication and continuity of care, the child's records must detail a full holistic and wound assessment, the recommended dressing regime and an evaluation of planned care. The psychological impact on the child and family should also be included. The use of wound assessment charts is strongly recommended to ensure continuity and consistency of information recorded.

Surgical wounds should be assessed at every dressing change and measured at least on a weekly basis. For the vast majority of wounds the simple measuring devices such as tracing or measuring are adequate and provide enough information to demonstrate the impact of the treatment regime.

## CONCLUSION

In order to promote good surgical wound care for babies and children it is important that all of the multiprofessional team are involved and aware of current best practice. The field of wound care is an ever changing arena and relies on the professionals themselves to keep up-to-date and apply the new evidence to their current practice. Surgical wound healing is a complex process and relies on environmental and physical factors as well as professional practice. Children often have difficulty understanding the complexity of medical and nursing practice and many feel very frightened by untoward interventions. The role of the nurse therefore extends beyond just the application of wound dressings and involves providing psychological support for both the child and family throughout the whole episode of care. The use of a specialist wound care nurse could help to support the more complex cases where healing is compromised by a number of factors.

The majority of surgical wounds in babies and children will heal rapidly without complications. However, where wound breakdown occurs the primary goal is to heal the wound with minimal disruption, and to ensure that scar tissue is minimised as the scar can be a visual reminder for children of their experience. Surgical wound care needs to be carefully managed by competent, confident practitioners who are trained to care for the specific needs of children and their families as well as having the knowledge and skills to perform high standards of wound care.

## References

Adzick HS, Harrison MR, Glick PL 1985 Comparison of foetal and adult wound healing by histological enzyme – histochemical and hydroxide proline determinations. Journal of Paediatric Surgery 20(4): 315–319

Benbow M 1995 Parameters of wound assessment. *British Journal of Nursing* 4(11): 647–651

Bond MR 1979 Pain. Its nature, analysis and treatment. Churchill Livingstone, Edinburgh

Briggs M 1997 Principles of closed surgical wound care. Journal of Wound Care 6(6): 288–292

Chrintz H, Vibits H, Corditz TD 1989 Need for surgical wound dressings. British Journal of Surgery 76: 204–205

Cruse PJ, Foord R 1980 The epidemiology of wound infection. Surgical Clinics of North America 60(1): 27–40

Dealey C 1999 The care of wounds, 2nd edn. Blackwell Science, London

Flanagan M 2000 Essential wound healing. Part 4: Wound infection. EMAP Healthcare, London

Forester JC, Zederfeldt BH, Hunt TK 1969 A bioengineering approach to the healing wound. Journal of Surgical Research 79: 927

Gilchrist B 1990 Washing and dressings after surgery. Nursing Times 86(50): 71

Graham-Rowe D 2003 Drug smooths the way to healing. New Scientist 2400: 14, 21 June

Heifetz CJ, Lawrence MS, Richards FO 1952 Comparison of wound healing with and without dressings. Archives of Surgery 65: 746–751

Lawrence JC 1997 Wound irrigation. Journal of Wound Care 6(1): 23–26

Lindsay WK, Birch JR 1964 Thin skin wound healing. Canadian Journal of Surgery 7: 297–308

Lock PM 1980 The effects of temperature on mitotic activity at the edge of experimental wounds. In: Lundgren A, Soner AB (eds) Symposium on wound healing: plastic surgical and dermatological aspects. Molndal, Sweden

Marks J, Harding KG, Ribeiro CD 1985 Pilonidal sinus excision – healing by open granulation. British Journal of Surgery 72: 63–640.

Morison M, Moffatt C, Bridel Nixon J, Bale S 1997 Nursing management of chronic wounds, 2nd edn. Mosby, London

Moy LS 1993 Management of acute wounds. Wound Healing 11(4): 759–760

National Institute for Clinical Excellence 2001 Guidance on the use of debriding agents and specialist wound care clinics for difficult to heal surgical wounds. NICE, London

Partridge C 1998 Influential factors in surgical wound healing. Journal of Wound Care 7(7): 350–353

Rossiter G 1997 Paediatric wound care. (Editorial) Journal of Wound Care 6(6): 255

Smith and Nephew Healthcare 1999 Iodoflex product information sheet. Hull

Turner T 1985 Which dressing and why in wound care. William Heinemann Medical Books,

Wall PD, Melzack R 1995 Textbook of pain. Churchill Livingstone, London, p 377–378

Williams C 1999 Wound irrigation techniques: new Steripod normal saline. British Journal of Nursing 8(21): 1460–1462

Winter GD 1962 Formulation of the scab and the rate of epithelialisation in the skin of the domestic pig. Nature 193: 293–294

# Chapter 5

# Care of the child in the operating theatre

Sue Harris

## INTRODUCTION

The care of the child in the operating theatre needs to be a continuation of the nursing care on the ward, using the same or a similar model of nursing. The difference is that care is taking place at a critical time of the child's hospital stay. The child will be rendered unconscious and have surgery, major or minor, lasting only a few minutes or many hours.

A paediatric philosophy of care (Royal College of Nursing 1996) needs to reflect treatment of the child as an individual, recognition of the rights of the child, and the nurse acting as an advocate, ensuring dignity, safety and confidentiality during the child's stay in theatre, along with the child's right to have age appropriate information (Perry 1994).

The child's family needs to be involved and family-centred care should be practised (see Ch. 1) so that the child and the family receive the best possible care in the operating theatre (Campbell et al 1993, Brown 1997).

It is imperative that all equipment in the operating department is correctly serviced and maintained and that the local infection control policies are observed for the safety of the child (Unerman 1994).

## PLANNING THE CARE OF THE CHILD IN THE OPERATING THEATRE

The most effective way of planning the care for the child in the operating theatre is to carry out a preoperative visit (Wicker 1995), the most appropriate staff to undertake this visit being the anaesthetic or recovery nurse.

Informal ward visits also help to remove the impression that theatre nurses are only involved with painful and unpleasant procedures, and it is helpful for children to see the theatre staff wearing scrub suits and being normal human beings.

When carrying out formal preoperative visits, before actually meeting the family it is useful to check through the medical notes and the nursing care plan to see if there is anything pertinent that the theatre staff need to know, for example:

- Is the child asthmatic?
- Does the child have any allergies?
- What is the child's family environment? For example, does the child have step-parents known by names other than Mummy or Daddy?
- Does the child use a hearing aid or wear glasses?
- Do the child's parents speak English or is an interpreter being used?
- Does the child have special needs?

During the preoperative visit, assessment of the child's behaviour should take place:

- Is the child being very quiet because of nervousness and perhaps fear?
- Is the child being very boisterous and loud, again to disguise anxiety?

Children may behave in either of these ways to try and cope with events that they do not understand.

Reassurances need to be given to the child and the family, and perhaps further information about what is going to happen, but definite fears will need to be addressed before coming to the operating theatre. The nurse should give an explanation about exactly what will happen in the anaesthetic room, the operating theatre and recovery room, in words that are appropriate for the child's understanding and development. The family and child should have been part of the preoperative preparation (see Ch. 1), which should include ensuring that the patient knows what is going to happen. Children still come into hospital unaware of what is going to happen because their parents either cannot or will not tell them the truth.

Preparation needs to take place to ensure that the children know exactly what to expect after the operation when they wake up; for example, their legs may feel numb because of a caudal epidural, they may have intravenous lines or drains, they may even have a plaster cast on. They must know what to expect and explanations must be given.

Counselling of the parents as to the part they will play in their child's care in the operating theatre is necessary to gain their cooperation. It is usually recommended that only one parent accompanies the child to the anaesthetic room to provide a quiet reassuring presence (see Fig. 5.1) (Turner 1989) (see Ch. 1).

Normally, parents will be invited to the recovery room as soon as the child is stable and starting to wake up. Sometimes grandmother or another relation comes with the child instead of a parent. It has been known for a young person, with her parent's permission, to have her boyfriend accompany her into the anaesthetic room.

Communication is essential between the theatre nurse and the child to build up a relationship and rapport. The nurse also needs to discover how to pronounce the child's name. This is especially important when dealing with children and families from different ethnic groups (Hewitt 2000).

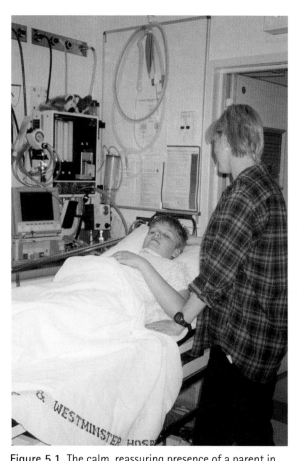

Figure 5.1 The calm, reassuring presence of a parent in the anaesthetic room.

The theatre nurse should also establish the need for any special equipment or apparatus required to keep the child safe. Finally, honest and truthful answers must be given to any of the questions asked by the child and family, with reassurance and encouragement. If there are any questions to which nurses do not know the answer then they should ensure that someone gives the family the information that they require.

Communication between the ward staff and theatre staff is also a very necessary part of providing the best possible care for the child (Harris 1991). The ward staff may know if the child has a fear of needles, or of waking up during the operation. All these things need to be addressed before the child comes to the operating theatre and the theatre nurse is often the best person to give reassurances to the child and his family.

A theatre care plan needs to be devised to enable the staff to plan and record the care received by the child whilst in the theatre. This needs to be user friendly but also comprehensive and compatible with the care plans that are used on the children's wards so that continuity of care is maintained and the philosophy and model of care in use is reflected. This document also becomes a useful tool for teaching and at handover to ensure that everything is communicated to the ward staff. All this information about the needs of each individual child and family must then be communicated to the rest of the theatre staff (Lewis 1994).

## THE ANAESTHETIC ROOM

The anaesthetic room needs to be appropriately decorated with lots of colourful pictures on the walls and ceilings, and toys around for distraction purposes. Music playing softly also helps to provide a calm, normal atmosphere. The anaesthetic room should be fully prepared with all the necessary equipment and drugs before the child enters the room. There is nothing more frightening for small children than to have to watch syringes and needles being prepared before their very eyes.

A full check needs to be carried out to ensure that the right child gets the right operation, that the child has been starved for the correct time (see Ch. 1), that all allergies are noted, correct limbs marked and the consent form has been signed (Cormack 1998). All these should be documented on the theatre care plan and all other appropriate documentation should accompany the child (National Association of Theatre Nurses 1997).

It is at this time that there may be a disagreement between the child and parents; for example, the parents may have signed the consent form but the child does not want to have the operation and will not cooperate (Radford 2000) (see Ch. 3). A protocol or guideline needs to be in place so that the staff know how to manage this situation. Is it a life saving operation or one that could be delayed until the child is older and will have a better knowledge and understanding? Sometimes returning to the ward to allow time for everyone to calm down, and administering a premedication with the child's consent, resolves the problem.

Physical restraint of a child in order to administer an anaesthetic without the child's consent is a last resort and should not be the first line of intervention. Health professionals must be aware of the rights of the child (United Nations 1989) and the point at which restraint becomes an assault (Royal College of Nursing 1999) (see Ch. 3).

Children who are especially afraid of needles or particularly nervous or frightened should be referred to the hospital play specialist for therapeutic play (see Ch. 1). It may also be possible for them to visit the anaesthetic room together where the play specialist may provide distraction therapy (Chandler 1994).

Even for confident children who have had Emla or Ametop skin analgesia applied to their hands, it is a good idea to perform venepuncture out of the child's sight, behind the parent's back if the child is sitting on the parent's lap (see Fig. 5.2). Most people seeing a needle advancing towards them would feel apprehensive and the expectation of pain could become a reality, with or without skin analgesia.

It is unnecessary to remove children's glasses or hearing aids before they have gone to sleep. They may not be able to see properly or to hear what you are saying to them; this is very frightening to a child and it is unnecessary to put them through this extra stress.

If possible, children should be offered some choices; for example, how they would like to travel to the operating theatre (carried by mum or dad, riding on a trolley or walking) (see Fig. 5.3). Would they like to go to have their special sleep on mum's lap or lying on the trolley? Would a small toddler like the 'magic wind' (anaesthetic gas) or 'magic milk' (propofol and anaesthetic induction agent given intravenously)? This gives children a sense of

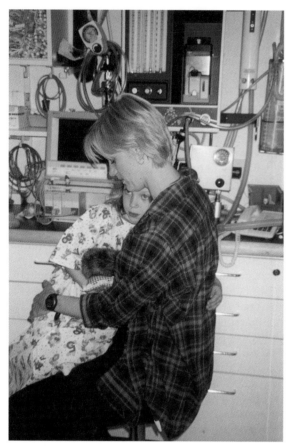

**Figure 5.2** Hand for cannulation out of sight behind mum's back.

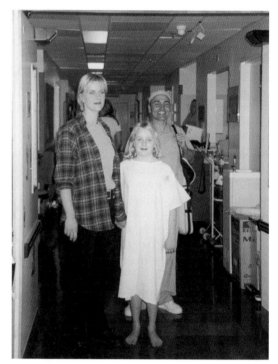

**Figure 5.3** Walking to theatre.

having some control over things and feeling that they are not being treated like objects who have no say in the way things are done. Children will often cooperate if they are consulted and agreements reached.

The intravenous cannula should be treated as a surgical wound and have a sterile dressing applied. All airway maintenance devices, endotracheal tubes and laryngeal mask airways should be securely fixed, taking into account any allergies that the child may have to sticking plasters and ensuring that undue pressure is not applied to the side of the mouth or nostril, causing a pressure ulcer. All monitoring equipment needs to be applied well out of the way of the surgical field. The eyes should be protected by taping them shut, and lubricating gel can be used to keep the eyes moistened.

Moving from the anaesthetic room into the operating theatre should only be undertaken when the anaesthetist is ready, along with all appropriate

equipment and the child is completely anaesthetised and stable. Any operating table supports of extra pillows or support foam pieces should be to hand.

The local manual and handling policy should be adhered to when moving the child onto the operating table, thereby ensuring the safety of the patient and the staff. Special day surgery trolleys are available for children, which means that the children do not have to be moved onto the operating table and off again.

## PARENTS IN THE ANAESTHETIC ROOM

It is usual practice for one parent or family member to accompany their child into the anaesthetic room. Any deviation from this should be discussed with the anaesthetist before the child arrives in the theatre department. Occasionally, the parent does not wish to accompany the child into the anaesthetic room and for whatever reasons this should be accepted. The nurse or a play specialist would be a suitable substitute with the child's consent. It is just as wrong to coerce a parent to go into the anaesthetic room, if they don't want to, as it is to bar a parent from going. Each family must be treated individually (see Ch. 1).

There is no need for the parent to dress up with hats, gowns or overshoes. This can be very frightening to young toddlers, especially if they have been premedicated, making them slightly dozy. There is no evidence that the parents in normal clothing pose an infection risk in any way, but there is evidence that overshoes are a definite infection risk if not removed correctly and the hands washed thoroughly afterwards (Carter 1990).

Once the child is asleep the ward nurse should take the parent out of the anaesthetic room and should be there to offer support and a shoulder to cry on if necessary. The opportunity to get a cup of tea or do some shopping should be encouraged, and an approximate time for being available to go to the recovery room given. It is becoming good practice to issue parents with pagers for this purpose (see Ch. 1).

## THE OPERATING THEATRE

The theatre should be completely ready to receive the patient (National Association of Theatre Nurses 1998a). The temperature and humidity should be at the correct level depending on the patient and the procedure to be performed. A small neonate will require a very warm, humid atmosphere, especially until the operation is under way and the patient's condition stabilised (see Ch. 9), whereas a young person who is normally fit and well will only require a comfortable temperature and humidity. The controls of the heating in the theatre should be easy to use and effective in order to provide children with the best environment for their needs.

Children are susceptible to pressure ulcers and prevention is an essential element of nursing care. Preterm or low birth weight infants with very thin skin and virtually no underlying fat are very prone to pressure damage (Dimond 1994). The child needs to be lying with all limbs in a neutral position so that nerves are not damaged during surgery.

All monitoring leads and intravenous lines must be positioned safely alongside the patient, not lying on top or underneath, where they could cause damage to the skin. The breathing circuits should not rest on the patient but be supported by foam, swabs or a tube holder. A diathermy plate must be applied according to the manufacturer's instructions and the lead safely positioned away from the child. The

child may also be kept warm by the use of heating pads or convection heaters with the appropriate blanket for the surgery taking place. These devices must be applied with care and the child's temperature monitored continuously. The use of wet swabs should be kept to a minimum because they will cause the child to lose heat due to convection. The skin preparation solution can also be warmed before being applied to the child, again a measure to prevent the child losing heat.

The scrub nurse and circulating nurse must check the consent form against the child's name band and any allergies the child may have to ensure that the correct child has the correct operation to the correct site which should have been marked preoperatively and is not given anything to which the child is allergic. Spirit based skin preparation solution brings particular risks of possibly burning the child, either by conducting the electrical current from the diathermy or causing a chemical burn if pooling occurs and the solution is in contact with the skin for any length of time. Unnecessary pooling will also contribute to the loss of heat of the child due to evaporation.

The scrub nurse needs to ensure that the child is not at risk of harm from the weight of the drapes, or from the application of any surgical instrument being applied incorrectly or laid down on top of the child. Blood loss needs to be accurately measured, especially in neonates or small children as their circulating volume is very small (see Table 5.1).

The family of any child having a surgical operation will naturally be very anxious and, as part of family-centred care, regular communication with them through their ward nurse regarding the progress of the operation is very reassuring, especially if the surgery is major or lengthy or is taking longer than was originally planned. In some units if the parents are going to leave the hospital during a long operation then the theatre receptionist's telephone number could be given to the parents so that they can enquire after their child.

At the end of surgery a simple adhesive dressing pad will be applied taking into account the allergy

Table 5.1 Blood volumes

| Age of child | Volume |
| --- | --- |
| Neonate | 85 mL per kg body weight |
| Age 1–2 years | 75 mL per kg body weight |
| Age 2–16 years | 72 mL per kg body weight |

status of the patient. The disconnection of all monitoring or the transportation of portable monitoring needs to be managed safely and the child transferred to the recovery room under the auspices of the anaesthetist or the recovery team.

## THE RECOVERY ROOM

The recovery room should be child friendly with lots of pictures and toys. If the child brought any toys, clothes, a dummy or cuddly toy, glasses or hearing aid with them to theatre then they should be there, waiting for the child. The staff should be appropriately experienced, preferably with Registered Sick Children's Nurse (RSCN) or Registered Nurse (RN) (Child) qualification. Appropriate analgesia should be administered before the child leaves the operating theatre (see Ch. 6).

During the early stages of recovery from anaesthesia, the maintenance of the airway and protection against children injuring themselves should they be very restless are paramount. Routine observations, i.e. heart rate, respiration rate and blood pressure, should be carried out and recorded. Also, there should be frequent checks of intravenous lines, drains and catheters, and circulation of limbs should be checked if a plaster cast has been applied.

In the recovery room the child can be cleaned of skin preparation solution and/or plaster of paris; all lines, catheters and drains should be securely fixed and made as child-proof as possible, remembering any allergies the child may have to plasters. Children left to recover from the anaesthetic in their own time, in a peaceful and quiet environment, are usually much calmer than if actively stimulated to wake up. As soon as the airway is secure and the patient beginning to wake then the parents can be sent for. Many recovery rooms can accommodate both mum and dad (Edwards 1998).

The recovery staff must ensure that the parents will be around to come to the recovery room. There is nothing more distressing for a child than having been promised that mum will be called, then to find that Mum has had to attend an appointment somewhere else. This is not fair on the child and indicates a lack of communication between the ward and theatre.

Children can also return to their own beds, which are much more comfortable than theatre trollies, and often they return to sleep. The recovery nurse should be able to give the parents all the information they require, but if this is not the case

then the surgeon and/or anaesthetist can see the family in the recovery room. The parents have a captive audience in the nurse caring for their child in the recovery stage, and may express concerns and anxieties about the child, for example anxieties about discharge and how they are going to manage. These worries can then be communicated to the ward staff at hand-over and can be addressed before the patient is discharged. If at all possible parents should be encouraged to have the children on their laps for a cuddle; this is the place where most small children feel secure and safe. If appropriate, the child should be given a drink from the breast, bottle or cup. Many mothers are very anxious that their babies will not breast feed after surgery and putting the baby to the breast as soon as possible will not only reduce the baby's starvation time but also reassure mum that all is well.

Pain management of the child should be regularly assessed and appropriate action taken if the child is in pain (see Ch. 6).

Some children, for example those with special needs or very restless ones, are sometimes nursed more easily on play mats, on the floor, as they feel more secure. In recovery rooms where play mats have been kept for this purpose nurses can get down on the floor to observe the child's recovery and the parents can do the same when they arrive. In special circumstances the patient's siblings may be allowed into the recovery area to be reassured about their brother or sister; they may also have some questions that the recovery staff are well qualified to answer. Individual evaluation of each patient and of the patient's family needs to be made by the recovery nurse.

Once children have woken up, they will often return to sleep if comfortable and reassured by the presence of parents. If their pain is well managed and the observations are satisfactory, then the child's ward nurse may be called and transfer back to the ward initiated.

Hand-over to the ward staff should be verbal and written; the theatre care plan should reflect everything that has happened to the child whilst in the operating theatre suite and ensures that communication is thorough and complete.

## CHILDREN WITH SPECIAL NEEDS

Extra care needs to be taken with the children with special needs to ensure that they understand as much as they are able about what is going to happen to them. Parents and carers should be listened to and their help elicited, as they know their children so well. Children with severe disabilities also have a much greater risk of pressure ulcers. These children should be thoroughly assessed and their skin examined for any evidence of potential pressure ulcers, and measures should be taken to protect these areas with a dressing, e.g. Tegaderm, applied before surgery begins (see Ch. 4). They should also have their limbs and back well supported by pillows and various sized pieces of foam. Because children with special needs are known far more intimately by their carers than by the nurses, it is often helpful to have them in the recovery room just before the child wakes up. They can communicate with their child, they know if the child is in pain and are generally better able to console and support the child in this unusual, and perhaps frightening, situation.

## CONCLUSION

The best possible care of the child in the operating theatre requires psychological preparation, planning for each individual's specific needs, and good communication between the child, the family, the ward staff and the theatre nurses, with all the potential risks to the child being safely managed (National Association of Theatre Nurses 1998b). When all these things are successfully managed, then the best outcome for children and their families will be achieved.

## References

Brown V 1997 The child in theatre: should the parents be involved? British Journal of Theatre Nursing 7(8): 5–7

Campbell S, Kelly P, Summersgill P 1993 Putting the family first. Child Health Aug/Sep: 59–63

Carter R 1990 Ritual and risk. Nursing Times 86(13): 63–64

Chandler K 1994 Play preparation for surgery. Surgical Nurse 7(4): 14–16

Cormack K 1998 Audit of consent forms. British Journal of Theatre Nursing 8(9): 14–16

Dimond B 1994 Pressure sores: a case to answer. British Journal of Nursing 3(14): 721–727

Edwards J 1998 Parents in recovery: a paediatric recovery nurse's view. British Journal of Theatre Nursing 8(6): 5–6

Harris S 1991 The role of the theatre nurse. Paediatric Nursing 3(1): 13–15

Hewitt D 2000 Child centred care: ethnofriendly or ethnocentric? Paediatric Nursing 12(6): 6–8

Lewis M 1994 Communication in theatres. Surgical Nurse 7(1): 27–29

National Association of Theatre Nurses 1997 Safeguards for invasive procedures: the management of risks. National Association of Theatre Nurses, Harrogate

National Association of Theatre Nurses 1998a Nursing the paediatric patient in the adult peri-operative environment. National Association of Theatre Nurses, Harrogate

National Association of Theatre Nurses 1998b Principles of safe practice in the peri-operative environment. National Association of Theatre Nurses, Harrogate

Perry J 1994 Communicating with toddlers in hospital. Paediatric Nursing 6(5): 14–17

Radford M 2000 The child's right to refuse surgery. British Journal of Anaesthetic and Recovery Nursing 1(1): 16–21

Royal College of Nursing 1996 Paediatric nursing: a philosophy of care. Issues in Nursing and Health (10) (Leaflet). Royal College of Nursing, London

Royal College of Nursing 1999 Restraining, holding still and containing children: guidance for good practice. Royal College of Nursing, London

Turner L 1989 Creating the right atmosphere. Nursing Times 85(32): 16–17

Unerman E 1994 Infection control in the operating theatre. Surgical Nurse 7(1): 31–34

United Nations 1989 The United Nations convention on the rights of the child. United Nations, Geneva

Wicker P 1995 Pre-operative visiting – making it work. British Journal of Theatre Nursing 5(7): 16–19

Chapter **6**

# The assessment and management of postoperative pain

## Alison Twycross and Vanessa Unsworth (nee Peden)

## INTRODUCTION

Many nurses consider that children who have had a surgical procedure are inevitably going to experience pain during their hospital stay and while convalescing at home. However, pain can be preempted, and if we know that a child is going to be in pain we should be taking steps to manage the pain effectively. Unrelieved pain has both physical and psychological consequences and so it is important that nurses manage children's pain effectively. Unrelieved pain and chronic pain can cause personality and mood changes (Beales 1986). Morton (1998a) identifies the consequences of unrelieved pain as:

- rapid shallow breathing which can lead to alkalosis
- inadequate expansion of lungs which can lead to bronchiectasis and atelectasis
- inadequate cough which can lead to retention of secretions
- increased heart rate and tissue ischaemia
- the child will not move spontaneously and will not ambulate
- increased fluid and electrolyte losses, resulting in rapid respiration, increased perspiration and an increased metabolic rate
- psychological consequences resulting in nightmares about pain and surgery – the child will be less cooperative in the future and will have increased anxiety.

Poor pain management has a number of adverse effects and children's nurses need to ensure that pain is managed appropriately. Furthermore, as the child's advocate, the nurse has a responsibility to ensure that pain is managed effectively. The aim of this chapter is to provide the underpinning knowledge with which to manage children's pain. It will present definitions of pain and discuss methods of assessing pain in children. Methods of managing pain will then be identified and some guidance will be given on managing pain in children of all ages.

McCaffery (1972) defines pain as whatever the experiencing person says it is, existing wherever the person says it does. Pain has also been defined as an unpleasant sensory and emotional experience with actual or potential tissue damage, or described in terms of such damage. Pain is always subjective. Each individual learns the application of the word through experiences related to injury in early life (International Association for the Study of Pain 1979). These definitions of pain suggest that pain is both subjective and an individual experience. It is therefore not surprising that the assessment and management of pain, especially children's pain, can be difficult.

## COGNITIVE DEVELOPMENT AND PERCEPTION OF PAIN

An understanding of how children develop a concept of illness will enhance the quality of care that

nurses provide. It has been shown that most healthcare professionals do not approach children according to their developmental level, but rather address all children as if they were in Piaget's concrete operational stage (Perrin & Perrin 1983). Knowledge about how a child's understanding of illness develops will mean that age-appropriate explanations can be given to children, thus reducing the anxiety and psychological distress children suffer during hospitalisation.

Muller et al (1986) suggest that if nurses have knowledge about a child's level of understanding they will be able to:

- improve explanations of illness and hospitalisation
- provide sensitive reassurance for children
- gain greater understanding of what the child is saying to them
- gain some insight into how the child is interpreting all the strange occurrences that can accompany illnesses.

## DEVELOPMENT OF UNDERSTANDING ABOUT THE CAUSE AND EFFECT OF PAIN

Thompson & Varni (1986) state that pain is an abstract concept and for the young child in the early stages of cognitive development, the term 'pain' may be meaningless. Children's cognitive level may, therefore, have a significant effect on their perception and report of pain. Consequently, in order to assess children's pain, the nurse needs to have an understanding of how children of different ages and developmental levels perceive pain. Linguistic immaturity may prevent some children from adequately expressing the pain they are feeling but just because these children cannot tell the nurse that they are in pain does not mean that they are not experiencing pain. Young children demonstrate behavioural cues that indicate that they are experiencing pain. These non-verbal clues should always be considered when assessing pain.

Hurley & Whelan (1988) found that a child's perception of pain appears to progress through the cognitive levels described by Piaget (see Table 6.1). Jeans (1983) found that during the preoperational stage (4–7 years approximately) the child begins to use language to express pain. Although the vocabulary may be limited, the child can understand simple instructions. Gaffney & Dunne (1986) found an

**Table 6.1** How children perceive the cause and effect of pain (adapted from Hurley & Whelan 1988)

| Piaget's Stage of Development | Perception of Pain |
|---|---|
| *Preoperational* (2–7 years approximately) | • Pain is primarily a physical experience<br>• Child thinks about the magical disappearance of pain<br>• Not able to distinguish between cause and effect of pain<br>• Pain is often perceived as punishment for a wrong doing or bad thought (Gildea & Quirk 1977) particularly if children do something they were told not to do immediately before they started experiencing pain<br>• Children's egocentricity means that they hold someone else responsible for their pain and, therefore, are likely to strike out verbally or physically when they have pain<br>• Children are apt to tell a nurse who gave them an injection, 'You are mean' (McCaffery 1972) |
| *Concrete operational* (7–11 years approximately) | • Relate to pain physically<br>• Able to specify location in terms of body parts<br>• Increased awareness of the body and internal organs means that fear of bodily harm is a strong influence in their perception of painful events<br>• Fear of total annihilation (body destruction and death) enters their thinking (Alex & Ritchie 1992; Schultz 1971) |
| *Transitional formal* (10–12 years) | • Have a perception of pain which is not quite as sophisticated as formal operational children<br>• Their perception of pain is not as literal as would be expected in children who are in the concrete operational stage of development<br>• Children in the transitional formal stage are beginning to understand the concept of 'if . . . then' propositions |
| *Formal operational* (12 years and above) | • Begin to solve problems<br>• Do not always have required coping mechanisms to facilitate consistent mature responses<br>• Imagine the sinister implications of pain (Muller et al 1986) |

increasing use of semi-abstract ideas in children's definitions of pain, with a lessening of concrete definitions in a relationship with increasing age, and concluded that the changes corresponded to Piaget's stages of cognitive development. So it would appear that a child's perception of the cause and effect of pain mirrors the stages of cognitive development described by Piaget. While Piaget's work has been criticised in recent years, it remains a useful framework to work from. However, care needs to be taken to assess each child's perceptions of pain on an individual basis.

## HOSPITALISATION AND PERCEPTION OF PAIN

Children's experiences of illness and hospitalisation may affect their perception of and ability to cope with pain. As children's understanding of the cause and effect of pain develops, it is important to consider whether sickness and/or hospitalisation have any effect on children's perception of pain. Unrah et al (1983) found that suffering from chronic pain may result in a child having a more mature perception of the cause and effect of pain than would normally be expected. McCaffery (1972) cited studies demonstrating that frequent exposure to painful stimuli does not desensitise subjects but, instead, increases their sensitivity to the pain. Thus, contrary to common belief, children do not become accustomed to pain (Wong & Baker 1988). Under the stress of illness, regression to an earlier developmental stage may occur, with an associated decrease in a child's ability to verbalise about pain (Gaffney & Dunne 1986). Savedra et al (1982) found that children aged 9–12 years who had been hospitalised described pain differently from children who had not been in hospital. Nurses need to remember that children who have undergone repeated painful procedures may be more sensitive to pain than other children, and that their perception of pain may differ from what might normally be expected. Individuals differ in their responses to pain, so as well as taking into account a child's level of cognitive development, all children should have their perception of pain individually assessed.

## THE ASSESSMENT OF PAIN IN CHILDREN

Determining the level of pain a person may be experiencing is one of the most common and most difficult tasks for nurses to accomplish (Bradshaw & Zeanah 1986, Franck et al 2000). Knowing how much pain a child is experiencing is the first step towards offering appropriate treatment for the pain (Price 1994). When assessing a child's pain the nurse must consider the child's age and level of cognitive development and use a method of assessment that is appropriate to the child's age. Pain should be assessed in order to intervene appropriately to control and manage the pain. Pain assessment also involves evaluating the effectiveness of pharmacological and non-pharmacological.

### HOW TO ASSESS PAIN

The QUESTT tool encompasses many of the important features of pain assessment (Baker & Wong 1988). The nurse needs to:

Question the child
Use pain-rating scales
Evaluate behaviour and physiological changes
Secure parents' involvement
Take the cause of pain into account
Take action and evaluate results.

### Question the child

Ideally this should happen before any painful episodes occur. The nurse should ask about the child's past experiences of pain and ascertain whether there are any specific words the child uses for pain. The nurse will then understand how the child perceives pain and what coping mechanisms have been used to cope with pain in the past. Involving children in their pain assessment also increases their feelings of control.

### Use pain–rating scales

Pain assessment tools enable the nurse to acquire a clear perspective on a child's pain (Ellis 1988,

Franck et al 2000). The child should be allowed to choose an appropriate scale. The nurse must then explain the use of the tool to the child, preferably before the child is experiencing pain.

### Evaluate behaviour and physiological changes

Observing the child's non-verbal cues is an important part of pain assessment. Physiological changes in pulse and blood pressure can, in acute pain, be useful indicators of whenever a child is in pain (Gadish et al 1988, Royal College of Nursing 1999a). However, they should be used in conjunction with other methods of assessing pain because after a period of time physiological adaptation occurs.

### Secure parents' involvement

Parents are the best source of information about how their child behaves when in pain. However, they may be stressed and have little experience of seeing their child in severe pain (Eland 1985a) and therefore may be unable to focus on their child's pain. Further, parents also expect nurses to know when their child is in pain (Woodgate & Kristjanson 1996) and so nurses need to encourage parents to be involved in their child's pain management and to inform them if they believe that their child is in pain.

### Take the cause of pain into account

Nurses should have some knowledge of different conditions and the type and amount of pain that results from them and use this knowledge to give an indication of how much pain a child is likely to experience.

### Take action and evaluate results

The nurse should administer analgesic drugs, utilise appropriate non-pharmacological methods and, having given time for the analgesics to take effect, evaluate the effectiveness of interventions.

Assessment of pain should be a continuous process and the methods that are used should enable the accurate evaluation of nursing interventions as well as suggesting changes in these interventions (Price 1994). When assessing pain it is, therefore, important to record its frequency, duration and intensity on a flow chart. The pain relieving interventions used, and their effectiveness, should also be recorded.

## THE ROYAL COLLEGE OF NURSING (RCN) CLINICAL GUIDELINES

The clinical guidelines for the recognition and assessment of pain in children were developed by the RCN (Royal College of Nursing 1999a) with the help of children, parents and healthcare professionals. This document reviews the literature and research findings about children's pain management and makes nine key recommendations. The strength of the evidence to support these recommendations varies. Grade I indicates a generally consistent finding in a majority of multiple acceptable studies. Grade II is either evidence based on a single acceptable study, or a weak and inconsistent finding in multiple acceptable studies. Grade III indicates limited scientific evidence which does not meet all the criteria of acceptable or absence of directly applicable studies of good quality. This includes published and unpublished opinion.

The recommendations are given below, with their gradings.

### WHEN CHILDREN'S PAIN SHOULD BE ASSESSED

- Healthcare professionals should be vigilant for any indicators of pain (III).
- Pain should be assessed and recorded at regular intervals (III).
- Unexpected intense pain, particularly if sudden or associated with altered vital signs such as hypotension, tachycardia or fever, should be immediately evaluated (III).
- Children's pain should be assessed when undertaking other routine assessments to avoid unnecessary distress or disturbance (III).

### INDICATORS OF CHILDREN'S PAIN

- Changes in children's behaviour, appearance, activity level and vital signs should be noted as these may indicate a change in the pain intensity (I).
- Physiological measures (e.g. heart and respiratory rates) can be used to assess pain but only in addition to self-report and behavioural measures (II).

### INDIVIDUAL DIFFERENCES

- A pain history should be obtained from each child and his parents at the time of admission

and nurses should learn what words the child uses for pain (e.g. baddie, hurt, etc) (II).
- The importance of cultural factors should be considered and healthcare professionals should seek to identify whether they may affect the assessment of pain (II).

### PAIN ASSESSMENT TOOLS

- Pain assessment should include the use of a validated pain assessment tool. The tool should be used in conjunction with children's self-report, with parents' assessments and the healthcare professional's own assessment of a child's pain (I).
- Self-report tools should be used whenever the child can communicate (II).

### THE RECOGNITION AND ASSESSMENT OF PAIN IN NEONATES AND INFANTS

- Recognise that it is possible to measure the level of pain in premature infants (II).
- Behavioural measures can reliably and validly indicate that infants are experiencing pain. These measures include: crying, facial expressions, motor responses, body posture, activity, undue quietness, restlessness and appearance (I).
- No pain assessment tools should be used in isolation: the overall status and gestation age of infants, parental views and the environment must be taken into account (II).

### HOW SHOULD PAIN IN YOUNG CHILDREN BE RECOGNISED AND ASSESSED?

- Behavioural and/or self-report tools should be used to assess pain in young children. The tool used should be determined by a child's age, development and clinical condition (II).
- Behaviour should be observed for the following pain indicators: crying facial expression, motor responses, body posture, activity and appearance (III).
- Observation of behaviour should include and note blunted behaviour, which may be due to severe pain in addition to depression, fatigue, extreme illness or the use of sedatives or hypnotics (III).
- Self-report tools are appropriate for most children of 4 years and older and provide the most accurate measure of children's pain (II).

- Provide enough time for children to complete pain assessments (III).

## HOW SHOULD PAIN IN OLDER CHILDREN AND ADOLESCENTS BE RECOGNISED AND ASSESSED?

- Use a pain assessment tool appropriate for the child's developmental level, personality and condition (III).
- Older children and adolescents should be offered one of the recommended pain assessment tools and encouraged to use the one they feel is most appropriate (III).
- Provide enough time for older children and adolescents to complete pain assessments (III).

## PARENTS/CARERS/FAMILIES

- Children's families should be encouraged to contribute to the assessment of their pain (II).
- Parents' assessment of their child's pain should not override the child's self report. However, when children are unwilling or unable to give a self-report, family reports of pain should be used (II).
- Parents need adequate information to be able to contribute to the assessment of children's pain (II).
- Before discharge, methods of assessing pain and their effectiveness should be reviewed with the child and family and information provided about conducting pain assessment effectively at home.

## HEALTHCARE PROFESSIONALS

- Healthcare professionals should be trained to recognise and assess pain (II).

## WAYS OF ASSESSING PAIN IN CHILDREN

There are a number of ways of assessing pain in children. The nurse can:

- Ask the child
- Use the child's non-verbal cues
- Use physiological indicators
- Ask the parents.

## ASK THE CHILD

The RCN guidelines suggest that a child's self-report of pain should be considered the *gold stan-*dard. There are a number of pain assessment tools that can be used with children who can verbally communicate. The use of pain assessment tools enables a systematic approach to be taken to pain assessment and measurement. Assessment tools help children to indicate their pain intensity. The selection of a pain assessment tool should be based on the child's age and cognitive ability. The pain assessment tools used most commonly in clinical practice are the faces scale, the simple descriptive scale, the numerical scale and the visual analogue scale.

There are several faces scales for pain rating. The most frequently used is the Wong & Baker Faces Scale (Wong & Baker 1988). It can be used with children aged 3–18 years. There are six faces depicting expressions from smiling to neutral to total misery (Carter 1994). The nurse explains to the child that the smiling face is smiling because the person has *no hurt at all* and that the crying face is crying because the person has *as much hurt as they could possibly imagine.* (It is important to emphasise to the child that you do not have to be crying for your pain to be represented by the crying face; rather, it is how the child feels *inside.*) However, recent research has suggested that faces pain rating scales, such as that developed by Bieri et al (1990), with a neutral *no pain face* and non-cartoon like faces are a more valid way of measuring pain (Chambers et al 1999).

The simple descriptive scale is a horizontal or vertical 100 mm line with descriptors written along the line starting at the left with 'no pain' and progressing to 'worst possible pain' on the right. This scale can be used for children from 9 to 15 years (Taylor 1998). The numerical scale is a 100 mm horizontal line numbered 0–10 or 0–5, with 0 representing *no pain* and 5 or 10 representing *the worst pain imaginable.* In order to use the scale children need to be able to count, which excludes most children under 5 years.

The visual analogue scale (VAS) is a 100 mm horizontal or vertical line with a mark at either end with 'no pain' on the left and 'worst pain possible' on the right. Children mark the position along the line that indicates their pain intensity. The VAS is useful for children with limited language skills but the child needs a cognitive ability to translate experience into analogue format and to be able to understand proportionality (McGrath et al 1995). It can therefore only be used with the older child.

For a pain assessment tool to measure a child's pain effectively, it must be reliable and valid. Reliability refers to the consistency, stability and repeatability of measurements (Sellitz, Wrightsman et al 1976). Validity refers to the appropriateness, applicability and representativeness of using measurements as a 'true' finding (Morse 1989).

The authors of the tools have undertaken a number of studies into the effectiveness of pain assessment tools, consequently the potential of bias in the findings must be considered. Therefore many of the pain assessment tools described require further studies to establish validity and reliability. Even so, it is better to use any pain assessment tool in practice than not to use one at all.

## NON-VERBAL CUES

Children demonstrate a number of non-verbal pain behaviours. Some of these are identified in Box 6.1.

## PHYSIOLOGICAL SIGNS

Physiological signs can be used to establish whether a child is in pain but are most useful when combined with other data about pain involving behaviours and pain producing pathology (Eland 1990). If pain persists over a period of time, adaptation may occur and there is less increase in the sympathetic responses. Physiological signs should be used in conjunction with other methods of assessing pain.

### Box 6.1 Non-verbal pain behaviours

- Changed behaviour
- Irritability
- Unusual posture
- Reluctance to move
- Aggressiveness
- Increased clinging
- Unusual quietness
- Loss of appetite
- Restlessness
- Sobbing
- Lying 'scared stiff'
- Lethargy
- Banging head
- Pulling ear
- Refusal to move limbs

## ANALGESIC DRUGS

There are two main types of pain relieving interventions: analgesic drugs and non-pharmacological methods. Analgesics must be given regularly to control pain. Moriarty (1998) suggests that there are four main drugs that are used to manage pain in children: paracetamol, diclofenac, codeine phosphate and morphine. Paracetamol is effective for mild pain and is only available as suppositories and in oral form. Diclofenac, a nonsteroidal anti-inflammatory drug (NSAID) is effective for mild to moderate pain. It is available in dispersible tablets (which make small doses easy to administer) as well as rectally. It can also be given intramuscularly, but this route should not be used for children. Another commonly used NSAID is ibuprofen. The use of aspirin, or aspirin compounds, is not recommended in children under the age of 16 years because of an association with Reye's syndrome (British National Formulary 2004).

Codeine phosphate is a weak opioid and works well when administered in conjunction with paracetamol or a NSAID for moderate pain. Codeine phosphate cannot be given intravenously as it may cause apnoeic episodes. It is available in oral, suppository and intramuscular preparations. Dihydrocodeine, another weak opioid, is not widely used in children. Morphine is a strong opioid and is used for the treatment of severe pain. It is available in oral, intravenous, intramuscular and subcutaneous preparations. The use of intramuscular injections to administer analgesics to children should be minimised and many children's wards are now intramuscular injection-free zones.

## PHARMACOLOGY OF ANALGESIC DRUGS

Knowledge of the pharmacology of analgesic drugs helps the nurse understand how the different drugs interact.

### NSAIDs

All NSAIDs have an anti-inflammatory, anti-pyretic and analgesic action and inhibit/block the action of cyclo-oxygenase, an enzyme necessary in the formation of prostaglandins (Russell 1992, Day 1997). This decreases pain as prostaglandins sensitise the pain receptors and thus make them more likely to become activated by other chemicals released during trauma (Walsh 1997). Prostaglandins occur naturally and are released by cell damage, and are involved in the production of pain impulses. As well as sensitising pain receptors they are responsible for many of the features of inflammation, such as swelling and redness (Atkinson & Atkinson 1987).

## OPIOIDS

Opioids act on the body's opioid receptors, which are found throughout the central nervous system (Day 1997). Most opioid drugs are agonists, resulting in stimulation of the receptor. However, partial agonists, such as buprenorphine, also exist. They have dual action, partially stimulating and partially blocking the receptor. Antagonists, such as naloxone, work by blocking the receptor sites and reversing the action of opioids. Opioids act on very specific sites in the brain – the opioid receptors (Russell 1992). Opioid analgesics bind to these receptors and activate them, mimicking the effect of the endogenous enkephalins (Atkinson & Atkinson 1987). Opioid agonists (e.g. morphine) are drugs that combine with tissue receptors to elicit a positive response. Opioid antagonists (e.g. naloxone) are drugs that produce no response but nevertheless possess receptor affinity. They block the action of an opioid because they have a greater affinity than the opioid for the receptor site. Opioid partial agonists (e.g. buprenorphine) readily bind to receptor sites but elicit only a partial response. They may antagonise the effects of more potent pure agonists by occupying the same binding sites. For this reason, drugs such as buprenorphine and morphine should not be given together (Russell 1992).

## ANALGESIC TECHNIQUES

### EPIDURALS

The use of epidural analgesia in children has become more widespread over the last few years and is a well established method of pain relief for neonates, infants and children postoperatively (MacIntyre & Ready 1996). Epidural analgesia is produced by injecting or infusing local anaesthetic and/or and opioid into the epidural space. Opioids administered epidurally are thought to block the release of substance P when they bind to opioid receptors in the dorsal horn. This action affects the transmission of pain impulses to the cerebral cortex (Rosen & Calio 1990). The analgesic effect provides a segmental block of the nerve impulses across the spinal nerves innervating in the surgical area (Ochsenreither 1997). Local anaesthetics bind to the sodium channels of the neurones, preventing depolarisation and thereby blocking the conduction of the nerve impulses. Local anaesthetics may be given alone and this works well in children. However, it has been reported that a combination of local anaesthetics and opioids can produce a synergistic effect, allowing the reduction of their respective doses and concentrations and therefore achieving a good level of analgesia, with minimal side effects (Al-Shaikh 1997, Ochsenreither 1997).

When children are receiving analgesia via an epidural infusion a number of observations need to be carried out on an hourly basis. These are identified in Table 6.2.

An ice cube can be used to assess the level and extent of the motor block by detecting loss of cold sensation. The point at which the child perceives cold sensation is the level of the block. If a bolus of analgesia is given the child should be more closely monitored.

While these children require high dependency nursing, it is possible to manage them effectively in the ward situation. Continuous monitoring using an oxygen saturation monitor will help by ensuring that blood oxygen levels and pulse can be seen at a glance. In the ward situation, it is recommended that an acute pain service is available for expert advice. If the child's mobility is affected because of the epidural it is important to carry out regular pressure area care, with careful observation of at risk areas such as the child's heels. The epidural line and syringe must be clearly labelled, and local training should include the management of epidural analgesia in babies and children as well as the changing of epidural syringes in order to reduce the fatal risk of local anaesthetic being accidentally delivered by the intravenous route.

### PATIENT CONTROLLED ANALGESIA

Patient controlled analgesia (PCA) is widely used for the postoperative pain management of children. PCA was developed to meet the need for analgesia to be tailored to the individual child's requirements and refers to the intravenous administration of small bolus doses of an opioid drug which is triggered by the child pressing a button (Lloyd Thomas

**Table 6.2** Observations required when an epidural infusion is in situ

| Observation | Rationale |
| --- | --- |
| Pain intensity | • To ensure effective pain relief is being provided |
| Pulse | • Surgical requirement |
| Respiratory rate and oxygen saturation levels | • To detect respiratory depression (due to the opioids; may increase if child's pain not adequately controlled)<br>• To detect rostral spread of local anaesthetic which would cause respiratory failure |
| Temperature | • Epidural infusions pose a potential infection risk |
| Blood Pressure | • Epidural infusions can cause hypotension – this is uncommon in children younger than 8 years |
| Level of block | • To ensure the block is not unilateral or too high |
| Sensation | • Indicates the level of the block |
| Motor movement | • Tested alongside the level of the block<br>• Indicates any problems with mobility |
| Site of epidural | • To check for leakage and inflammation |
| Sedation | • A possible side effect of opioids |
| Side effects of drugs | • Epidural infusions may cause nausea and vomiting or pruritis<br>• Local anaesthetic toxicity – circum oral tingling followed by a rapid decrease in blood pressure, confusion and fitting |
| Volume infused used | • To ensure that the epidural infusion is running as prescribed |
| Patency of IV cannula | • To ensure IV access if required |

1993). The use of PCAs in children has a number of psychological benefits. It allows children to control their own pain and to prepare themselves for painful procedures. Most children aged 5 years and older are able to use the PCA effectively and the analgesia provided compares favourably with continuous morphine infusions in the older child (Morton 1998b). Some younger children are also able to use the PCA system; this depends on the ability of the individual child. Children require a detailed explanation on how the lockout system works. PCA is usually commenced intra-operatively and the commonest opioid used is morphine.

Children receiving PCA should be monitored closely and have hourly observations of pulse rate, respiratory rate, the volume delivered, oxygen saturation, pain score, sedation score and nausea and vomiting. Parental education is important, as their support is essential to the child in the postoperative period. Parents need to be informed of the set up of the PCA system and any fears they may have must be addressed. Many children's wards and units provide written information for both the child and parents. It is important that parents understand that they must not press the button for the child.

## NURSE CONTROLLED ANALGESIA (NCA)

In children under 5 years of age the use of NCA has become popular (Lloyd-Thomas & Howard 1994).

This is a morphine infusion with the ability to administer controlled boluses of the drug at times of increased pain. To prevent an overdose of morphine, a longer lockout time is employed; however, if the child is in pain at the start of NCA a loading dose must be administered to ensure an adequate drug level in the body. Nurses should consult the child and parents about the need for extra analgesia, but it is the responsibility of the nurse to *press the button* (administer the drug). The same observations are carried out when using PCA.

## INTRAVENOUS INFUSION OF OPIOID DRUGS

Some children will have a continuous infusion of an opioid drug following surgery. The concentration of drugs used varies in different hospitals; however, the Alder Hey *Guidelines on the Management of Pain in Children* provides a useful framework (Alder Hey Royal Liverpool Children's NHS Trust 1998). Again, hourly observations of pulse rate, respiratory rate, volume delivered, oxygen saturation, pain score, sedation score and nausea and vomiting should be recorded. It may be necessary to adjust the rate of the infusion up or down to maintain the child in a pain free state. This is best accomplished by the prescription being written as a sliding scale.

## SUBCUTANEOUS CANNULA

In areas where it is not possible to use PCAs or epidurals, a butterfly or Y-can can be placed subcutaneously or intramuscularly at the time of the operation (Lloyd-Thomas 1993). This allows for intermittent boluses of opiate analgesia to be administered without having to give an intramuscular injection. It is important to check the needle site regularly for signs of infection or displacement. When weaning a child from any of the above methods it is important to ensure that oral medication is prescribed and administered before the effect of the intravenous/subcutaneous medication has worn off. The aim of pain management is to maintain children in a pain free state rather than waiting for them to be in pain before administering analgesia.

## NON-PHARMACOLOGICAL METHODS OF PAIN RELIEF IN CHILDREN

Non-pharmacological methods of pain control are probably most effective as coping strategies rather than for actual reduction of the intensity of pain. Although there are exceptions to this statement, such as the use of heat and cold packs, the most likely outcome of techniques such as relaxation and distraction is that pain will be more tolerable, not necessarily less severe in intensity (McCaffery & Wong 1993). Many non-pharmacological techniques can be taught or facilitated by nurses so that children and families can take over this part of pain management (Carter 1994), giving them some control over the management of their pain. Non-pharmacological methods of pain control may be overused or even abused with certain children or in selected circumstances. It is important to remember that children who are using distraction techniques and other non-pharmacological methods of pain relief may not look as if they are in pain. Nurses need to remember that non-pharmacological methods do not take away the pain, they dull the child's perception of the pain. Non-pharmacological methods should, therefore, be used in conjunction with analgesic drugs. Some of the more commonly used non-pharmacological methods are described below.

## DISTRACTION

Distraction is most effective when used to manage pain of relatively short duration, such as procedural pain (Carter 1994). It does not relieve pain but makes it more tolerable or bearable by putting pain at the periphery of awareness (McCaffery & Beebe 1989), with attention being focused on the distracter rather than on the pain. When using distraction with children, it is necessary to determine an effective distraction strategy; this should be planned with the child and parents and should identify what is particularly interesting to the child (McCaffery & Wong 1993).

## RELAXATION

Relaxation does not reduce the intensity of pain but reduces the distress associated with pain (Carter 1994). A patient cannot be relaxed and anxious concurrently, therefore pain tolerance should be increased if the patient is relaxed (Weisenberg 1980). Relaxation is an effective coping strategy for procedural, chronic or ongoing pain. However, for pain that lasts most of the day a relaxation technique may be performed several times a day. When caring for children in pain, the presence of a parent is useful in helping to reduce distress associated with pain for all age groups (McCaffery & Wong 1993). To ensure the effectiveness of relaxation techniques they should ideally be taught prior to painful procedures.

## IMAGERY

Imagery involves the use of imagination to modify the response to pain (Doody et al 1991) Sensory images are used to modify the pain to make it more bearable by substituting a pleasant image in place of pain (McCaffery & Beebe 1989). Imagery can be used in a guided way so that children imagine something about their pain which will help reduce it; for example, children who have pain can picture the pain flowing out of their bodies (Carter 1994).

## AROMATHERAPY

Aromatherapy is a holistic form of healing using essential oils extracted from aromatic plants, and is being used increasingly as a means of reducing stress, relaxing, treating symptoms and providing relief from pain. Aromatherapy promotes healing on different levels – physical, emotional and mental – and should only be practised by a trained practitioner (Carter 1995).

Nurses and parents can use many of the non-pharmacological methods with very little training. Other methods, such as aromatherapy and hypnosis, require a recognised qualification to be obtained and, if practised as part of holistic nursing care, the Director of Nursing must be informed in order to ensure that vicarious liability is accepted by the Trust. It is important that nurses do not implement methods of which they have little or no knowledge. Utilising the skills of the multidisciplinary team is important; play specialists and clinical psychologists can play a vital role in implementing non-pharmacological methods.

## SPECIAL CONSIDERATIONS

### NEONATAL PAIN

Neonatal pain management and assessment has been a neglected area (Carlson et al 1996). This is due, at least in part, to the fact that many healthcare professionals felt that neonates did not feel pain (Owens 1984, Tatman & Johnson 1998). This myth was perpetuated because of the belief that incomplete nerve pathways meant that pain could not be felt (Langdon 1995). A number of studies demonstrate that infants and premature infants are capable of experiencing pain and they can display a range of different responses (Anand & Hickey 1987, Grunau & Craig 1987). Facial expression in the infant or neonate has been the most studied behavioural pain assessment measure and has been referred to as the gold standard of behavioural responses in the infant (Craig 1998). Grunau and Craig (1987) discuss the facial expressions of infants experiencing acute pain. These include the following characteristics: eyes forcefully closed, brows lowered and furrowed, nasal roots broadened and bulged, deepened nasolabial furrow, a square mouth, and a taut, cupped tongue.

A number of pain assessment tools have been developed for use with preterm babies and infants. A summary of these scales can be seen in Table 6.3. The RCN (1999a) guidelines recognise that it is possible to measure the level of pain in premature infants and confirm that behavioural observation is the main parameter used to assess pain in the non-verbal child. However, relying solely on behavioural measures can be misleading; the infant may, for example, be incapable of crying or have restricted body movement (Johnston et al 1995). It also important to consider the environment and

other factors that can help to reduce pain. The careful coordination of painful procedures and elimination of unnecessary noise and environmental stimuli all contribute to the non-pharmacological variables that can help to reduce pain and discomfort for the neonate and infant (Mann et al 1986). The use of sucrose solutions prior to painful procedures has also been shown to reduce the pain reaction in neonates (Stevens et al 1999). In recent years swaddling, positioning and rocking have been used to reduce pain in neonates.

### INFANTS AND TODDLERS

Infants and toddlers have a limited cognitive ability and also limited verbal skills which make pain assessment and management in the age range a difficult task for all healthcare professionals (Bieri et al 1990). The pain behaviour exhibited by young children when expressing their pain may, therefore, be different from that in older children. Nurses then have problems with interpreting the differing behaviour children exhibit. This can lead to difficulties and mismanagement within pain assessment and pain management.

Many children aged 3 years can differentiate the presence or absence of pain. It is therefore paramount that language is used that is appropriate to the child's age and cognitive ability. Often children do not understand the word pain and respond to other terms such as 'poorly', 'hurts' and 'ow'. This essential information can be gained from the parents or carers during the preoperative assessment or throughout the child's stay. A number of tools have been devised for this age group and they are summarised in Table 6.4. Young children may not be able to tell you where their pain is and Franck et al (2000) discuss how children can be asked to make a mark to indicate an area of pain on a body outline.

### PAEDIATRIC INTENSIVE CARE UNIT

Children in the intensive care unit (ICU) are liable to experience pain from a number of sources including:

- wounds
- fractures
- indwelling tubes and catheters
- procedures
- immobility
- underlying condition. (Henning 1997)

Table 6.3 Pain assessment tools for neonates (0–1 months)

| Tool and Reference | Validated | Indicators | Advantages/Disadvantages |
|---|---|---|---|
| NFCS (Neonatal Facial Coding System) (Grunau et al 1990) | | Bulging brows, eyes squeezed tightly shut, deepening of nasolabial furrow, open lips, mouth stretched, taut tongue | • anatomically-based system for assessing facial expression |
| CRIES (Crying, Requires $O_2$ for saturation above 95, Increased vital signs, Expression and Sleeplessness) (Krechel & Bildner 1995) | | Cries, oxygen saturation, heart rate/blood pressure, expression, sleeplessness | *Advantages* <br>• easy to remember and use <br>• valid and reliable down to 32 weeks gestational age <br>• reliable between observers <br>• tracks pain and the effect of analgesics <br>*Disadvantages* <br>• uses oxygenation as a measure which can be affected by many other factors <br>• BP measurements may upset babies |
| NIPS (Neonatal Infant Pain Scale) (Lawrence et al 1993) | | Facial expression, cry, breathing patterns, arms, legs, state of arousal | *Disadvantages* <br>• uses 6 categories, 2 of which are similar <br>• hard to remember <br>• cannot be used in intubated or paralysed patients |
| COMFORT (Ambuel et al 1992) | | Alertness, calmness/agitation, respiratory response, physical movement, blood pressure, heart rate, muscle tone, facial tension | *Disadvantages* <br>• complicated <br>• 8 categories and many sub-categories <br>• cannot be used in intubated or paralysed patients |
| LIDS (Liverpool Infant Distress Score) (Hogan & Choonara 1996) | | Spontaneous movements, spontaneous excitability, flexion of fingers and toes, facial expression, quantity of crying, sleep pattern and amount | *Advantages* <br>• assesses postoperative pain <br>• 0–5 point scale |

**Table 6.4** Pain assessment tools for infants and toddlers (1 month–3 years): behavioural and physiological signs of pain and distress

| Tool and Reference | Validated | Indicators | Advantages/Disadvantages |
|---|---|---|---|
| CHEOPS (Children's Hospital of Eastern Ontario Pain Scale) (Barrier et al 1989, McGrath et al 1985) | | Alertness, calmness/agitation, respiratory response, physical movement, blood pressure, heart rate, muscle tone, facial tension | *Disadvantages*<br>• complicated behavioural scale<br>• may not track postoperative pain well in 3–7 year olds as pain behaviour inhibited<br>• 10 categories, 4 of which are similar<br>• confusing (high score = low pain)<br>• cannot be used in intubated or paralysed patients |
| TPPPS (The Toddler/Pre-Schooler Postoperative Pain Tool) (Tarbell et al 1992) | | Verbal pain, complaint/cry, groan/moan/grunt, scream, open mouth, squint, brow bulge, restless motor behaviour, rub/touch | *Advantages*<br>• suitable for age 1–5 years<br>• tracks pain relief and effects of analgesia<br>• correlates with nurse and parental pain assessments<br>*Disadvantages*<br>• 7 categories to score |
| FLACC (Face, Legs, Activity, Cry, Consolability) (Merkel et al 1997) | | Face, Legs, Activity, Cry, Consolability | • behavioural scale<br>• postoperative pain<br>• easy to use in practice |

In conjunction with this there are a number of factors which make pain management in ICU difficult, including:

- communication difficulties
- severity of illness
- treatments
  - — sedatives
  - — muscle relaxants
  - — artificial ventilation
- fear
- guilt
- absence of parent. (Henning 1997)

Pain management for children in the ICU is therefore complicated. Effective analgesia has been shown to reduce post-surgical stress response and complications such as cardiovascular instability and raised intracranial pressure (Hazinski 1999). Children's physical condition can affect their response to pain. Children may have difficulty in expressing pain due to the alteration of their level of consciousness, sedation, intubation or nature of their injury and so when assessing pain in children in ICU the nurse needs to use a combination of physiological and behavioural measures (Coffman et al 1997). The presence of the family also reassures the child. Parents are important to consider in relation to pain assessment; they have valuable information about their child's previous response to pain. However, parents can be under enormous stress in this type of environment.

## CHILDREN WITH SPECIAL NEEDS

Children with special needs are at an increased risk of experiencing pain. A child with special needs may have medical problems that may cause pain and many children with special needs may require various surgical procedures. Various levels of behavioural limitations, such as an inability to communicate verbally, have the potential to mask the expression and experiences of pain (McGrath et al 1998). It should be remembered that every child can communicate in some way and a pain history should be taken on admission to identify pain behaviours. Examples of questions that can be asked can be seen in Table 6.5.

Assessing children with any degree of developmental delay or special needs poses difficulties for all health professionals. There is a limited amount of literature available on pain assessment with children with special needs, although recently there has been increasing interest in this area of paediatrics and recognition that pain assessment in relation to the child with special needs is an area in urgent need of development. It is suggested that what is painful to an able-bodied child is as painful to a child with special needs unless otherwise proven, and it is essential that this should underpin nursing practices. For further information on the pain assessment and management of the child with special needs see Twycross et al (1999).

## PROCEDURAL PAIN

UNICEF (1999) in the UK has launched a charter for children in hospital which draws upon the *United Nations Convention on the Rights of the Child* (United Nations 1989).

It states that: 'All invasive procedures in the conscious child must be accompanied by adequate

**Table 6.5** Pain experience history (adapted from Hestor & Barcus 1986)

| Child Form | Parent Form |
|---|---|
| Tell me what pain is | What word(s) does your child use in regard to pain? |
| Tell me about the hurt you have had before | Describe the pain experiences your child has had before |
| Do you tell others when you hurt? If yes, who? | Does your child tell you or others when he is hurting? |
| What do you do for yourself when you are hurting? | How do you know when your child is in pain? |
| What do you want others to do for you when you hurt? | What do you do for your child when he is hurting? |
| What helps the most to take your hurt away? | What does your child do for himself when he is hurting? |
| Is there anything special that you want me to know about when you hurt? (If yes, have child describe) | What works best to decrease or take away your child's pain? |
| Are there any signs/communication aids which you use to let people know that you are hurting? (If yes, have child describe) | Is there anything special that you would like me to know about your child and pain? (If yes, describe) |

analgesia and when systematic analgesia is used, personnel experienced in the resuscitation of children should be immediately available.'

Children in hospital often undergo painful procedures. It is important that these are managed effectively. The use of a local anaesthetic cream such as EMLA or Ametop prior to cannulation or venepuncture is very effective – as long as the cream is left in situ for long enough. Analgesia can also be administered prior to a painful procedure, remembering to allow enough time for the analgesia to take effect.

When healthcare professionals perform procedures on children and have to hold the child down to do so, they often try to convince themselves that they are not hurting the child, however, this is *not* the case. This is a coping mechanism used by nurses and doctors and this rationale should not be used to deny pain relief to any child. Procedures are easier to manage on cooperative children. It is more appropriate to use chemical restraints, such as analgesics, than physical restraint (Eland 1985b). This concurs with the guidance from the Royal College of Nursing (1999b) on restraining, holding still and containing children.

## ENTONOX

Entonox is a gaseous mixture of 50% nitrous oxide and 50% oxygen. The use of Entonox (nitrous oxide) has led to an improvement in the quality of care for children undergoing painful procedures (Vater & Hessell 2000). Entonox is a powerful inhalation analgesia that has pain-relieving properties similar to that of a dose of morphine. Onset of action is fast, within 2–3 breaths, and lasts as long as the child continues to inhale the gas. Its fast onset and offset makes it a suitable agent for providing analgesic procedures for a child undergoing painful procedures of short duration. In order to use Entonox, children should be old enough to understand how to operate the valve (the child needs to suck on the mouthpiece) and to understand the instructions given by the nurse on how to use the equipment. It is recommended for use in children over 5 years; however, any child who can drink through a straw can potentially use Entonox via the mouthpiece. Entonox can be used as an adjunct to opioid analgesia for the types of procedures suggested in Box 6.2; however, care should be taken if an opioid has been administered in the past hour as the Entonox may

> **Box 6.2 Some Indications for the use of Entonox (Bruce & Franck 2000, Vater & Hessell 2000)**
>
> - Acute trauma
> - Removal of pins or K wires
> - Change of plaster
> - Removal of drains
> - Dressing changes
> - Orthopaedic procedures – e.g. pinsite care
> - Application of traction and plaster of paris

increase its effectiveness; the patient should be observed for signs of sedation or respiratory depression. Some of the contraindications for the use of Entonox can be seen in Box 6.3.

Nitrous oxide is known to inactivate vitamin $B_{12}$ and prolonged or repeated use may affect folate metabolism, impairing DNA synthesis and causing megaloblastic changes in the bone marrow (Amos et al 1994, Nunn 1987). It is recommended, in the light of this, that those patients using Entonox more frequently than every four days should have a regular full blood count (BOC 1995). Before administering Entonox to a patient it is necessary for nurses to have undertaken the relevant training and have had their competence assessed.

> **Box 6.3 Contraindications for the use of Entonox (Bruce & Franck 2000, Vater & Hessell 2000)**
>
> - **Air embolism** – Entonox is a space occupying gas
> - **Existing pneumothorax** – Entonox is a space occupying gas
> - **Acute head injury** – possible loss of consciousness
> - **Middle ear occlusion** – Entonox is a space occupying gas
> - **Maxillofacial injuries** – will be unable to use the mouthpiece or mask
> - **Gross abdominal distension** – Entonox is a space occupying gas
> - **Intoxication** – may be vomiting or unable to use the mouthpiece or mask

## CONCLUSION

Unrelieved pain has a number of undesirable consequences and so there is a need to assess and manage pain in children effectively. Pain assessment tools allow nurses to quantify a child's pain intensity. An appropriate pain assessment tool should be used to assess pain in children of all ages. Once pain has been assessed nurses should use both analgesic drugs and non-pharmacological pain relieving interventions to manage a child's pain. After an appropriate length of time the effectiveness of these interventions should be evaluated.

When communicating with children about their pain it is important to consider their level of cognitive development and what their perception is regarding the cause and effect of pain. Nurses should also use a child's parents to help manage pain. However, it is important to give parents sufficient information to do so. It is only when nurses work in partnership with parents and other healthcare professionals to implement the treatments described within this chapter that children's pain will be managed effectively.

## References

Alder Hey Royal Liverpool Children's NHS Trust 1998 Guidelines on the management of pain in children. Alder Hey Royal Liverpool Children's NHS Trust, Liverpool

Alex JA, Ritchie MR 1992 School-aged children's interpretation of their experience with acute surgical pain. Journal of Pediatric Nursing 7(3): 171–180

Al-Shaikh B 1997 Epidural analgesia in ICU. Care of the Critically Ill 13(3): 20–24

Ambuel B, Harnlett KW, Marx CM et al 1992 Assessing distress in pediatric intensive care environments: the COMFORT Scale. Journal of Pediatric Psychology 17(1): 95–109

Amos RJ, Amess JA, Nancekievill DG et al 1984 Prevention of nitrous oxide induced megaloblastic changes in bone marrow using folinic acid. Journal of Anaesthesia 56(2): 103–107

Anand KJS, Hickey PR 1987 Pain and its effects in the human neonate and fetus. New England Journal of Medicine 317(21): 1321–1329

Atkinson R, Atkinson C 1987 Introduction to psychology. Harcourt Brace Jovanovich, London

Baker C, Wong D 1988 QUESTT: a process of pain assessment in children. Orthopaedic Nursing 6(1): 11–21

Barrier G, Attia J, Mayer MN et al 1989 Measurement of postoperative pain and narcotic administration in infants using a new clinical scoring system. Intensive Care Medicine 15(Suppl 1): S37–S39

Beales JG 1986 Cognitive development and the experience of pain. Nursing 3(11): 408–410

Bieri D, Reeve RA et al 1990 The faces pain scale for the self assessment of the severity of pain experienced by children: development, initial validation and preliminary investigation for ratio scale properties. Pain 41(2): 139–150

British National Formulary 2004 British national formulary. BMA and RPS, London

Bradshaw C, Zeanah P 1986 Pediatric nurses' assessments of pain in children. Journal of Pediatric Nursing 1(5): 314–321

BOC 1995 Medical Gases. Entonox Datasheet. BOC, Manchester

Bruce E, Franck L 2000 Self administered nitrous oxide (Entonox) for the management of procedural pain. Paediatric Nursing 12(7): 15–19

Carlson KL, Clement BA, Nash P 1996 Neonatal pain: from concept to research questions and a role for the advanced practice nurse. Journal of Perinatal and Neonatal Nursing 10(1): 64–71

Carter B 1994 Child and infant pain: principles of nursing care and management. Chapman and Hall, London

Carter B 1995 Complementary therapies and the management of chronic pain. Paediatric Nursing 7(3): 18–22

Chambers C, Gresbrecht K, Craig KD 1999 A comparison of faces scales for the measurement of pediatric pain: children's and parents' ratings. Pain 83(1): 25–35

Coffman S, Alvarez Y, Pygolil M et al 1997 Nursing assessment and management of pain assessment in critically ill children. Heart and Lung 26(3): 221–228

Craig KD 1998 The facial display of pain. In: Finlay GA, McGrath PJ (eds) Progress in pain research and management vol 10. IASP Press, Seattle, p 103–122

Day R 1997 A pharmacological approach to acute pain. Professional Nurse 13(1): S9–S12

Doody SB, Smith C, Webb J 1991 Non-pharmacological interventions for pain management. Critical Care Nursing Clinics of North America 3(1): 69–75

Eland J 1985a Myths about pain in children. The Candlelighters' Childhood Cancer Foundation V(1): 1–4

Eland J 1985b The child who is hurting. Seminars in Oncology Nursing 1(2): 116–122

Eland J 1990 Pain in children. Nursing Clinics of North America 25(4): 871–884

Ellis J 1988 Using pain scales to prevent undermedication. The American Journal of Maternal/Child Nursing 13(3): 180–182

Franck LS, Greenburg CS, Stevens B 2000 Pain assessment in infants and young children. Pediatric Clinics of North America 43(3): 487–512

Gadish HJ, Gonzalez JL et al 1988 Factors affecting nurses' decisions to administer pediatric pain medication postoperatively. Journal of Pediatric Nursing 3(6): 383–389

Gaffney A, Dunne EA 1986 Developmental aspects of children's definitions of pain. Pain 26(1): 105–117

Gildea J, Quirk T 1977 Assessing the pain experience in children. Nursing Clinics of North America 12(4): 631–637

Grunau RVE, Craig KD 1987 Pain expression in neonates: facial action and cry. Pain 28(3): 395–410

Grunau RVE, Johnston CC, Craig KD 1990 Neonatal facial and cry responses to invasive and non invasive procedures. Pain 42(3): 295–305

Hazinski MF 1999 Management of pediatric critical care. Mosby, St Louis

Henning R 1997 Pain in the intensive care unit. In: McKenzie I, Gaukroger PB, Ragg P et al (eds) Manual of acute pain management in children. Churchill Livingstone, Melbourne

Hesor NO, Barcus CS 1986 Assessment and management of pain in children. Pediatrics Nursing Update 1(14): 1–8

Hogan M, Choonara I 1996 Measuring pain in neonates: an objective score. Paediatric Nursing 8(10): 24–27

Hurley A, Whelan EG 1988 Cognitive development and children's perception of pain. Pediatric Nursing 14(1): 21–24

International Association for the Study of Pain (IASP) 1979 Pain terms: a list with definitions and notes on usage. Pain 6: 249–252

Jeans ME 1983 The measurement of pain in children. In: Melzack R (ed) Pain measurement and assessment. Raven Press, New York

Johnston CC, Stevens BJ, Yang F et al 1995 Differential response to pain by very premature neonates. Pain 61(3): 471–479

Krechel SW, Bildner J 1995 CRIES: a new neonatal postoperative pain measurement score. Initial testing of validity and reliability. Paediatric Anaesthesia 5(1): 53–61

Langdon J 1995 Neglect of essential right: perspectives on pain management in children. Child Health 3(1): 10–13

Lawrence J, Alcock D, McGrath P et al 1993 The development of a tool to assess neonatal pain. Neonatal Network 12(6): 59–65

Lloyd-Thomas AR 1993 Postoperative pain control in children. Current Paediatrics 3(4): 234–237

Lloyd-Thomas AR, Howard RF 1994 A pain service for children. Paediatric Anaesthesia 4(1): 3–15

McCaffery M 1972 Nursing management of the patient in pain. Lippincott, Philadelphia

McCaffery M, Beebe AB 1989 Pain: clinical manual for nursing practice. Mosby, St Louis

McCaffery M, Wong D 1993 Nursing interventions for pain control in children. In: Schechter NL, Yaster M, Berde C (eds) Pain in infants, children and adolescents. Williams and Wilkins, Baltimore

McGrath PJ, Johnson G, Goodman JT et al 1985 CHEOPS: a behavioral scale for rating postoperative pain in children. In: Fields HL (ed) Advances in pain research and therapy. Raven Press, New York, p 395–402

McGrath PJ, Unrah AM, Finley GA 1995 Pain measurement in children. Pain: Clinical Updates 3(2): 1–4

McGrath PJ, Rosmus C, Canfield C et al 1998 Behaviours caregivers use to determine pain in non verbal cognitively impaired individuals. Developmental Medicine and Child Neurology 40(5): 340–343

MacIntrye DE, Ready LB 1996 Acute pain management: a practical guide. WB Saunders, London

Mann NP et al. 1986 Effect of night and day on pre-term infants and newborn infants: randomised trial. British Medical Journal 293: 1265–1267

Merkel S, Voepel-Lewis T, Shayevitz JR et al 1997 The FLACC: a behavioral scale for scoring postoperative pain in children. Pediatric Nursing 23(3): 293–297

Moriarty A 1998 The pharmacological management of acute pain. In: Twycross A, Moriarty A, Betts T (eds) Paediatric pain management: a multi-disciplinary approach. Radcliffe Medical Press, Oxford

Morse J 1989 Qualitative nursing research: a contemporary dialogue. Sage, London

Morton NS (ed) 1998a Acute paediatric pain management: a practical guide. WB Saunders, London

Morton NS 1998b Prevention and control of pain in children. Pain Reviews 5(1): 1–15

Muller DJ, Harris PJ, Wattley L 1986 Nursing children: psychology, research and practice. Harper and Rowe, London

Nunn JF 1987 Clinical aspects of the interaction between nitrous oxide and vitamin $B_{12}$. British Journal of Anaesthesia 59(1): 3–13

Ochsenreither J M 1997 Analgesia in infants. Neonatal Network 16(6): 79–83

Owens ME 1984 Pain in infancy: conceptual and methodological issues. Pain 20(3): 213–230

Perrin EC, Perrin JM 1983 Clinicians' assessments of children's understanding of illness. American Journal of Disease in Childhood 137(9): 874–878

Price S 1994 Assessing children's pain. British Journal of Nursing 3(20): 1046–1048

Rosen HF, Calio M 1990 An epidural program – balancing risks and benefits. Critical Care Nursing 10(8): 32–41

Royal College of Nursing 1999a Clinical guidelines for the recognition and assessment of acute pain in children. Recommendations. Royal College of Nursing, London

Royal College of Nursing 1999b Restraining, holding still and containing children: guidance for good practice. RCN, London

Russell K 1992 Pharmacology of pain. Surgical Nurse 5(6): 18–22

Savedra M, Gibbons P, Tesler M et al 1982 How do children describe pain? A tentative assessment. Pain 14(2): 95–104

Schultz NV 1971 How children perceive pain. Nursing Outlook 19(10): 670–673

Sellitz C, Wrightsman L et al 1976 Research methods in social relations. Rinehart and Winston, New York

Stevens B, Johnston C, Franck L et al 1999 The efficacy of developmentally sensitive interventions and sucrose for relieving procedural pain in very low birth weight neonates. Nursing Research 48(1): 35–43

Tarbell SE, Cohen IT, Marsh JL 1992 The toddler-preschooler postoperative pain scale: an observational scale for measuring postoperative pain in children aged 1–5: preliminary report. Pain 50(3): 273–280

Tatman A, Johnson P 1998 Pain assessment in preverbal children. In: Twycross A, Moriarty A, Betts T (eds) Paediatric pain: a multi-disciplinary approach. Radcliffe Medical Press, Oxford

Taylor A 1998 Pain assessment in children. In: Twycross A, Moriarty A, Betts T (eds) Paediatric pain: a multi-disciplinary approach. Radcliffe Medical Press, Oxford

Thompson KL, Varni JW 1986 A developmental cognitive–biobehavioral approach to pediatric pain assessment. Pain 25(3): 283–296

Twycross A, Mayfield C, Savory J 1999 Pain management for children with special needs: a neglected area? Paediatric Nursing 11(6): 43–45

UNICEF 1999 Global millennium targets: UNICEF child-friendly hospital initiative. Paediatric Nursing 11(10): 7–8

United Nations 1989 The United Nations convention on the rights of the child. United Nations, Geneva

Unrah A, McGrath P, Cunningham SJ, Humphreys P 1983 Children's drawings of their pain. Pain 17(4): 385–392

Vater M, Hessell D 2000 Nitrous oxide and acute procedural pain. Paediatric and Perinatal Drug Therapy 4(2): 3–12

Walsh D 1997 TENS: clinical applications and related theory. Churchill Livingstone, Edinburgh

Weisenberg M 1980 Understanding pain phenomenon. In: Carter B 1994 Child and infant pain: principles of nursing care and management. Chapman and Hall, London

Wong D, Baker C 1988 Pain in children: a comparison of assessment scales. Pediatric Nursing 14(1): 9–17

Woodgate R, Kristjanson L 1996 A young child's pain: how parents and nurses "take care". International Journal of Nursing Studies 33(3): 271–284

# Chapter 7

# The nutritional care of infants and children undergoing surgery

## Carolyn Patchell and Chris Holden

## CHAPTER CONTENTS

## INTRODUCTION

Appropriate nutrition in infancy and childhood is essential to ensure optimal growth and development. The development of improved surgical techniques, specialised enteral feeds and parenteral feeding has revolutionised the care of children who are surgical patients. Enteral feeding is used for children who have a functional gastrointestinal tract (see Table 7.1) while parenteral nutrition is reserved for babies and children with severely compromised gut function (see Box 7.1).

The nutritional care of surgical patients requiring nutritional support involves many different professional disciplines. Cooperation and pooling of expertise among those involved in the care of children offer the greatest opportunity for more rational, safe and effective provision of nutritional support. A multidisciplinary team approach is therefore essential. The benefits of multidisciplinary care teams have been well documented (Sexton et al 2000) and are represented in Box 7.2.

Reported benefits of teams have been demonstrated in the increased use of enteral feeding, instead of parenteral nutrition, whenever possible, and the reduction in central venous catheter sepsis, mechanical catheter complications, metabolic complications of parenteral nutrition, average length of the course of parenteral nutrition and expenditure of parenteral nutrition (Booth 1995). Dietetic, nursing and surgical protocols must be in place to ensure nutrition is delivered in a safe effective manner.

**Table 7.1** Indications for enteral nutrition of the surgical patient (after Holden et al 2000)

| Indications | Examples |
| --- | --- |
| Inability to suck or swallow | • Neurological handicap and degenerative disorders<br>• Severe developmental delay<br>• Trauma<br>• Ventilated child |
| Increased nutritional requirements | • Malabsorption syndromes; for example short gut syndrome<br>• Congenital heart disease |
| Congenital abnormalities | • Trachea–oesophageal fistula<br>• Oesophageal atresia<br>• Malrotation<br>• Gastroschisis<br>• Oro-facial malformation<br>• Hirschsprung's disease |
| Post surgery | • Short bowel syndrome<br>• Malrotation<br>• Duodenal atresia<br>• Cleft lip and palate repair |

---

**Box 7.1 Indications for parenteral feeding for the surgical patient**

- Possible prevention of necrotising enterocolitis
- Pseudo-obstruction
- Postoperative abdominal surgery. Parenteral nutrition is always required postoperatively for the following conditions:
    - intestinal failure
    - gastroschisis
    - duodenal atresia
    - malrotation
    - short gut syndrome.

N.B. Enteral feeds are commenced as soon as possible when gut function is improved and ileus is resolved.

---

**Box 7.2 The role of teams has resulted in:**

- Early detection of surgical patients at risk
- Development of nutritional assessment and documentation–in surgical, dietetic and nursing notes
- The provision of specialised nutritional support
- Clinical and biochemical monitoring
- Audit
- Education
- Research.

---

Key points in the nutritional management of surgical patients include:

- A precise knowledge of the pathophysiology of the condition
- Use of the gut whenever possible, even if the amount of nutrients tolerated are nutritionally insignificant, to prevent atrophic effects upon the gut
- Malnutrition damages the gut
- Nutritional care needs a multidisciplinary approach involving surgeons, dietitians, nurses, speech therapists, physiotherapists, pharmacists, biochemists and microbiologists.

## NUTRITIONAL REQUIREMENTS

In order to calculate nutritional requirements of infants and children undergoing surgical procedures, some form of nutritional assessment is necessary. There are a number of methods available, but no one measure gives an overall picture of nutritional status for all nutrients. Table 7.2 lists the main methods which should be available in most centres.

Measurements of height or length and weight give the best assessment of overall status. The measurements should be plotted on centile charts (Tanner et al 1966). Weight and height should not differ by more than two percentiles.

**Table 7.2** Nutritional assessment

| Type of assessment | Method of assessment |
| --- | --- |
| Dietary intake | • Food diary/recall |
| Anthropometry | • Weight |
| | • Height/length |
| | • Head circumference |
| | • Mid/upper arm circumference |
| Biochemistry | • Albumin |
| | • Serum vitamins |
| | • Haemoglobin |
| | • Ferritin |
| | • Total iron binding capacity |

## Expected weight gain

Normal infants will exhibit weight loss in the first 5–7 days of life, whilst feeding on full volumes is established. This weight loss should be regained by day 14. Thereafter, expected weight gains are as in Table 7.3.

During the second year weight gain should be around 2.5 kg per year, reducing to 2 kg per year until puberty.

## Dietary Reference Values (DRVs)

The Department of Health report on dietary reference values (Department of Health 1991) provides figures for nutritional requirements for a range of nutrients and energy (see Tables 7.4a and 7.4b). The DRVs are based on normal healthy populations. Requirements will be increased for sick children (see Table 7.5). When estimating requirements for children, energy and nutrient intake should be based on actual body weight and not expected body weight. The latter may lead to a proposed intake which is too high for an underweight child. In some circumstances height age rather than chronological age may be used for children who are severely stunted in growth.

**Table 7.3** Expected weight gain

| Age | Weight gain |
| --- | --- |
| 0–3 months | 200 g per week |
| 3–6 months | 150 g per week |
| 6–9 months | 100 g per week |
| 9–12 months | 50–75 g per week |

## ORAL FEEDING

### Infants

Many infants post surgery will be able to feed orally by breast, bottle, cup or syringe.

### Infants over 2.5 kg birth weight

Fluids should be offered at 150–200 mL/kg/24 hours. Feed should be offered every 2–3 hours. Breastfed infants will regulate their own intake. For most infants a normal formula is suitable, however, in infants who have increased requirements, or in whom catch-up growth is required, feeds may be fortified or high energy infant formula offered (see Table 7.5).

### Infants less than 2.5 kg birth weight

Most low birth weight infants will require 130–160 mL/kg, but have a high energy requirement of approximately 130 kcal/kg. This can be easily achieved by feeding the infant either fortified expressed breast milk or a specially designed low birth weight formula (see Box 7.3).

## BREAST FEEDING

Breast feeding is the most appropriate method of feeding the normal infant and may be suitable for sick infants. Demand breast feeding ensures that a healthy infant gets the right volume of milk. If the infant is too ill to feed, the mother may express her milk and feed the infant by continuous or bolus tube feeding. Expressed breast milk may be modified to suit the sick infant's requirements by the addition of a breast milk fortifier. This will increase the energy density of expressed breast milk to 83 kcal/100 mL by the addition of 2.7 g carbohydrate and 0.7 g protein/100mL. Examples of breast milk fortifiers include Eoprotin (Mead Johnson), Nutriprem Breast Milk Fortifier (Cow & Gate) and SMA Breast Milk Fortifier (SMA Nutrition).

### Expressing breast milk

If an infant is unable to feed orally, the mother must be instructed on the correct technique for expressing her breast milk. Breast milk may be expressed by hand or pump, either electric or hand pump, into a sterile container. It should be stored refrigerated at 2–5°C until required. If the milk will not be used immediately, it may be necessary to terminally heat

Table 7.4a  Selected nutrient requirements for infants and children (male) (Department of Health 1991)

| Age | Weight kg | Fluid mL/kg | Energy (EAR)[a] kcal/day | Energy (EAR)[a] kcal/kg/day | Protein g/day | Protein g/kg/day | Sodium mmol/day | Sodium mmol/kg/day | Potassium mmol/day | Potassium mmol/kg/day |
|---|---|---|---|---|---|---|---|---|---|---|
| 0–3 m[b] | 5.1 | 150 | 545 | 115–100 | 12.5 | 2.1 | 9 | 1.5 | 20 | 3.4 |
| 4–6 m | 7.2 | 130 | 690 | 95 | 12.7 | 1.6 | 12 | 1.6 | 22 | 2.8 |
| 7–9 m | 8.9 | 120 | 825 | 95 | 13.7 | 1.5 | 14 | 1.6 | 18 | 2.0 |
| 10–12 m | 9.6 | 110 | 920 | 95 | 14.9 | 1.5 | 15 | 1.5 | 18 | 1.8 |
| 1–3 y[c] | 12.9 | 95 | 1230 | 95 | 14.5 | 1.1 | 22 | 1.7 | 20 | 1.6 |
| 4–6 y | 19.0 | 85 | 1715 | 90 | 19.7 | 1.1 | 30 | 1.9 | 28 | 1.6 |
| 7–10 y | – | 75 | 1970 | – | 28.3 | – | 50 | – | 50 | – |
| 11–14 y | – | 55 | 2220 | – | 42.1 | – | 70 | – | 80 | – |
| 15–18 y | – | 50 | 2755 | – | 55.2 | – | 70 | – | 90 | – |

[a]Estimated Average Requirement
[b]months
[c]years

Table 7.4b  Selected nutrient requirements for infants and children (female) (Department of Health 1991)

| Age | Weight kg | Fluid mL/kg | Energy (EAR)[a] kcal/day | Energy (EAR)[a] kcal/kg/day | Protein g/day | Protein g/kg/day | Sodium mmol/day | Sodium mmol/kg/day | Potassium mmol/day | Potassium mmol/kg/day |
|---|---|---|---|---|---|---|---|---|---|---|
| 0–3 m[b] | 4.8 | 150 | 515 | 115–100 | 12.5 | 2.1 | 9 | 1.5 | 20 | 3.4 |
| 4–6 m | 6.8 | 130 | 645 | 95 | 12.7 | 1.6 | 12 | 1.6 | 22 | 2.8 |
| 7–9 m | 8.1 | 120 | 765 | 95 | 13.7 | 1.5 | 14 | 1.6 | 18 | 2.0 |
| 10–12 m | 9.1 | 110 | 865 | 95 | 14.9 | 1.5 | 15 | 1.5 | 18 | 1.8 |
| 1–3 y[c] | 12.3 | 95 | 1165 | 95 | 14.5 | 1.7 | 22 | 1.7 | 20 | 1.6 |
| 4–6 y | 17.2 | 85 | 1545 | 90 | 19.7 | 1.7 | 30 | 1.7 | 28 | 1.6 |
| 7–10 y | – | 75 | 1740 | – | 28.3 | – | 50 | – | 50 | – |
| 11–14 y | – | 55 | 1845 | – | 42.1 | – | 70 | – | 70 | – |
| 15–18 y | – | 50 | 2110 | – | 45.4 | – | 70 | – | 70 | – |

[a]Estimated Average Requirement
[b]months
[c]years

**Table 7.5** Oral requirements in sick children

| Nutritional requirements | Infants 0–1 year (based on actual weight) | Children |
|---|---|---|
| High energy | 130–150 kcal/kg/day | 120% estimated average requirement (EAR) |
| Very high energy | 150–220 kcal/kg/day | 150% EAR |
| High protein | 3.0–4.5 g/kg/day | 2.0 g/kg/day |
| Very high protein | 6.0 g/kg/day | |
| High sodium | 3.0 mmol/kg/day | |
| Very high sodium | 4.5 mmol/kg/day | |
| High potassium | 3.0 mmol/kg/day | |
| Very high potassium | 4.0–5.0 mmol/kg/day | |

---

**Box 7.3  Low birth weight and infant formulas**

**Low birth weight formulas**
Nutraprem RTF (Cow & Gate)
Osterprem (Farleys)
Premcare Powder (Farleys)
Pre-Aptamil (Mead Johnson)
SMA Gold LBW RTF (SMA Nutrition)

**Whey dominant infant formulas**
SMA Gold (SMA Nutrition)
Farleys First (Farleys)
Cow & Gate Premium (Cow & Gate)
Aptamil First (Milupa)

**Casein dominant infant formulas**
SMA White (SMA Nutrition)
Farleys Second (Farleys)
Cow & Gate Plus (Cow & Gate)
Aptamil Extra (Milupa)

---

treat and freeze the milk until it is required. Once defrosted, the milk should be used within 12 hours. Ideally, fresh raw expressed milk should be given. It is important that if milk has been expressed and stored, it is fed to the infant in chronological order with the colostrum and early milk being given first.

The volume of milk expressed in a 24-hour period should match approximately the volume required by the infant. The mother should be discouraged from over-production, as when the infant is ready to breast feed, there will be an excess of milk being produced, which could lead to engorgement and mastitis.

In addition, if the mother is producing too much breast milk, the infant may not empty the breast and will not receive the energy-rich hind milk and may fail to thrive as a result. Mothers should be encouraged to express milk every 3–4 hours, including at least once at night, to maintain a good milk supply.

## DIETARY SUPPLEMENTS

Wherever possible, children should be encouraged to feed orally. If appetite is poor, they should be encouraged to eat little and often. Favourite foods should be offered and between-meal snacks encouraged. If there is an increased requirement for nutrients, or existing failure to thrive, dietary supplements should be encouraged. The nurse should be aware of the developmental stage of the child to ensure that appropriate nutrition is given (Coad & Maloney 2000) (see Appendix 1).

A range of supplements is available (see Box 7.4). They should be given at an appropriate volume and after meals so that they supplement oral nutrition, but do not suppress appetite. For example, a child of 4–6 years will be expected to take 400 kcal from dietary supplements and a 7–12 year old 600 kcal supplements.

Some children may require total nutrition via a nasogastric, gastrostomy or jejunostomy tube. Others may require nutritional support to supplement their poor oral intake, or to meet their increased nutritional requirements (Holden et al 2000). Choosing a suitable feeding regimen is essential to ensure the nutritional requirements of the surgical patient are met.

## ROUTES OF FEEDING

The main routes of feeding into the gastrointestinal tract include oral, nasogastric, nasojejunal,

Box 7.4  Selected dietary supplements available in the UK

**Fortified milkshakes**
- Ensure Plus (Ross)
- Fortisip (Nutricia) not suitable for children under 3 years
- Entera (Fresenius)
- Fortini (Nutricia)
- Fortini Multi Fibre (Nutricia)
- Fresubin (Fresenius)
- Paediasure (Ross)
- Paediasure Plus (Ross)
- Paediasure Fibre (Ross)

**Fortified juice drinks**
- Clinutren Fruit (Nestlé)
- Enlive plus (Ross)
- Fortijuce (Nutricia)
- Provide Extra (Fresenius)

**Glucose polymer drinks**
- Polycal (Nutricia)
- Maxijul liquid (SHS International)

**Glucose polymer powders**
- Maxijul (SHS International)
- Caloreen (Clintec)
- Polycal (Nutricia)

**Milkshake powders for use with fresh milk**
- Scandishake (SHS International)

gastrostomy, gastrojejunal and jejunal feeding. Appendix 2 identifies the advantages and disadvantages of each route. Appendix 3 gives an overview of feeding tubes and devices (Holden & MacDonald 2000). Large studies have reviewed, in particular, gastrostomy feeding, which appears to be on the increase (Khatlak et al 1998, Sullivan 2000).

## PSYCHOLOGICAL PREPARATION OF FAMILY FOR SPECIALISED FEEDING

In particular, it is important that both the parents and child or infant are prepared psychologically if specialised feeding is required. Holden et al (2000) have identified that the social and emotional impact of tube feeding is often overlooked or grossly underestimated. It is therefore essential that we focus upon the effectiveness of the information we provide. Parents should receive information about their child's feeding regimen in both verbal and written format.

Play specialists have a valuable role to play in preparing children for feeding. Parents/carers have commented that play specialists helped their children through play by providing them with an outlet for aggression and anger. Pictorial teaching aids and videos are increasingly being used to inform parents about the process of feeding.

## CHOOSING A SUITABLE FEEDING REGIMEN

Tube feeding can be given continuously via an enteral feeding pump, as boluses or in a combination of both. A regimen should be chosen to meet the individual needs of the surgical patient (see Table 7.6).

Feeding problems in children are common. It is, therefore, important that the causes of feeding difficulties are identified so that appropriate medical and nutritional treatment is offered (see Table 7.7). Alliot (2000) identifies some of the common causes of feeding problems the nurse may encounter.

## MONITORING

Children commenced on enteral feeding require regular monitoring. Goals should be set regarding improvement in symptoms, oral intake or nutritional status. Children requiring long term enteral nutrition will need their feeding regimen reviewed regularly to take into account changes in nutritional requirements and in the child's daily routine. Intolerance to the feed may be a problem, particularly as the feed is being first introduced. Symptoms such as vomiting, nausea, diarrhoea or feed aspiration may be controlled by changing the type of feed or the administration rate or method of administration. Table 7.8 outlines possible solutions to common problems associated with feed intolerance.

### Maintaining oral feeding skills

All children, except those with an unsafe swallow, should have opportunity to feed orally to enable them to experience tastes and textures. It is particularly important in infants as oral skills may easily be

**Table 7.6** Types of feeding regimen

| Regimen | Examples of and reasons for |
|---|---|
| Bolus top-up feeding | The child's feed is offered orally. If the child is unable to complete it, the remainder of the feed is given via tube. Examples of children who would benefit from this form of feeding include children with cleft lip and palate. They may be unable to complete feeds due to functional immaturity, breathlessness and poor suck |
| Exclusive bolus feeding | Giving boluses 3–4-hourly throughout the day via the nasogastric or gastrostomy tube. This mimics a physiologically normal feeding pattern<br>Post fundoplication bolus feeding is recommended for children who have had:<br>a surgical anti-reflux procedure and are often unable to vomit<br>Large volumes of feed from a continuous infusion can accumulate in the stomach and remain undetected in children who have gastric stasis or poor gastrointestinal motility. This can lead to gastric rupture. Bolus feeding with a gravity feeding pack will prevent overfilling of the stomach |
| Combination of bolus and continuous feeding | • Children with an oesophagostomy who are sham-fed should, preferably, receive bolus feeds to coincide with their oral feeds<br>• Enteral feeds may interfere with the absorption of medication. Bolus feeding can be provided for a period of time before and after the medication to allow optimal absorption |
| Overnight feeding | • Transitional phase related to postoperative care of the surgical patient from continuous to bolus and then oral feeding<br>• May be used to supplement oral feeding when there are problems achieving catch up growth |
| Continuous feeding | • Infants and children with malabsorption will benefit from a continuous infusion of feed. This will slow transit time and may improve symptoms of diarrhoea, steatorrhoea and abdominal cramps, and help to promote adequate weight gain<br>• Infants and children, post gut surgery, for example for short bowel syndrome, will benefit from continuous feeding<br>• Feeds given via a jejunostomy should always be delivered by continuous infusion. The stomach acts as a reservoir for food in the normally fed child, regulating the amount of food that is delivered to the small intestine. Feed given as bolus into the jejunum can cause abdominal pain, diarrhoea and dumping syndrome, resulting from rebound hypoglycaemia<br>• Inability to tolerate bolus feeds, for example:<br>– short gut syndrome<br>– ventilated child<br>– malabsorption<br>– hypoglycaemia |

lost and will often be difficult to regain. Small amounts of foods with different tastes and textures should be offered wherever possible.

## Anthropometry

Weight gain is usually the best short term indicator of improvement in nutritional status. Infants should be weighed daily in hospital. Older children will require twice weekly weighing. This allows inadequate or excessive weight gain to be recognised early and the feeding regimen to be adjusted. Children requiring longer term enteral nutrition should have their length or height monitored. Mid-upper arm circumference may be used, particularly in severely disabled children when height measure-

ments may be difficult, or in a child in whom weight is not an accurate measure of nutritional status, e.g. children with organomegaly or solid tumours.

## Dietary assessment

Records of food intake should be kept so that intakes of nutrients from foods can be considered when adjusting the feeding regimen.

## Blood monitoring

Enteral feeds are designed to be nutritionally complete. However, children with increased requirements or on long term feeding will require an

**Table 7.7** Feeding difficulties (after Alliot 2000)

| Type of problem | Problem | Result |
| --- | --- | --- |
| Neurological | Inability to move food around the mouth with the tongue | Bolus of food is not formed. If a bolus of food is formed, it may not be moved efficiently to the back of the mouth to trigger the swallow reflex. Food may be stored in the cheeks or roof of the mouth |
| | Uncoordinated swallow | Choking on food or fluids. Swallowing of air. |
| | Delayed feeding as part of global developmental delay | |
| Anatomical | High roof of the mouth | Food storage in the roof of the mouth. This can then 'fall down' when the child is not expecting it and cause the child to choke |
| | Unusual dentition | Absence of normal bite, making chewing more difficult |
| | Large tongue | Difficulty in moving food around the mouth. Where tongue thrust is present, there is also difficulty keeping food in the mouth |
| | Poor lip closure | • Difficulty in swallowing food |
| | | • Fluid loss from the mouth |
| | | • Difficulty in using a cup |
| | | • Difficulty in removing food from a fork or spoon |
| Physiological | Fatigue, e.g. due to congenital heart problems, anaemia, chronic under-nutrition or medication | Child is too tired to continue eating a meal, so stops eating before satisfying nutritional requirements |
| | Taste alterations, e.g. due to trace element deficiency or medication | Food may not taste as the carer expects, so more or less seasoning may be required |
| | Lack of appetite due to illness or constipation | Poor nutritional intake |
| Communication | Poor communication skills | Inability to express food preferences, hunger or satiety until a simple communication method has been developed to suit the child |
| | Prolonged enteral/parenteral feeding in the early months of life due to prematurity, medical or physical problems | Feeding development may be significantly delayed. Oral stimulation techniques can reduce this effect |
| Behavioural | Fear of choking or vomiting from previous experience | The child may refuse to open mouth, or may store food in the cheeks rather than swallowing it. Behavioural problems may also develop due to other areas covered in this table |
| | Hypersensitivity of the mouth or surrounding areas | The child may startle or gag or appear to be in discomfort when these areas are touched |

Table 7.8 Feed intolerance

| Symptom | Cause | Solution |
|---|---|---|
| Diarrhoea | Unsuitable feed in children with impaired gut function | Change to hydrolysed or modular feed |
| | Excessive infusion rate | Slow infusion rate and increase as tolerated to provide required nutrition |
| | Intolerance of bolus feeds | Frequent, smaller feeds or change to continuous infusion |
| | High feed osmolarity | Build up strength of hyperosmolar feeds and deliver by continuous infusion |
| | Microbial contamination of feed | Use sterile, commercially produced feeds wherever possible and prepare other feeds in clean environments |
| | Drugs (e.g. antibiotics, laxatives) | Consider drugs as a cause of diarrhoea before feed is stopped or reduced |
| Nausea and vomiting | Excessive infusion rate | Slowly rate of feed |
| | Slow gastric emptying | Correct positioning and drugs |
| | Constipation | Maintain regular bowel motions with adequate fluid intakes and laxatives |
| | Medicines given at the same time as feeds | Allow time between giving medicines and giving feeds or stop continuous feed for a short time when medicines are given |
| Regurgitation and aspiration | Gastro-oesophageal reflux | Correct positioning, drugs, feed thickener, fundoplication |
| | Dislodged tubes | Secure tube adequately and test position of tube regularly |
| | Excessive infusion rate | Slow infusion rate |
| | Intolerance of bolus feeds | Smaller, more frequent feeds or continuous infusion |

analysis of albumin, electrolytes, haemoglobin, vitamin, mineral and trace element levels on a 6–12 monthly basis.

## CHOICE OF FEEDS

There is a wide range of polymeric nutritionally complete feeds available for use in paediatrics. The appropriate feed must be chosen to meet the requirements of the individual child. The choice of feed will depend on several factors, including:

- Age
- Dietary restrictions
- Specific nutrient requirement
- Gut function
- Route and method of administration
- Cost
- Prescribability if the feed is to be continued in the community.

Standard polymeric feeds are available to use as well as more specialist feeds, e.g. for lactose intolerance, gastrointestinal disease, metabolic disorders etc. Table 7.9 summarises the choice of feeds available.

### Standard enteral feeds

Infants and children who require enteral feeding due to an inability to eat or poor dietary intakes, will normally tolerate a whole protein standard feed: for infants, either breast milk or normal formula; and for pre-school children, Paediasure or Nutrini. It may be necessary, if the child needs to gain weight or is fluid restricted, to give an energy-dense formula. In this case a high energy infant feed (Clarke et al 1998) for infants or a 1.5 kcal/mL paediatric feed for 1–6 year olds would be the feed of choice. Children over 6 years of age or over 20 kg body weight should be given a feed designed for older children (Tentrini range – Nutricia) which are available with an energy density of 1.0 kcal/mL or l.5 kcal/mL children over 12 years of age or over 45 kg body weight will require an adult feed. Some adult feeds have a high protein content and care must be taken when using these feeds to ensure excessive protein intakes are not given. Enteral feeds enriched with fibre are available in the full range of feeds. These may be used for children who have constipation and may be the feed of choice for children who are likely to require full enteral feeding in the medium to long term.

### Hydrolysed protein feeds

Infants and children with impaired gut function may benefit from the use of a hydrolysed whey feed. These feeds have a lower allergenicity and are cow's milk protein and lactose free. Peptijunior has a proportion of the fat as medium chain triglyceride (MCT) which is beneficial in children with fat malabsorption, liver disease and short gut syndrome. A hydrolysed protein feed is also preferred if the feed is to be given via a jejunostomy, as in this situation the feed is being administered distal to the action of pancreatic enzymes and bile.

### Modular feeds

In some circumstances, a commercially available formula may not be tolerated by the infant or child. In this situation a modular feed may be used comprising separate protein, fat and carbohydrate sources. This affords greater flexibility to meet the dietary restrictions and nutritional requirements for individual children. Modular feeds are time-consuming to prepare, expensive, and mistakes may be made during preparation. There is also greater risk of bacterial contamination. For this reason modular feeds should only be used when a standard feed is not tolerated. The use of a modular feed must always be supervised by a paediatric dietitian.

### Gastro–oesophageal reflux

Gastro-oesophageal reflux (GOR) is common in infants and children with neurological disease. Feed thickeners may help in controlling vomiting. A number of thickeners are available, many of which can be added to enteral feeds. Most are stable and do not change consistency over time. All will provide additional energy, ranging from 2.5 to 4.0 kcal/g, with the exception of Nestargel (Nestlé). Examples of feed thickeners are Carobel (Cow & Gate), Nestargel (Nestlé), Thixo D (Sutherland Health) and Thick'n Easy (Fresenius).

## PARENTERAL NUTRITION

Parenteral nutrition is indicated when gastrointestinal function is compromised by malformation, disease or immaturity. The aim of treatment, however, should be to attain full enteral nutrition as soon as possible (Puntis et al 1987). The following is a brief overview of some of the key issues related to parenteral nutrition. An in-depth analysis is beyond

Table 7.9  Specialist feeds

| Age | Normal gut function | Impaired gut function |
|---|---|---|
| 0–12 months | Breast milk +/– fortifier, normal infant formula follow-on milk, or high energy formula, e.g. Infatrini (Cow & Gate) or SMA High Energy (SMA Nutrition) | Hydrolysed protein feeds e.g. Peptijunior (Cow & Gate), Nutramigen (Mead Johnson) +/– energy supplements or Neocate (SHS) |
| 1–6 years (8–20 kg) | Polymeric, ready-to-use paediatric feeds, e.g. Nutrini (Nutricia), Paediasure (Ross) 1 kcal/mL, or Nutrini Energy (Nutricia) 1.5 kcal/mL or Nutrini Multi Fibre (Nutricia) 1 kcal/mL or Paediasure with Fibre (Ross) 1 kcal/mL | Hydrolysed protein feed +/– energy supplements, e.g. Pepdite 1+, MCT Pepdite 1+ (SHS), or Modular feed |
| 7–12 yrs (21–45 kg) | Tentrini, Tentrini Multi Fibre, Tentrini Energy, Tentrini Energy Multi Fibre | Hydrolysed protein or elemental feeds +/– energy supplements, e.g. Pepdite 1+ (SHS), Nutrison Pepti (Nutricia), or Modular feed |
| 12 yrs + (>45 kg) | Standard polymeric ready to use feed, e.g. Nutrison Standard (Nutricia), Ensure Plus (Ross), Osmolite (Ross), Nutrison Energy Plus (Nutricia), Fortisip (Nutricia), Nutrison with Fibre or Fortisip Multifibre (Nutricia) | Hydrolysed protein or elemental feeds +/– energy supplements, e.g. Pepdite 1+ (SHS), Nutrison Pepti (Nutricia) or Modular feed |

the remit of this chapter. Ball et al (1998) provide us with more detailed prescribing information about the delivery of parenteral nutrition. He emphasises the need for a multidisciplinary experienced team to monitor the care of children and babies requiring parenteral nutrition.

## COMPOSITION OF PARENTERAL NUTRITION

### Basic principles

Parenteral nutrition support provides the baby/child with sufficient energy and protein to support metabolic activity and sufficient volumes of fluid to allow waste excretion and replacement of insensible losses. It is easiest to think of parenteral nutrition solutions as having separate and distinct parts, i.e. energy, protein, water volume, electrolytes, minerals and vitamins which are necessary for an ongoing metabolism. Table 7.10 gives a brief overview of components of parenteral nutrition.

## MONITORING AND DELIVERY

An overview of central venous devices and equipment for the administration of parenteral nutrition is detailed in Appendix 4. Bravery (1999) has written a comprehensive review of intravenous therapy in paediatric practice. Ongoing assessment of the child's response to parenteral nutrition is part of the nurse's responsibility of care.

### Administration of parenteral nutrition

In any clinical situation parenteral nutrition is only justified if the benefits outweigh the hazards. The safety of the technique depends on available resources and expertise. Intensive medical and nursing care and biochemical monitoring are essential to ensure safe delivery of feeds.

Monitoring of children requiring parenteral nutrition should include the following:

- Daily weight
- Weekly nutritional assessment to include skinfolds, a reflection of energy stores and mid-arm circumference indication of muscle mass
- 4-hourly temperature, pulse, respirations and blood pressure
- Blood glucose monitoring
- Daily urinalysis
- Collection of urine for biochemistry
- Accurate assessment of fluid balance and cumulative fluid balance

- Review of central venous exit site
- Recording care in nursing profile.

It is important that written guidelines and policies on catheter management are readily available and should include catheter insertion and setting up of parenteral nutrition, changing parenteral nutrition bags and giving exit site and dressing changes.

Procedures should also be available for the management of:

- air in the administration set
- catheter occlusion
- catheter damage
- catheter sepsis
- obtaining blood cultures.

## COMPLICATIONS

Catheter-related sepsis remains an unsolved problem. The prevalence of catheter-related sepsis in infants has been reported from 8% to 45%, while staff training plays a key role in prevention. *Staphylococcus epidermis* and *staphylococci aureus* are the most common causes of infection. It is important that precautions to minimise the risk of sepsis are undertaken.

The following programmes must be in place to ensure patient safety:

- Ongoing educational programmes for nursing and medical staff
- Central venous catheters to be placed in strict aseptic conditions
- Multidisciplinary protocols adhered to for the management of insertion and care of central venous catheters, prescribing, making and monitoring of parenteral nutrition
- The manipulation of the central venous catheter hub must be kept to a minimum
- Single lumen catheters to be used for parenteral nutrition whenever possible
- Holden et al (2003) have developed pictorial teaching guidelines for the care of babies and children, which can be used at the bedside (see Appendix 5).

### Catheter occlusion

Catheter occlusions occur frequently with the long term usage of central venous access devices. Parenteral nutrition solutions used may contain more calcium and phosphorous, which may lead to

Table 7.10 Components of Paediatric Parenteral Nutrition (After King 1998)

| Component | Use | Deficiency | Complications |
|---|---|---|---|
| Water | Vehicle for delivery of nutrients. Helps meet daily requirements | Fluid deficit: decreased skin turgor, decreased weight, decreased tears, decreased central venous pressure, lower temperature, increased heart rate, increased respirations | Fluid excess, dilutional hyponatraemia |
| Calories | Meet energy needs to promote growth and development (anabolism) | Catabolism – negative nitrogen balance, negative growth and development | |
| Glucose (1 g = 3.4 kcal) most important macronutrient | • Maintain positive nitrogen balance (anabolism)<br>• Preferred energy source of central nervous system and red blood cells | Protein catabolism, negative nitrogen balance | Phlebitis, diuresis, hyperglycaemia, hypoglycaemia, hyperosmotic, hyperglycemic nonketotic acidosis |
| Protein (1 g = 4.0 kcal)<br>Essentials: Lysine, Leucine, Isoleucine, Methionine, Phenylalanine, Threonine, Tryptophan, Valine, Arginine, Histidine<br>Non-Essentials: Proline, Alanine, Serine, Tyrosine, Glycine, Cystine | • Growth and tissue synthesis<br>• Provide energy if shortage of glucose and fat<br>• Buffer in the extra-cellular and intra-cellular fluids | Kwashiorkor: Oedema, anemia, fatty degeneration of liver, scaling dermatitis, infection confirmed by serum transferrin<br>Morasmus: Adipose and skeletal muscle atrophy, weight loss, depressed skin test react reactivity to antigens, lethargy, dehydration<br>Mixed Disorder: Kwashiorkor and Morasmus | Azotemia, hyperammonaemia, abnormal plasma aminograms, hepatotoxicity |
| Fats (1 g = 9 kcal)<br>Components: Soybean or safflower oil<br>Fatty acids: Linolec, palmitic, oleic, steric acid, egg yolk, phospholipids, glycerol | Energy – prevent fatty acid deficiency and provide concentrated caloric source | Mild diarrhoea, dry and thickened desquamated skin, hair loss, brittle osteoporotic bones, thrombocytopenia | Altered pulmonary functions, deposition of pigmented material in macrophages, kernicterus, coronary artery disease, spurious hyperbilirubinemias, spurious hyponatraemia<br>Adverse reactions: Fever, chills, shivering, chest pain or back, warmth, vomiting |
| Potassium | • Tissue synthesis<br>• Transports glucose and amino acids across cell membranes<br>• Regulates heart rhythm<br>• Nerve impulses | Fatigue, drowsiness, decreased muscle tone, gastrointestinal obstruction, paresthesias | Hyperkalaemia, tissue sloughing and necrosis if infiltration, hypokalaemia, cardiac arrhythmias |
| Chloride | Acid base balance | Excessive sweating, diarrhoea, clouded sensorium, hypotonicity of muscles, tetany, decreased respirations | Hyperchloraemia, hypochloraemia, metabolic acidosis/alkalosis |

precipitate occlusions, particularly in neonates (Reed & Phillips 1996). Other causes of catheter occlusions are mechanical problems, thrombosis formation, lipid deposition, drug, mineral or electrolyte precipitate and fibrin sheath formation.

## Catheter damage

This can occur as a result of catheter fatigue and persistent twisting. It is important that nursing staff are aware of complications and ensure that the weight of the catheter is taken off the exit site and secured firmly to prevent damage or dislodgement.

## References

Alliot L 2000 Feeding children with special needs. In: Holden C, Macdonald A (eds) Nutrition and child health. Harcourt, London, p 143–160

Ball PA, Booth IW, Holden CE et al 1998 Paediatric parenteral nutrition. Pharmacia and Upjohn, Milton Keynes

Bannister T, Wills B 2000 Guidance on feeding for babies with cleft lip and/or palate. Prepared by the Cleft Nurses Special Interest Group and the Clinical Standards Advisory Group Services for Cleft Lip and Palate. The Stationery office, London

Booth IW 1995 The nutritional management of gastro-intestinal disease in childhood. In: Davis DP (ed) 1995 Nutrition in child health. Royal College of Physicians of London and Laveham Press, London, p iii, 121

Bravery K 1999 Paediatric intravenous therapy in practice. In: Docherty L, Lamb J (eds) Intravenous therapy in nursing practice. Harcourt, London

Clarke SE, MacDonald A, Booth IW 1998 Impaired growth and nitrogen deficiency in infants receiving an energy supplemented standard infant formula. Proceedings of the Royal College of Paediatrics and Child Health annual Spring meeting. Abstract G132 2: 75.1

Coad J, Maloney A 2000 Nursing assessment of children's nutritional status during illness. In: Holden C, MacDonald A (eds) Nutrition and child health. Harcourt, London, p 77–196

Department of Health 1991 Dietary reference values for food, energy and nutrients for the United Kingdom. Report on Social Subjects No. 41. HMSO, London

Holden C, Sexton E, Gray J et al 2003 Central venous catheter-related sepsis (CRS) in children receiving parenteral nutrition (PN). In house publication. Princess Diana Children's Hospital, Birmingham

Holden C, Johnson T, Caney D 2000 Nutritional support for children in the community. In: Holden C, MacDonald A (eds) Nutrition and child health. Harcourt, London, p 177–220

Holden C, MacDonald A (eds) 2000 Nutrition and child health. Harcourt, London

Khatlak IU, Kimber C, Kiely EM et al 1998 Percutaneous endoscopic gastronomic in paediatric practice – complications and outcomes. Journal of Paediatric Surgery 33(1): 67–72

King C 1998 Parenteral nutrition for the pre-term infant: optimal levels of key nutrients. Journal of Neonatal Nursing 4(4):12–15

Puntis JWL, Ball PA, Booth IW 1987 Complications of neonatal parenteral nutrition. Intensive Therapy and Clinical Monitoring 8: 48–56

Reed T, Phillips S 1996 Management of central venous catheter occlusions and repairs. Journal of Intravenous Nursing 19(6): 289–294

Sexton E, Holden C, Abel G 2000 A team approach to nutritional support. In: Holden C, MacDonald A (eds) *Nutrition and child health*. Harcourt Publishers, London

Sullivan P 2000 Gastrostomy feeding in the disabled child. Archives of Disease in Childhood 82: 428

Tanner JM, Whitehouse RH, Takish M 1966 Standards from birth to maturity for height weight, height velocity and weight velocity in British children. Archives of Disease in Childhood 41: 454–471

## Useful Address

Cleft Lip & Palate Association
235-237 Finchley Road, London
NW3 6LS
Tel: 020 7431 003
Fax: 0207 431 8881
Email: clapa@cwcom
Net website: http://clapa.mcmail.com
Registered charity 277842

## CASE SCENARIOS

This section contains two case studies which illustrate aspects of nutritional care.

### CASE STUDY 7.1 RAEESAH

Raeesah was born at term with congenital malrotation and ileal atresia. Her birth weight was 2.8 kg (9th centile) and her length 50 cm (50th centile). Raeesah's head circumference was 34.5 cm (50th centile). She had a corrective surgery (Ladds procedure) and an ileostomy, and a central venous feeding line was inserted. Postoperatively she had 7 days of parenteral nutrition. She started enteral feeding on day 7 and was gradually weaned down from parenteral nutrition as feeds were tolerated.

### Question

Think about Raeesah and answer the following questions:

1. What nursing interventions and monitoring would you undertake for this baby?
2. What administration method might you use for enteral feeding?
3. What enteral feed would you choose?

### Answers

1. It is essential that the following information is monitored to ensure that Raeesah's care is undertaken safely.

   a. Large sodium losses should be accounted for due to ileostomy output; check urinary electrolytes weekly.
   b. Ileostomy output must be tested for reducing substances. Feeds can then be altered if positive reducing substances are obtained. Extra sodium may be added to the feed to ensure adequate growth.
   c. Biochemical monitoring of electrolytes, urea and trace elements should be undertaken routinely.
   d. Raeesah's nutritional status should be monitored by daily measurement of weight, weekly measurement of head circumference and monthly measurement of length

   e. She is receiving parenteral nutrition via a central venous line. Vital signs, e.g. temperature, pulse and respirations, should be undertaken 4-hourly

2. Try oral bolus feeds with tube top-ups as necessary. This is helpful to ensure oral skills are maintained, but ensures Raeesah completes all her feeds. Consider continuous feed, if there is evidence of feed intolerance, for example vomiting excess watery ileostomy output which is positive for reducing substances, or failure to gain weight despite the child completing all bolus feeds.

3. Offer expressed breast milk if it is available, or offer normal formula milk, but change to hydrolysed protein feeds if there is evidence of malabsorption, for example increased stoma output, or stoma output that is positive for reducing substances.

## CASE STUDY 7.2 MEGAN

Megan was a full term baby, born with Pierre Robin Syndrome and a cleft palate. Her birth weight was 4 kg (91st centile), her length 55 cm (91st centile), and her head circumference 34 cm (25th centile). At birth she was put onto continuous feeding and given a normal infant formula at 150 mL/kg. At 3 weeks of age her growth was faltering.

### Questions

1. How would you modify Megan's feeding in view of poor growth?
2. How would you progress from continuous to oral/bolus feeding?
3. What guidelines are you aware of for supporting children with cleft lip and palate?

### Answers

1. Continuous feeding was initiated as Megan was extremely breathless when feeding. In view of poor weight gain, the volume of feed was increased. An additional trial of high energy feed, such as Infatrini or SMA High Energy formula, was given due to her need for additional calories because of the increased respiratory effort.

2. It is always advisable to use nasogastric feeding where breathing difficulties are immediately evident at birth. Deterioration in respiratory function may result following the introduction of oral feeding. Nasogastric feeding may be required in the immediate neonatal period to support the emergence of oral skills, but where problems persist it may continue for a few months.

Long term difficulties with oral feeding are usually related to other associated anomalies where the ability to swallow or breathe effectively fails to develop. Bannister & Wills 2000, in conjunction with the Cleft Lip and Palate Association (CLAPA) have produced detailed guidelines for feeding babies with a cleft lip and palate. They suggested

that non-nutritive sucking during nasogastric feeding encourages development of oral feeding skills. They suggest that the introduction of oral feeds may involve nutritive sucking using swabs of milk only.

3. Guidance on feeding for babies with cleft lip and/or palate have been produced by the Cleft Nurses Special Interest Group and the Cleft Lip and Palate Association (Bannister & Wills 2000). They emphasise that the immediate aims of feeding a baby with a cleft lip are the same as for any other baby. These are to provide a feeding method that respects parental preference and that is as close to normal as possible, maximising continued oral development, resulting in a happy, well-nourished infant. It is recommended that specialist care be provided by a multidisciplinary team as recommended in Bannister & Wills (2000).

We wish to thank Annie Cole, Cleft Lip and Palate clinical nurse specialist, of the Diana Princess of Wales Children's Hospital, Birmingham for her help with this chapter.

APPENDIX 7.1    Developmental considerations to facilitate nutritional assessment of children during illness (from Coad & Maloney 2000)

| Baby | <ul><li>Birth weight is directly linked to maternal nutritional status and the required energy intake of a baby is higher than that of an adult.</li><li>Infants are reliant on the parents/carers for all their nutritional needs.</li><li>Rhythms and daily cycles, including eating, are established very early.</li><li>Questions should be centred towards the parents and main carers. Examples of questions may include:<ul><li>What type of feeding is currently used (breast/bottle)?</li><li>What is the 'normal' pattern of feeding for the infant?</li><li>How much food is taken at each feed/meal?</li><li>At what stage of motor development is the infant? (such as holding objects, including food pincer grip)</li><li>At what stage of social development is the child? (such as attempting to feed with fingers or spoon)</li><li>Does the infant make any sound associated to mealtimes?</li><li>Has the child's normal pattern of feeding changed in the last few days?</li><li>Any vomiting or 'cough' during meals?</li><li>Ask specifically about any changes, such as less milk taken or gone off weaning and only wants milk.</li></ul></li></ul> |
|---|---|
| Preschool | <ul><li>Pre-school children (2–6 years) are growing rapidly, both physically and socially. During hospitalisation, the food they like should be available in the hospital and reassurances are needed that the admission is not a punishment.</li><li>Questions should be directed at the child, but these may need phrasing in simplistic sentences. Example of questions to include:<ul><li>Do you like?</li><li>What do you not like? (choose foods to prompt in both cases)</li><li>Are you hungry now?</li><li>Do you use a cup (plate, spoon, chair)?</li><li>Do you use a spoon (plate, cup) to eat with?</li><li>Do you have a favourite spoon (plate, cup)?</li><li>Can you show me how you eat/drink?</li></ul></li></ul> |
| School | The nutritional status affects the rate of puberty. Therefore, an energy-dense diet may be required. Children of 7–12 years are also developing social understanding (equity, fairness) and logical reasoning. They need appropriate explanation to overcome their fears about why you are asking the questions. Thus, phrasing should be open to allow them to build up a rapport with the nurse. Examples of questions might include:<ul><li>What did you eat today?</li><li>What do you like?</li><li>What don't you like?</li><li>Have you any 'special' foods?</li><li>What meal do you like (breakfast, dinner, tea)?</li><li>Ask about preferences of equipment and eating places.</li></ul> |

*(Continued)*

**APPENDIX 7.1** Developmental considerations to facilitate nutritional assessment of children during illness (from Coad & Maloney 2000)—cont'd

| Adolescent | Adolescents are able to problem-solve systematically. They may exhibit rebellious tendencies or possess idealistic values, including media images such as thinness being ideal. The nurse should encourage them to discuss their preferences and how an illness episode might affect their diet. They may also form strong opinions regarding their nutritional needs or practices and this must be fully respected in the assessment. Examples of questions might include:<br><br>– Do you want to fill out the care plan, showing your own food preferences?<br>– When do you normally like your meal times?<br><br>*Note*: Cultural special dietary requirements must always be considered for all age groups. |
| --- | --- |

**APPENDIX 7.2** Enteral feeding routes (after Holden & MacDonald 2000)

| Method | Advantages | Disadvantages |
| --- | --- | --- |
| Nasogastric | Short term feeding | Tube re-insertion may:<br>• be distressing to the child/family/nurse<br>• easily be removed by the child/baby<br>• increase risk of aspiration<br>• cause discomfort to nasopharynx<br>• have psychosocial implications |
| Nasojejunal | • Less risk of aspiration<br>• Short term feeding | • Difficulty of insertion<br>• Radiographic check of position required<br>• Risk of perforation<br>• Abdominal pain and diarrhoea will occur unless continuous feeding is used<br>• Discomfort to nasopharynx |
| Gastrostomy | • Cosmetically more acceptable to some children and families<br>• Easily hidden<br><br>• Long term feeding (Khatlak et al 1998) | • Reflux of bile is facilitated<br>• Increases reflux if already present<br>• Local skin irritation<br>• Infection<br>• Granulation tissue<br>• Leakage<br>• Gastric distension<br>• Stoma closes within a few hours if accidentally removed<br>• Precipitation of bile into stomach |
| Gastrojejunal | • Facilitates placement beyond ligament of Trietz<br>• Reduced risk of aspiration<br>• Long term feeding | • Regular gastric aspiration required<br>• Surgical/radiology procedure<br>• Risk of perforation. Continuous feeding must be used<br>• Bacterial overgrowth<br>• Dumping syndrome can occur |

**APPENDIX 7.3    Ideal feeding tubes and devices (from Holden & MacDonald 2000)**

Nasogastric Tube
- Conforms to British Standards BS 6314 (should have a male luer and anti intravenous female connection)
- Small FG with a large internal diameter
- Comfort/cosmetically acceptable
- Tip: soft with no dead space; scooped end to avoid suction of the tip onto the stomach wall; aids aspiration and reduces blockage
- Guidewires should be stiff to ensure easy insertion; flexible to avoid damage to the tube and should not coil
- Connectors should be durable and fit any giving set or syringe with or without a suitable adapter
- Radiopaque

Nasojejunal Feeding Tube
- Tube and guidewire should be radiopaque to help confirm position
- Biocompatible polyurethane tube Tungsten weighted may be helpful
- Open distal end promotes good fluid flow
- Comfort/cosmetically acceptable

Percutaneous Endoscopic Gastrostomy Tube (PEG Tube)
- Bumper bar and tube should be made of pliable, biocompatible silicone. This material easily passes down the oesophagus and helps maintain a healthy stoma
- Bumper bar helps to resist inadvertent removal and migration into stoma tract
- Connections compatible with external feeding systems to minimise separation and leakage

Gastrostomy Tube
- Medical grade silicone material, biocompatible and flexible for patient comfort
- Y-Port connector to allow easy flushing and giving of liquid medication without disconnecting feeding sets
- Centimetre graduations to allow assessment of potential tube migration
- Securing disc lifts easily for cleaning of stoma site/prevents tube migration
- Translucent to facilitate assessment of stoma
- Holes to promote airflow for a healthy stoma site
- Gastric balloon expands evenly to maintain a secure, comfortable fit and to minimise leakage
- Balloon inflation port is safely marked with the maximum balloon volume and the words 'inflation' to prevent accidental over-inflation and administration of medicines
- Open distal end promotes good fluid flow

Gastrostomy Button
- Low profile device makes it suitable for children or adults, who may be self-conscious of standard gastrostomy tube
- Anti-Reflux valve prevents leakage of feed when tube is not in use
- Balloon inflation to facilitate removal/replacement

Stoma Measuring Devices for Buttons
- Depth of tract required is measured by a stoma measuring device
- Measuring device packed separately to the button

Transgastric Jejunal Feeding Tube
- Facilitates placement of tube beyond the ligament of Trietz for endoscopic and radiologic procedures
- Provides gastric decompression while simultaneously feeding into the jejunum
- Multiple feeding ports improve flow of feed and minimise clogging
- Sliding ring balloon system prevents the tube migrating and controls gastric leakage
- Built-in universal connectors help minimise feeding set disconnections

Jejunal Feeding Tube
- Flexible medical grade clear silicone to minimise site irritation
- Radiopaque allows verification of tube position

APPENDIX 7.4    Central venous access devices and equipment for the administration of parenteral nutrition (Diana, Princess of Wales Children's Hospital, Birmingham)

| Device | Description | Advantages | Disadvantages |
|---|---|---|---|
| Partially implantable devices<br><br>For example:<br>Broviac Line | Silicon, radiopaque, flexible catheter with open or closed ends<br><br>The dacron cuff on catheter tissue facilitates tissue growth to secure the line | • Dacron cuff<br>• Easy to use<br>• Easily removed<br>• Able to be repaired | • Requires regular heparin flushes (weekly)<br>• Must be clamped at all times |
| Totally implanted devices<br>For example:<br>Port-a-cath<br>Vascuport | Totally implantable metal or plastic device<br>Consists of self-sealing injection port with pre-connected or attachable silicon catheter that is placed in a large blood vessel | • Reduced risk of infection<br>• Placed completely under the skin<br>• No limitations on most physical activity<br>• No dressing required<br>• Increased patient acceptance | • More difficult to access<br>• Must pierce skin for access<br>• Removal more complex<br>• Catheter may become dislodged from port |
| | Peripherally inserted central venous catheter | • Can be inserted on ward<br>• No general anaesthetic required | • Block more easily |
| Intravenous feeding lines and equipment | | | |
| | In-line Filters | Use of inline filters offer protection against;<br>• Inadvertent particulate matter<br>• Air embolism<br>• Precipitates<br>• Inadvertent fungal infections | |
| | Closed IV connection systems –for example Interlink (Becton and Dickinson), Bionnector (Vygon UK Ltd.) | • Can reduce sampling port and fluid contamination<br>The prevention of catheter related sepsis is achievable by having the development of sound policies for the handling of different catheter types which will help to minimise potential problems.<br>• Protocols for care of central venous catheters should be based upon current research and catheter type<br>• Trained nursing staff should care for these lines | |

APPENDIX 7.5    Best practice guidelines to prevent infections and complications of central venous feeding lines (Diana, Princess of Wales Children's Hospital, Birmingham)

The Birmingham Children's Hospital NHS
NUTRITIONAL CARE DEPARTMENT NHS Trust
Parenteral Nutrition (PN)
Best practice Guidelines to Prevent infections and Complications of Central Venous Feeding Lines

| Designated Line Must Be Identified For PN | Line violation must be minimised | No proven septicaemia – antibiotics via other route<br>Proven septicaemia – antibiotics via PN Line |
|---|---|---|
| Handwashing | • Ayliffe hand washing technique must be used<br>✓ Using soap<br>✓ Dry hands thoroughly<br>✓ Use alcohol gel, allow to dry | |
| Aseptic Technique<br><br>Do not rush the procedure<br>Take one step at a time | • Adhere to BCH policy for setting of parenteral nutrition<br>✓ Use of a non-touch technique<br>✓ Use of sterile gloves | |
| Patient Safety | ✓ Knowledge of line placement/ position/type -should be recorded in the notes<br>✓ Check patient identity and prescription<br>✓ Check concentration of dextrose<br>✓ Label central venous PN lines<br>✓ Ensure lipid rates are less than amino acids<br>✓ Never give more than on pharmacy prescription | Amino Acid Mix        Lipid |
| Equipment | ✓ Pumps must be serviced and cleaned regularly<br>✓ Expert knowledge of pump required<br>✓ Equipment training must be undertaken regularly re infusion pumps, use of filters and closed systems | Reduction of connections ensures best practice<br>Integral intravenous sets which include closed IV system is recommended |
| Closed Intravenous Systems | ✓ To reduce hub manipulation | Reduce manipulations |
| Filters | ✓ To be used to prevent formation of endotoxins, particulate matter and air from the infusions<br>✓ Label filter to include date and time of next change | |
| Covered Line | ✓ Lines must be supported, well anchored and taped<br>✓ Connections to be covered with gauze whenever possible | |

*(Continued)*

APPENDIX 7.5    Best practice guidelines to prevent infections and complications of central venous feeding lines (Diana, Princess of Wales Children's Hospital, Birmingham)—cont'd

| Dressings | ✓ Dressings to be used to anchor and cover the lines<br>✓ Record date, time and any changes during dressing change<br>✓ ? Site problems send a swab to Microbiology<br>✓ Observe catheter site daily for signs of infection<br>✓ Clean site weekly, daily if infected | |
|---|---|---|
| Monitoring Documentation | ✓ Prescriptions details must be clear and signed by medical staff<br>✓ Monitor temperature, pulse, respirations and blood pressure<br>✓ Rate of infusion must be documented accurately/Strict fluid balance<br>✓ Blood Glucose Monitoring (BM)<br>✓ Daily Weight<br>✓ Height<br>✓ Head Circumference (Children under 2)<br>✓ Urinalysis   } Record and plot on Centile Chart | Record and Plot:<br>• Height    • Weight<br>• Head Circumference |

## Chapter 8

# Day care surgery

Tracy Morse

## INTRODUCTION

Benefits of paediatric day care surgery have been documented for many years; however, increased activity is a relatively recent development. As far back as 1909, Nicoll performed thousands of orthopaedic surgical procedures on children as day cases. He believed that avoiding overnight admission to hospital was less traumatic for the child. Despite this, the majority of children continued to be admitted the day prior to minor surgery and to remain in hospital on the night following surgery. Wider recognition of the need to reduce the time spent in hospital occurred in the 1950s, when it was suggested that children suffered long term effects due to maternal deprivation when separated from their main carer.

The Platt Report (Department of Health 1959) was also influential in reducing the time children spent in hospital, as this highlighted associated psychological effects hospitalisation might have on the child. However, it was not until much more recently that this concept has been widely accepted and adopted by health professionals. A marked increase in day case surgery has been noted following the Royal College of Surgeons Report (1992), in which they wholeheartedly recommended day case surgery.

Historically, children undergoing day care surgery were nursed within adult orientated areas, included on general surgical operating lists, and frequently were not cared for by children's trained nurses. As the dangers of this were recognised, there was pressure to ensure children were nursed on general paediatric wards and efforts were made to segregate day cases from inpatients.

As the benefits of day care surgery have been recognised, provision of specialist day surgical units has increased. This includes anaesthetic rooms, ward and recovery areas within close proximity of each other.

Day care provision is now incorporated as part of ambulatory rather than inpatient care. The needs of children using this service differ from inpatient needs, as the children are not perceived to be ill and therefore should not be nursed with ill children. This reduces potentially frightening experiences which the child may face, and reduces the risk of exposure to hospital acquired infection. Standards are needed to maintain a quality service and ensure that day cases are not seen to be in less need of resources than acute or longer term health problems.

Standards have been adopted by many day care units following Thornes' report *Just for the Day* (1991). This set 12 quality standards for paediatric day case admissions (see Box 8.1). Since this was first published, many adult orientated surgical units have realised the importance of providing separate facilities for children, and employing experienced registered children's nurses. Nurses working within this area should also be experienced in day care surgery. Changes introduced with the introduction of clinical governance aim to increase the expertise of surgeons and anaesthetists involved with children's surgery. It is now the norm to have purely paediatric day surgery operating lists led by experienced surgeons and anaesthetists.

If day care surgery is to be a positive experience for the child and family, considerable assessment and planning are required. Admission and discharge should be planned to take place on the same day as the surgical procedure as, according to Thornes (1991), this will reduce the likelihood of potentially frightening experiences. The carer can also expect that a child admitted as a day case will

---

**Box 8.1  12 quality standards for paediatric day case admissions (Audit Commission 1992)**

1. Planned admissions to include pre-admission, day of admission and post-admission care.
2. Preparation offered before and during admission day.
3. Written information to enable parents to understand their responsibilities.
4. Admission to area designated for day care.
5. Children should not be admitted or treated alongside adults.
6. Children should be cared for by identified staff designated to the day case setting.
7. All staff should be trained and skilled in working with children and families and should have expertise in day case work.
8. Work should be planned and organised, and planned specifically for day cases, to ensure that the child is likely to discharge on the same day.
9. Buildings, equipment and furniture should comply with safety standards suitable for children.
10. The environment should be homely with a play area and activities suitable for children and young people.
11. Documentation should be completed before the child is discharged.
12. Nursing support should be provided once the child is transferred home.

---

safely recover at home, with minimal postoperative observation or treatment.

Day care surgery need not be a stressful time. To avoid this, the care setting must be child friendly, comfortable, have a relaxed, secure atmosphere, and be family orientated. This will include parents' facilities, play staff and a philosophy actively supporting the concepts of partnership and parental involvement in care. Children are best supported by those that they know and love, particularly if this takes place in a familiar environment. Transfer home will therefore be encouraged as soon as the carer is able to provide suitable care for the child with the support of an outreach service.

In accordance with the Department of Health (1991) recommendation that home is the best place to care for a child, time spent in hospital is kept to a minimum. A familiar environment enhances feelings of security for the child, but also parents may be less intimidated without being overlooked by professionals. Reducing the length of stay in hospital also causes less disruption to the family's routine. Day care surgery requires a holistic approach, which considers the family's needs from the pre-admission stage and includes aftercare. Day case surgery should not happen by accident, as skilled nursing assessment and careful planning must be carried out in conjunction with the child's carer for it to be successful.

Although resources are made available to allow early discharge, some parents feel unable to provide care for their child in the early stages after anaesthesia and surgery. Adequate time and knowledge are invaluable for the carer to plan aftercare. Without this, families who are offered the opportunity to go home considerably earlier than expected may panic and can confuse this with the hospital system pushing them out too quickly. The amount of time spent in hospital does not reflect the amount of advice and support required by carers. Parents need adequate opportunity to ask questions and discuss their fears. This facilitates a more equal relationship and empowers parents to care for their child during the recovery stage. Information and professional aftercare support are needed, as without this parents may fear the unknown and feel powerless and unprepared to care for their child when back in the home setting.

To avoid inappropriate early discharge and prevent families feeling they are unable to cope, it may be necessary in certain circumstances to delay discharge.

The increase in day care surgery activity reflects major advances in surgical and anaesthetic techniques. In recent years surgery has become less invasive, therefore requiring shorter time under anaesthetic, and pain can now be adequately controlled without sedation. Nursing theory and practice has undoubtedly adapted well to these changes, promoting a fairly rapid recovery. Parental education has facilitated parents' ability to care for their child at the earliest stage possible. Transition of care from hospital to home is usually a smooth, continual process. Currently, provision of paediatric care is undergoing major changes with the aim of continuing to reduce the number of inpatient beds. It is expected that increased efficiency and shorter stays in hospital will reduce waiting lists, increase patient satisfaction and have financial savings for health providers.

## SUITABILITY FOR DAY CARE SURGERY

The decision to allow a child to be treated as a day case rests on a number of considerations, such as the suitability of the surgery and the physical fitness of the child. Consideration of psychological and psychosocial needs, including the family's ability to cope, are just as significant. The Royal College of Nursing (1996), warns of problems related to the expansion of day surgery which may be harmful for carers who are expected to undertake a primary role in psychological preparation and provision of care following surgery. Various professionals will be involved in the screening process designed to ensure day care is the most appropriate option. During the initial outpatient consultation, the surgeon recommends if the procedure is suitable to be performed as a day case, and will then refer the child for preoperative assessment.

## PRE-ASSESSMENT – PRIOR TO DAY CARE SURGERY

Appropriate patient selection is a major factor in the success of day care surgery; therefore, many areas have introduced the practice of pre-assessing children prior to admission. During this assessment the medical practitioner is able to check the child's suitability for day care surgery and detect health problems which would contraindicate an anaesthetic. This provides opportunity to:

- consider social and psychological factors
- obtain a medical history (child's and parents')
- instigate any necessary investigations/X-rays/ blood tests
- explain the procedure
- obtain consent
- physically examine the child
- complete relevant paper work.

Pre-assessment usually takes place within 2 weeks of the planned surgery and reduces the risk of inappropriate admission and also accelerates the admission process on the day of surgery. Parents and children are given opportunity to ask questions and consider implications of surgery, in a non-threatening environment, which is necessary to allow informed consent.

All key personnel should be in agreement with patient selection as recommended by the Audit Commission (1992). Various medical conditions are contraindicated for day care surgery (see Box 8.2). It

Box 8.2  Contraindicated for day care surgery (Audit Commission 1992)

- Blood disorders
- Uncontrolled asthma
- Diabetes
- Renal problems
- Cardiac problems
- Hepatic problems
- Infants less than 6 months with a problematic neonatal period (risk apnoea)
- It would be unusual for any baby under 1 year to be treated as a day case
- Previous anaesthetic problems
- Obesity
- Infants less than 5 kg weight
- Growth retardation (risk hypoglycaemia/hypothermia)

is likely that a child not meeting the necessary criteria will be admitted overnight prior to surgery, for investigation and stabilisation. Well controlled asthma is not a contraindication for day surgery. Usual medication should be continued and extra bronchiodilators may be prescribed prior to anaesthesia, as a prophylactic measure.

Conditions which would postpone day surgery include:

- acute illness within the last 2 weeks – particularly pyrexia, upper respiratory tract infection (cough, cold, wheezing, and sore throat)
- gastroenteritis
- communicable/infectious disease.

Postponing surgery avoids the increased anaesthetic risks associated with these conditions.

Children with skin or hair infestations may still be operated on, in accordance with local infection control protocols.

If the child is planning to participate in an important event, such as a sporting event, competition or holiday, it may be sensible to postpone non-urgent surgery. This will reduce the likelihood of children returning to normal activities before they have fully recovered. Adolescents who are due to take any examinations soon after surgery may also be advised to postpone non-urgent surgery, as levels of concentration may be reduced during this time.

Nursing staff will advise parents at the pre-admission stage on the procedure if the child should become ill before the admission date. Policies on this increase consistency in care and treatment. Pre-assessment frequently avoids cancellation on the day of surgery, which consequently avoids emotional distress and inconvenience for the child and family. Inappropriate admissions and cancellations also have financial implications for the healthcare providers and increase waiting times for other users of the service.

## PRE-ADMISSION SCHEMES – PRIOR TO DAY CARE SURGERY

The success of day surgery does not rely totally on the surgery itself. The role of the nursing team cannot be underestimated, as they are frequently involved with the family before admission. Various types of pre-admission schemes (parties/visits/clubs) are currently successfully provided, aimed at preparing children and families for their stay in hospital. Pre-admission schemes assist in physical and emotional preparation for surgery, improve the quality of stay and reduce the time spent in hospital. Ideally, pre-assessment and pre-admission schemes should be held on the same day to avoid several visits to hospital. As with pre-assessment, pre-admission schemes act as a screening system, preventing inappropriate or unnecessary admission to hospital.

Motivation and commitment amongst nursing and support staff are required if a scheme is to be successful, as this service is time consuming and requires extra resources. Those involved must have effective communication skills and be knowledgeable practitioners. A positive attitude from staff and provision of necessary information will increase the family's confidence about the forthcoming admission. If at this stage it is noted that the child or family is not suitable to be treated as a day case admission, alternative arrangements can be made. More frequently, potential problems are detected and can be rectified before admission.

Psychosocial difficulties highlighted can be acted upon prior to admission. Frequently, these problems include a lack of transport, support at home or telephone access, or inadequate care arrangements for other children/dependents. If discharge is likely to be prolonged because of lack of facilities, it may be appropriate to contact the hospital social worker. All options should be considered, such as travel benefits, hospital transport and mobile phone loan schemes, to reduce social inequalities.

Pre-admission schemes usually take place within the month prior to surgery. Timing of this visit is important and determined by the individual child's age, cognitive abilities and coping mechanisms. If the visit is too far in advance, the child may experience difficulties in the uncertainties involved with admission and may suffer unnecessary distress. Younger children may lose the positive memories gained if the gap is too long. However, if children visit the hospital and then are not provided with adequate time to assimilate this information at their own pace, they may find this emotionally problematic. The child may then experience difficulties in retaining self-control when faced with the need to cooperate with care and treatment.

Attendance is not normally compulsory, but certainly should be encouraged, as it is known to have many benefits to the child and family. The thought of admission then becomes less threatening, which consequently improves the quality of the stay in hospital and eases the transition of care to the child's home.

Many parents fail to recognise the benefits of pre-admission schemes for a child undergoing day care surgery, as they assume the amount of time spent in hospital relates to the amount of trauma a child will suffer. This extra visit to the hospital may then be seen as unnecessary for their child. Another frequent reason for avoiding the pre-admission visit is parents' reluctance to inform their child about the planned surgery. Some parents prefer to delay discussion, thereby giving the child less time to worry. Another explanation is that some are unsure 'how' or 'what' to tell their child. Those utilising the pre-admission service benefit from increasing knowledge of the implications of surgery and familiarising themselves with the hospital routines.

Certain information should be provided, giving the child and family a logical explanation of the stay in hospital and the aftercare. They will then have a clear idea of who will be caring for them and the support mechanisms available. Photographs make a useful introduction to staff who are unable to be present during the pre-admission visit. Children also have the opportunity to familiarise themselves with the environment and play with equipment and hospital-related toys (Fig. 8.1). Parents will be actively encouraged to be involved in their child's care while in hospital, therefore they require realistic explanations of management and care. Verbal information provided at this visit should be based on written instructions, which should also be provided to non-attendees. Information is required at least 3 weeks before the admission date. This will include clear advice on:

- preoperative preparation (home and after admission)
- continuation of normal medication – bring in drugs with them
- suitable clothing
- personal belongings required during the stay (parent and child)
- postoperative management (providing realistic expectations of activities).

Literature must be appropriate for children, adolescents and parents.

The hospital play specialist will be involved in preparing the child for what to expect before, during and after the operation. Photographs, pictures and the use of play will assist explanation and preparation. Play specialists observe children's reactions and will use their specialist skills to deal with any fear that children may display.

As the time spent in hospital on the day of surgery is kept to a minimum, this reduces the opportunity to form a trusting relationship/partnership with the child and family. Pre-admission enhances the formation of a relationship, therefore reducing anxieties on the admission day. The nurse's expertise in the planned procedure and the likely consequences for the child and family can be discussed. With this information and the knowledge of their own child, parents are able to make an informed decision concerning informing their child. Hesitant parents should be supported in their attempts to tell their child about the forthcoming surgery, as children who are denied this preparation will suffer undue distress and are very likely to be distrusting in the future.

It is helpful if adolescents are allowed the opportunity to discuss aspects of management away from parents if they wish. They often have intense fears about surgery and need reassurance and advice about their lifestyle and the implications of surgery. It is particularly essential that this group is informed of consequences of their behaviour and the need to follow guidelines, such as not smoking for at least 24 hours prior to admission. Also, as adolescents frequently require a large degree of self-control and independence, they may reject parental advice and observation on returning home. They are likely to attempt returning to normal activities before medically advised. Others may be left to fend for themselves fairly rapidly, hence they require full knowledge of likely problems and rationales for adapted behaviour

## MANAGEMENT WITHIN THE DAY CARE SURGERY SETTING

It is evident that before the child's admission substantial planning is needed to promote a positive stay in hospital. This not only includes preparing the child and family but also the environment in which they will be cared for, and preparation with administrative tasks. A bed space should be identified and labelled, to include the child's, surgeon's and named nurse's names. A bedside cupboard should be cleared and age appropriate activities prepared. It is not necessary to have a bed/trolley bed in the ward area, as the bed will not be needed until the child arrives in the theatre complex. Many families find this concept strange as they expect to arrive in hospital, be given a bed and asked to get changed into their night clothes. This is thought to be unnecessary as children are generally more relaxed in their day clothes and should remain like this for as long as possible.

All emergency equipment, suction and oxygen will be checked before admission, and tissues and vomit bowls placed within easy reach to cover any eventuality. This planning and preparation certainly contributes to a safe and comfortable hospital experience.

Admission time should be planned, allowing at least 1 hour prior to surgery. Adequate time is necessary to assess needs and carry out physical and psychological preparation. This also allows time for children to relax and familiarise themselves with the environment. Carers appreciate a swift, organised service, which they can expect within the day care setting. They benefit from involvement in care and from not being rushed during the admission process. However, excessive waiting time prior to surgery should be avoided, as this is likely to cause necessary unrest. Staggered admission times can avoid this problem.

## THE ADMISSION DAY

On arrival the child and family will be welcomed to the area and allowed time to settle and meet staff and other families whose children are also undergoing day care surgery. Ideally, the child and family will be familiar with the named nurse, who they will have met at the pre-admission visit. Certainly, one of the rewarding aspects for nurses in this area of work is the opportunity to participate in holistic care from pre-admission up to and including aftercare. Many areas operate a 12-hour shift pattern to accommodate this, allowing continuity of care throughout the child's stay in hospital.

On admission, a nursing assessment will establish the child's and carers' understanding of surgery and its implications during the recovery period. Relevant health problems or behavioural difficulties should be highlighted. Effective communication links within the multidisciplinary team prevent unnecessary repetition or omissions of information.

Time utilised well at this stage in educating and preparing the child and carers, for example through role play, will enhance confidence and competence during the postoperative stage. Figure 8.1 shows a child acting out the role of a theatre nurse before surgery.

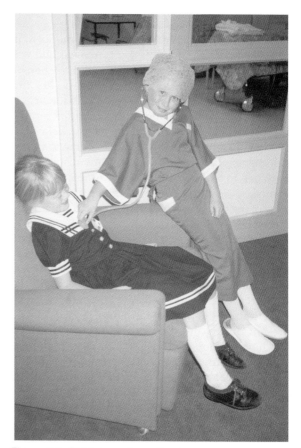

**Figure 8.1** Child dressed as a theatre nurse.

The level of physical, psychological and social preparation should be confirmed and it should not be assumed that instructions have been followed correctly. Various factors influence the ability or inclination of carers to carry out recommended preparation. It will be helpful to establish, at an early stage, the degree of parental involvement that can be expected. Carers should be encouraged to remain with their child throughout the stay and to participate as much as they are able. This not only provides opportunity for nursing staff to assess the carers' confidence and competence to care for the child at home, but also allows optimum use of time for education and demonstration. Children also benefit from experiencing parental care initially in a supportive, safe environment and are less likely to react negatively on returning home. Care will be planned and documented. Interventions should be recorded on a preoperative/preprocedure care plan (see Fig. 8.2) as this assists in checking that the child has been physically prepared for theatre.

## GENERAL HEALTH

The child's medical history, which has been taken during the pre-assessment stage, should be confirmed and any recent health problems identified.

Allergies should be recorded, and should include actual and suspected reactions to:

- Medications
- Plasters
- Latex
- Metal
- Food and drink (particularly egg – relevant to certain anaesthetic agents)
- House dust mite
- Pollens/grasses.

It is normal practice for the child to be seen by the surgeon on the day of surgery to discuss last minute concerns the child or parent may have. Occasionally it is decided that the operation is no longer required.

## NIL BY MOUTH

Confirmation that starving instructions have been followed is essential. Hitchcock and Ogg (1993) recommend children undergoing planned general anaesthesia should not eat for 6 hours prior to surgery but should have a final clear drink (150 mL) up to 3 hours before the planned surgery time. More recently, however, it is becoming increasingly common for clear fluids to be allowed up to 2 hours before surgery. A dextrose solution will be suitable for babies and young children, who are particularly prone to problems associated with prolonged starvation times such as hypoglycaemia and undetected metabolic disorders. Children who have been excessively starved will suffer unnecessary discomfort in feeling hungry and thirsty. They are also more likely to feel faint preoperatively, or nauseous postoperatively. Daborn et al (1994) suggest that this is particularly apparent with children having surgery in the afternoon who, despite receiving instructions, have not eaten since the previous day.

Eating or drinking after the recommended time is as common as prolonged starvation. Parents may not appreciate that sweets, snacks or milky drinks count as food and therefore may have allowed their child something to eat or drink. Also, some children have helped themselves, without their parents' knowledge. This situation is potentially hazardous as regurgitation of gastric contents and pulmonary aspiration may occur during induction of anaesthesia. Once starvation times have been established, a reminder to refrain from eating or drinking is necessary. Parents are often surprised how well infants and younger children adapt to this, as they expect this to be a challenging time. Incorrect starvation times may delay surgery and consequently delay discharge home. Education during the pre-admission stage greatly reduces the likelihood of this occurring.

## BASELINE OBSERVATIONS

Observations of temperature, pulse, blood pressure and respiratory rate will act as a screening mechanism, detecting abnormalities, and will provide comparison postoperatively. Urinalysis will be particularly useful to detect urinary infections for children undergoing urological surgery. If these are left untreated, postoperative infection may be problematic. Although it is unusual for children to display abnormalities of clinical observations at this stage, occasionally surgery is delayed to allow investigation or treatment.

Accurate measurement of weight will be necessary to calculate dose of anaesthetic agents and analgesia, and may identify growth abnormalities. Obesity is relatively uncommon in childhood but must be

Pre Operative / Pre-Procedure Care Plan

Name                                          Hospital

Date of Birth                                 Ward /Team

Address                                       Named Nurse

Hospital Number                               Speciality

*Problem*---------------------------------------------------------------------------------------------------------------

*Goal* ------------------------------------------------------------------------------------------------------------------

| | Checklist (interventions) | YES | NO | N/A |
|---|---|---|---|---|
| 1 | **Nil by Mouth from;** | | | |
| 2 | **Baseline observations**<br>**Pulse        Temp      Resp        BP** | | | |
| 3 | **Urinalysis recorded?**<br>**Abnormalities;** | | | |
| 4 | **Bath/Shower offered where appropriate?** | | | |
| 5 | **Wearing suitable clothing?** | | | |
| 6 | **Local anaesthetic cream applied?** | | | |
| 7 | **Local anaesthetic cream removed?** | | | |
| 8 | **Pre-medication prescribed?** | | | |
| 9 | **Pre-medication given?** | | | |
| 10 | **Identity band(s) in situ?** | | | |
| 11 | **Jewellery/Braces/Make up/Contact lens/Nail varnish removed?** | | | |
| 12 | **Potential hazards identified?**<br>**Loose teeth/hearing aids/ glasses** | | | |
| 13 | **Correct site marked by surgeon where relevant ?** | | | |
| 14 | **Allergies recorded?** | | | |
| 15 | **Blood/investigation results available?** | | | |
| 16 | **X-rays/ Photographs present?** | | | |
| 17 | **Notes present?** | | | |
| 18 | **Signed consent obtained?** | | | |
| 19 | **Individual needs relating to speciality?** | | | |
| 20 | **Pain assessment carried out?** | | | |
| 21 | **Patient identity checked?** | | | |

*Signature of Nurse responsible for final check;*---------------------------------------------

**Figure 8.2** Preoperative care plan.

identified, if it was not detected at the pre-assessment stage. Obesity may complicate induction of anaesthesia and therefore the child may not be suitable to be treated as a day case.

## HYGIENE

Hygiene needs should be assessed and a bath or shower made available for those children who have not carried this out before admission. Children having surgery to their feet should be encouraged to keep socks on until arriving in theatre to avoid getting their feet dirty. A last minute check prior to leaving for theatre will ensure hands are free from paint, glue and ink gained while playing before theatre. This will prevent foreign substances being introduced into the body during intravenous cannulation.

## TOPICAL SKIN ANAESTHETICS

As the preferred choice of induction of anaesthesia usually involves venepuncture, the application of a local anaesthetic cream will, in most cases, be advantageous. Ametop and EMLA cream are both in common use. An experienced practitioner should supervise application to prevent poor positioning. The non-dominant hand is the usual choice; if not, another visible vein may be used such as the anticubical fossa or foot. An occlusive dressing will be used to cover the cream after application. Use of a bandage over the dressing may also be beneficial in children who are at particular risk of breaking/removing the dressing and ingesting local anaesthetic.

Instructions for application must be strictly adhered to. Without adequate application the cream will be ineffective, giving the child a false sense of security. If it is left on in excess of the recommended times, vasoconstriction and severe skin irritations can occur. This will not only prevent desired sites from being utilised but will also cause the child discomfort or pain. Although the success of these creams is widely recognised, the child should not be promised that they will not experience pain. The perception of pain varies from individual to individual, and children frequently find that the restraint involved in undergoing intravenous access causes discomfort, even though the skin puncture itself may not. Sometimes it would appear that the cream has little effect in reducing pain, particularly when this is compounded by a large degree of anxiety.

## CLOTHING

Clothing worn during surgery should be clean, comfortable, non-threatening to the child and not compromise safety during anaesthesia. Increasingly, children are able to wear their own nightwear. This should be loose and made of cotton, to allow easy access and avoid static electricity. Front fastenings are ideal. A hospital theatre gown will be provided if the child's night clothes are unsuitable, particularly with infants to allow easy access to limbs and chest. Parents require clear instructions at the pre-assessment stage to avoid unnecessarily buying night clothes which may never be used again.

Bras, vests and crop tops should not be worn under nightclothes, although it is unnecessary for children to remove their pants. This is something children frequently fear as they find this embarrassing and intrusive. Pants can be removed once the child is asleep if the procedures necessitate this. Where possible, pants should be put back on before the child wakes up to reduce feelings of intrusion.

Some units have adopted the policy of allowing normal daytime clothing to be worn for minor procedures. If this is permitted, parents should be advised on suitable clothing and be aware of the need to bring a change of clothing in case of accidents or spillage. Needs of excretion should be met. For children still in nappies a clean nappy should be applied, and other children should be encouraged to urinate. All jewellery should be removed. If body piercing prevents this, jewellery should be securely covered with tape and theatre staff informed. Where possible hair should be tied back away from the face using non-metallic fabrics. Positioning of hair ties should occur in the area at the back of the neck. If positioned higher than this, pressure will be exerted on the head and the child's consciousness level may be compromised.

## PATIENT IDENTIFICATION

An identity band will be checked with the carer, child (if appropriate) and hospital records, and secured around the child's wrist or ankle in accordance with the hospital's policy. This must be carried out soon after admission; without correct identification the child's safety is compromised. The correct site for surgery should be marked by the surgeon where appropriate. Each hospital should have a policy for correct site marking.

## PREMEDICATION

It is unusual for a child to be prescribed a sedative premedication, although the nurse should assess each child and highlight children who may benefit from this preparation. Although premedication may reduce the child's fear occasionally, its only effect is to agitate the child preoperatively and induce deep sleep postoperatively. This in turn increases the period of hospitalisation. The decision to use a premedication should be made in partnership with the parents and child when appropriate.

Eye drops may be prescribed to dilate pupils before eye surgery. The prescription details should be followed strictly as the timing of giving these drops is important and they are usually given frequently over a short period of time. Bowel preparation is infrequently prescribed, but if it is required parents will administer the prescribed medication before admission to carry out this task.

## PAIN ASSESSMENT

A nursing assessment will be carried out to establish the child's experience of pain, expectations of the procedure and coping mechanisms the child is familiar with. Pain assessment tools may be used, although verbal advice is particularly useful, as time is limited for children to familiarise themselves with pain tools. As care within the day setting will be consistent and provided by a small team of people, assessment of pain will be carried out in partnership with the team, the child and the carer.

A preoperative visit and assessment from the anaesthetist will ensure the child and family have adequate understanding of pain management. This will also confirm that parents are prepared for their role in the anaesthetic room, and how their child may react when being anaesthetised.

## ANAESTHESIA

This is the part most parents dread and therefore if they are able to meet staff who will be responsible for the child in their absence they will find this immensely beneficial. Preoperative visits from anaesthetic and recovery nurses will assist in the preparation of the child and carer for the theatre experience. A visit to the anaesthetic and recovery areas should be offered if the child has not previously had this opportunity. After much work from professionals and pressure groups, it is now fairly accepted practice that a parent is permitted to accompany the child to the anaesthetic room. Separation from the parent should be avoided, particularly in the younger age group. It should be remembered that some parents feel unable to provide support for their child at this stage as they feel their own anxiety may be transferred to the child.

Occasionally carers will decline the invitation into the anaesthetic room, as they believe their child will be more cooperative without them.

To avoid parents feeling they are expected to remain with their child and to avoid last minute decision making, opinions should be discussed soon after admission. The child and carer will need prior explanation of what to expect when they get into this room. This reduces fears and allows events to proceed smoothly. Effective communication links between the ward and theatre areas will avoid the child experiencing long delays in the anaesthetic room. A suitable method of transportation will be arranged. This is likely to be a push along or battery operated car for younger children, or they may be carried in their parent's arms or go by foot. The younger age group usually look forward to a ride in the car (see Fig. 8.3). Ideally the anaesthetic room and theatre complex will be conveniently situated near the ward area. The anaesthetic room should be child friendly with age appropriate distractions

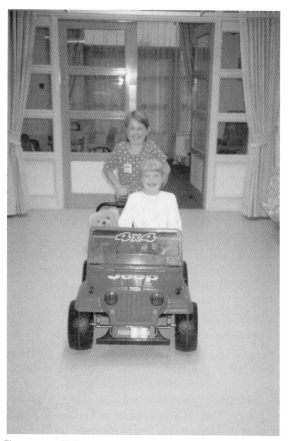

**Figure 8.3** Riding to the anaesthetic room.

such as toys, mobiles, music and room for the child's favourite comforter.

The child and carer will be met by a member of theatre staff who is known to them. Staff should be waiting to start, to avoid there being time for the child suddenly to panic in an unfamiliar place or to become bored. A team approach is needed, working together with the aim of safely anaesthetising the child in a way that is non-threatening for the child and carer. Many parents report that although they received good information prior to this stage, they had not imagined the degree of fear and helplessness actually experienced. Support for parents is necessary during induction and once they leave the theatre area. Parents should be encouraged to go and have something to eat and drink and get some fresh air, as it is likely they will have followed the same nil by mouth instructions as their child. An accurate estimation of when they will see their child again will be given. This allows parents to benefit from a break, and ensures that they are available for when their child asks for them. If the child is delayed for any reason, parents should be informed of this to avoid unnecessary worry.

## PROCEDURES COMMONLY PERFORMED AS DAY SURGERY

Types of procedures performed as day surgery continue to increase as advances in surgical technique continue to develop. The Royal College of Surgeons (1992) suggested that a day case procedure should last for approximately 30 minutes and not exceed 60 minutes duration. For this reason it is inadvisable for inexperienced anaesthetists or surgeons to carry out this work, as the procedure is then likely to exceed this recommended time. Since the Royal College of Surgeons (1992) recommendations (see Box 8.3) specifying procedures/operations suitable for day surgery, many more cases are successfully carried out.

A degree of postoperative care is universal, although specific advice is necessary according to the procedure carried out and the individual child's and family's needs and abilities.

## CIRCUMCISION

Circumcision is the surgical procedure used to excise the prepuce (penile foreskin) of the glans penis. It may be required as treatment for phimosis, paraphimosis, balanitis or injury, or for religious reasons.

---

**Box 8.3 Surgical cases suitable as day cases (Royal College of Surgeons 1992)**

**Dental surgery**

- Extractions
- Excision/biopsy of lesions and cysts
- Division of tongue tie

**Ear, nose and throat (ENT) surgery**

- Examination under anaesthetic of ears/ postnasal space
- Removal of foreign bodies
- Myringotomies
- Grommets
- Reduction of fractured nose
- Submucosal diathermy
- Electrocautery of epistaxsis
- Antrum washouts

**Ophthalmic surgery**

- EUA
- Correction of strabismus

**General surgery**

- Hernia repair – epigastric, umbilical, femoral, inguinal
- Hydrocele/varicocele – repair or ligation
- Circumcision
- Separation of preputial adhesions
- Minor hypospadias
- Cystoscopy
- Anal stretch
- Proctoscopy
- Sigmoidoscopy
- Excision of skin lesions
- Lymph node biopsy

**Orthopaedic surgery**

- Change of plaster
- Manipulations
- Release of trigger thumb
- Excision of ganglion
- Arthoscopy

## Complications

Reactionary and secondary haemorrhage and infection are not uncommon following this procedure.

Venous or arterial blood loss can be significant in young infants who may lose a considerable amount of the circulatory volume.

Initially, inability to pass urine may also be problematic. Occasionally, this is a side effect of the local anaesthetic block, used intraoperatively for pain relief. More frequently, problems are due to the child's fear of pain when urinating, or dislike of the appearance of the wound.

Haematoma formation can also lead to infection and consequently to secondary haemorrhage.

Local infection of the wound site may be detected within the first 2 or 3 days following surgery.

### Implications for practice

Frequent observation of the wound for signs of bleeding will be required. Parents should be advised to check the wound regularly during the first 24 hours postoperatively. Adolescents may find it embarrassing having these frequent checks and may wish to check their own wound site. If this is permitted at home, signs of infection should be clearly described. These include bleeding, discharge, pyrexia and increasing pain on urination.

Unless advised by the surgeon, dressings should be removed before discharge, as particular problems have been found in removing the dressing on the following day. At this point the dressing will adhere to the wound with dried exudate, and granulation of the wound will have already started to take place.

Clothing should be loose and comfortable. Cotton fabrics improve ventilation. Some boys prefer not to wear clothing on their lower half for the first few days, as they fear clothing touching the wound. Advice is needed that unclean hands and particles of food should be kept away from the wound.

A warm bath or shower twice a day will be comforting, cleansing and assist wound healing. Bubble baths or perfumed soaps can be irritating and should be avoided.

Strict hygiene is needed to keep the area clean. Baby cleansing products should not be used until complete healing has occurred. Nappies can be worn but must be changed regularly. Frequent observation of the wound is needed to avoid undetected bleeding into the nappy. For this reason a nappy with the minimum of absorbency is preferable. This also allows closer observation of urinary output.

Sutures are usually dissolvable; however, the child should be seen by the practice nurse 7 days following surgery to check the wound site. If the outcome of this visit is satisfactory the child may then return to playgroup or school. Strenuous activities such as games and sports should be avoided for up to 2 weeks following surgery. This includes cycling, climbing etc, which have added risks of trauma. Swimming is allowed once the wound is completely healed.

## ORAL SURGERY AND DENTAL EXTRACTIONS

Oral extraction or surgical excision may be needed to remove decayed or impacted teeth or as preparation for corrective orthodontic work to improve aliment and cosmetic effect.

Frenectomy is also commonly performed, in which the frenulum is excised. This fold of mucous membrane is situated under the tongue or between the lips and gums. If a problem with the frenulum is left untreated the child may develop speech defects and can experience difficulty with eating and drinking normally.

### Complications following surgery

Varying degrees of swelling, bleeding, discomfort and difficulty opening the mouth are likely following oral surgery. These problems should improve within 2–3 days.

Occasionally, infection and secondary bleeding can occur within the first 10 days following surgery.

### Implications for practice

During the first 6–10 hours following surgery, excessive saliva is produced which, when mixed with traces of blood, can be distressing for the child and cause nausea. The child and parent will need reassurance that this is normal. They also require insight into the appearance of fresh and stale blood and at what point they should seek further advice.

If bleeding occurs before discharge, a bite pad should be inserted into the mouth and held in position for at least 10–15 minutes. The child must at no point be left unattended with this in position as it can compromise the airway. Adequate pressure initially frequently prevents recurrent episodes of bleeding. Gloves should be worn in accordance with universal precautions.

If bleeding continues, gentle suctioning around the operation site prior to inserting a fresh bite pad can be tried. The pad should be soaked with sterile water before insertion, to ease removal and reduce the risk of further bleeding.

If bleeding occurs following discharge, the child should sit in a supported, upright position and bite onto gauze or a clean cotton handkerchief for 10–15 minutes. If this is not effective and bleeding recurs, parents should seek medical advice immediately.

Maintaining adequate hydration and nutrition can be problematic during the initial postoperative period due to pain, discomfort and unpleasant tastes.

Regular analgesia to control pain will be necessary following most procedures. Without this, the child is likely to be reluctant to talk, eat or drink.

Sutures and packs cause discomfort, and time is needed for the child to adapt to this. The lips should be kept clean and moistened with petroleum jelly or lip salve, giving particular attention to the outer aspects, which may be traumatised from stretching during surgery.

As the taste of dried blood can be off-putting and may prevent children regaining their appetite, tempting foods should be offered.

During the first 24 hours hot and sharp foods (e.g. toast, crisps) and drinks should be avoided. Suggestions of nourishing oral fluids and soft food should be given, as initially some children find eating very difficult. Drinking clear water regularly will remove traces of sugary drinks or food and assist wound healing.

Strict oral hygiene is necessary to assist wound healing, although mouth washing of any kind must be avoided for the first 24 hours postoperatively, to reduce the risk of interfering with clot formation and inducing haemorrhage.

After the first 24 hours a medicated mouthwash may be prescribed to reduce the risk of infection. Mouthwashes can be made successfully using a small amount of table salt or bicarbonate of soda in a cup of warm water.

Alternative advice should also be offered as many children find mouth washing impossible or refuse to participate in the routine. Brushing of teeth can be recommended after 24 hours, avoiding the operation site for 3 days.

Follow-up with the oral surgeon will be required within 1–2 weeks. Frequently, there will be sutures and packs to remove at this point.

All children require at least 1 day resting at home following a general anaesthetic and before attempting to return to school and normal activities. It is likely that a further 48 hours will be required to allow the swelling to settle and the child to be eating and drinking normally.

Oral surgery is particularly common during adolescence. This group is particularly conscious of the cosmetic effects of surgery and adolescents frequently prefer to remain at home for up to a week, by which time the swelling and bruising have resolved.

## MYRINGOTOMY, INSERTION OF VENTILATION TUBES AND EXAMINATION OF EXTERNAL AUDITORY CANAL UNDER ANAESTHESIA

Examination of the external ear is frequently required to remove foreign bodies and excessive impacted wax, which causes hearing loss, pain and infection. Non-invasive procedures that have not required a surgical incision will be relatively free from complications and are unlikely to require analgesia or a change of normal routine.

Myringotomy is a small surgical incision made in the tympanic membrane, allowing drainage of fluid or glue from the middle ear in cases of recurrent otitis media or glue ear. In childhood this is frequently carried out for children with hearing difficulties. Although some surgeons now favour conservative treatment such as antibiotics and use of hearing aids until the condition resolves itself, this procedure is still one of the most common surgical procedures carried out on children between the ages of 2 years and 10 years.

A small plastic tube may be inserted into the incision, allowing longer-term ventilation of the middle ear, to prevent pressure and fluid/glue accumulation. Several types are available, i.e. collar button tubes, grommets and 'T' tubes. Levels of hearing will be assessed preoperatively, to confirm the need to operate and to act as a comparison postoperatively.

### Complications

Discomfort is commonly experienced following these procedures, often associated with the pressure changes that occur within the middle ear following fluid drainage.

Infection may also occur, particularly within the first 7 days following surgery.

Parents should be warned that ventilation tubes are intended to stay in situ for a limited period of time (approximately 6–18 months). This avoids unnecessary distress if the parent finds they have fallen out earlier than expected.

Hearing improvement may be instantaneous, which can result in a miserable child who dislikes the sudden exposure to increased sound levels.

## Management/implications for nursing practice

Analgesia may be necessary for the first few hours after surgery but is rarely required after this. A small amount of bleeding from the ear is expected for the first 12–24 hours and a slight discharge for up to a week. Parents should be advised to seek advice if the child experiences increasing pain, unpleasant discharge or pyrexia, which may indicate infection.

The inside of the ear canal should not be cleaned or poked. Blood or other discharge on the external ear can be gently cleaned using a clean cloth and plain water. To assist the healing process and reduce the risk of infection the external canal should be kept dry. Various options are available to suit the individual children and their normal routines. When bathing, showering, washing hair or playing with water, cotton wool with a small amount of petroleum jelly placed in the outer ear canal will be effective to keep drops of water out of the ear. Earplugs or moulds may routinely be provided by the hospital; however, sports shops, chemists and hearing appliance shops will also be able to advise.

Most children will be ready to return to nursery or school after 24 hours. Swimming should be avoided for at least 2–6 weeks. During this time children should wear ear plugs and a close fitting cap and must not jump or dive into the water or completely immerse their heads under water.

## TONSILLECTOMY/ADENOIDECTOMY

This involves surgical removal of tonsils and adenoids which are situated on each side of the back of mouth and oropharynx. Although some children require both tonsils and adenoids to be removed, many will only require removal of either tonsils or adenoids. In health these vascular pads of lymphoid tissue protect the body from invading organisms. Many children, however, suffer with repeated infection, halitosis and difficulty swallowing and breathing. Frequently they suffer with repeated illness and absence from school.

It is increasingly common to carry out these procedures as day cases, despite known complications of reactionary haemorrhage. Surgery should be postponed if there is a history of recent infection as this increases the risk of haemorrhage.

## Complications

Haemorrhage within the first 4 hours is a major risk and can be life threatening if not detected and managed effectively.

Infection within the first 7–14 days following surgery may cause secondary haemorrhage.

Pain is recognised as a major complication that can hinder recovery.

## Management/implications for nursing practice

Initially nursing in a semi-prone position allows drainage of blood and secretions from the mouth and nose. Observations of pulse, respirations and temperature should be recorded regularly to detect abnormalities. General signs of restlessness and excessive swallowing may indicate bleeding. Concerns must be reported to medical staff without delay and the child closely observed. Every effort should be made to ensure the environment enhances rest and the child is comfortable and free from distress. Vomiting of blood can be alarming and unpleasant for the parent and child, so considerable reassurance is needed. Observation of vomit will include noting type (fresh/stale blood), quantity and frequency. Antiemetics are not advisable as these mask signs of bleeding. If bleeding continues, gargles may be prescribed to clean the tonsillar bed. Blood will also be grouped and cross-matched. Intravenous fluids will be given and the child will be given nil by mouth in preparation for a return to theatre if required.

It has become increasingly common to hydrate children undergoing this surgery with intravenous fluids, until they recommence oral fluids. Regular analgesia is paramount to assist a quick recovery and should be given approximately 20 minutes prior to meal times.

Introduction of a normal diet and effective oral hygiene can reduce the risks of infection. Snacks in between meals can also prevent the child having long gaps between eating, which can be very painful. Fluids must be encouraged regularly.

It is necessary to avoid smoky, crowded places and people with known infections for the first 14 days postoperatively. For this reason most children will require this length of time before returning to school and their normal activities.

## REALIGNMENT OF NASAL FRACTURE

This procedure involves manipulation and mobilisation of the nasal bones, frequently resulting from accidental and non-accidental trauma to the nose. The procedure may be required to ease breathing difficulties following a direct blow to the nose, or for cosmetic reasons.

## Complications

- Further trauma to unstable cartilage
- Bruising
- Pain
- Internal nasal swelling causing breathing discomfort
- Bleeding.

## Management/implications for nursing practice

A splint may be applied in theatre to be worn for 1 week. If this is not the case, advise the child to avoid school and sport.

Regular analgesia and rest will relieve discomfort.

Nose blowing and sniffing should be avoided for 2–3 days postoperatively to reduce the risk of bleeding.

## HERNIA REPAIRS, ORCHIDECTOMY AND ORCHIDOPEXY

A hernia is a protrusion of an organ or part of an organ through an opening in the cavity in which it is normally contained. This may be congenital or acquired. Different types include inguinal, umbilical, incisional and femoral. Both males and females may have hernias that require surgical repair to avoid strangulation, pain and disfigurement. Orchidopexy is mobilising an undescended testicle from the groin and fixing it in to the scrotum. This is usually carried out as a preventative measure after routine examination finds the testis has not fully migrated to the scrotum. This migration is required as without it the risk of infertility in later life will be increased and a mobile testicle is liable to become twisted. Orchidopexy and fixation will be required following acute torsion of the testes, because if left untreated the testicle can rapidly become gangrenous.

## Complications

These procedures are known to be particularly painful and are associated with complications of nausea and vomiting postoperatively.

Wound infections and bleeding are very rare.

## Implications for nursing practice

The child should be encouraged to rest and suitable amusements provided to encourage this. Loose, comfortable clothing will reduce rubbing or pressure on the wound. Nappies can be used as normal but if they are done up slightly loosely this will increase comfort and allow observation of the wound without unnecessary disturbance.

Dressings are not used in the scrotal area. Other wounds usually have some type of protective dressing. If a small pressure dressing has been used, this will be held in place with a clear waterproof dressing. In this case, and for children without dressings, they may bath as normal, although perfumed soaps or bathing products should not be added to the water.

If a collection of blood is noted under the dressing prior to discharge, the surgeon should be informed and pressure applied with a sterile dressing until this settles. If it occurs at home, the parents should seek advice to assist wound healing. Fluid should not be allowed to collect under the waterproof dressing.

If a dry dressing is used this should be kept dry for 4–7 days.

The family will be advised if sutures are dissolvable or require removal. All children should be seen 7 days postoperatively, when sutures would be removed if this is required.

Signs of infection such as redness around the wound, undue pain or swelling should be reported immediately.

Once children are walking normally, wearing clothes comfortably and the wound has healed, they may return to school and recommence gentle swimming. All other sports and strenuous activities must be avoided for at least 2–4 weeks following surgery. It is particularly important that younger children avoid riding on toys and all children should avoid cycling for the period following orchidopexy. During this period the testicles are particularly liable to migrate from the scrotum.

## ANAL STRETCH

Performed on children with long term constipation or small tears to the anal sphincter, this procedure allows inspection and may relieve painful episodes caused by these problems.

## Complications

Increased reluctance to have bowels open is rare as this procedure usually assists this process; however, immediate relief is not guaranteed.

## Management/implications for nursing practice

Extra oral fluids and a high fibre diet should be encouraged. Those children taking prescribed medication to soften stools will continue with this.

Analgesia may be required for the first 24 hours.

## CYSTOSCOPY

This procedure involves telescopic examination of the bladder in which the bladder is distended with sterile water. This is a diagnostic and therapeutic procedure for children with urinary incontinence or repeated urinary tract infections.

## Complications

Localised discomfort, which may be increased on voiding urine, is a problem.

Haematuria following trauma from instrumentation and introduction of air into the bladder can be a complication.

## Management/implications for nursing practice

Drinking plenty will dilute the urine and reduce discomfort, allowing the child to pass urine frequently. The first few times the child passes urine are likely to be uncomfortable. Regular analgesia may be given for the first 24 hours.

Urine should be observed to ensure bleeding is reducing. A slightly blood-stained urine is expected for the first 24–48 hours. Excessive bleeding can cause clotting and urinary retention.

## RECOVERY

Most parents and children are keen to be reunited as soon as possible following surgery. Parents should be welcomed into the recovery area and be encouraged to participate in care as soon as the child is safely awake (see Fig. 8.4). Time spent in this room is usually minimal, as recovery from anaesthesia is generally rapid. Parents should be warned the child might initially be unsettled. In younger children this usually relates to their inability to comprehend the events, their separation from carers and the unfamiliar environment. Older children can be tearful as the anxieties they had prior to surgery are released. This is particularly noted with all age groups if the induction was traumatic or long. Thirst, hunger and pressure or restrictions from equipment are other causes of discomfort, though pain from surgery is usually well controlled.

Oxygen is administered until the child is awake and pulse, oxygen saturation levels and blood pressure are monitored. Maintenance of airway will be a priority at all times. Removal of cannula, electrocardiography (ECG) stickers and medical devices should occur as soon as it is safe, to avoid unnecessary disturbance for the child. The nurse's skills of

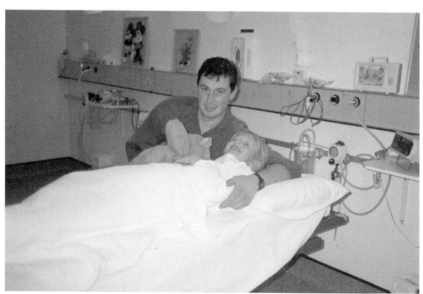

Figure 8.4 Reunited in the recovery room.

visual observation and assessment of condition will be paramount until discharge.

Children will be reunited with their carers as soon as possible. Transfer to the ward will be arranged as soon as they are safely awake. This takes place on the trolley bed or in a parent's arms if appropriate. The child will be continually monitored, although frequency of clinical observations such as pulse and respirations will depend on the child's condition.

## SLEEP

A child's reaction to the anaesthetic is variable. Most children are sleepy as they return from the recovery area. Parents will be given a brief overview of the procedure and reminded of the postoperative care. If the child is to have achieved expected goals before discharge, a lengthy sleep should be avoided. Parents frequently report an unsettled first night if the child has slept for too long during the day. Rest, however, is needed; this allows the body to recuperate and lowers the risk of haemorrhage. Studies have shown that increased periods of sleep reduce incidence of postoperative vomiting. However, if the child is allowed to sleep for too long discharge home will be delayed.

Another advantage of returning the child home as soon as possible after surgery is to allow a comfortable transfer home while still benefitting from intra-operative analgesia.

## PAIN MANAGEMENT

Pre- and postoperative pain assessment will assist the parent in deciding if the child is in pain, or is unsettled for another reason. Parents require advice on how to cuddle or move their child and on what clothing is required, as they are likely to fear hurting their child. Pain assessment also provides an opportunity to facilitate the parents' ability to carry out an adequate analgesia regimen at home. Various methods of analgesia are available to suit the child's needs and preference. Oral analgesia is usually very effective. Paracetamol suspension and ibuprofen syrup are both effective for minor surgical procedures and are familiar to parents, which eases administration. Careful consideration of the method of administration and gaining informed consent is necessary, particularly if rectal analgesia

is prescribed. Many children are fearful of this type of administration and consequently are reluctant to complain of pain or accept analgesia. Frequently parents are opposed to using rectal analgesia after discharge, as they see it as too invasive and fear they may harm their child during administration.

A combination of drugs such as voltarol and paracetamol may be prescribed for more invasive surgery which is associated with increased postoperative pain. Following oral surgery, a combination may also be prescribed, such as co-codamol with its anti-inflammatory properties.

Analgesia should be available for all procedures as even the less invasive procedures cause unnecessary discomfort for the child. Children suffering discomfort are less likely to eat, sleep and mobilise, and recovery will be delayed.

Local anaesthetic gels are useful after circumcision to apply before the child passes urine or during an acute painful episode.

Some children will be given a local anaesthetic injection, particularly those having hernia repairs, circumcision, orchidopexy and oral surgery. These will be administered while the child is asleep, either pre- or intra-operatively. Local anaesthetic abdominal and groin blocks can cause difficulty in standing and walking postoperatively. Someone should accompany the child in any walking for at least 8 hours postoperatively. As this wears off the child may complain of a feeling of pins and needles. Oral analgesia should be introduced prior to this.

Caudal epidurals are commonly used for orchidopexy and inguinal hernia repairs. Temporary urinary retention may be expected.

Prescriptions for analgesia required for discharge should be arranged promptly, avoiding unnecessary waiting when the child is ready to go home.

## EATING AND DRINKING

Fluids should be introduced with care, ensuring the child is fully awake and able to swallow. In most cases sips of water can be safely introduced within half an hour of waking. If the child is alert and has regained the swallowing reflex earlier, this time may be reduced. Gradually, normal fluids may be introduced as tolerated. Infants are likely to be particularly hungry on awaking and will quickly settle after having a feed. Once the child is tolerating fluids, oral analgesia may be administered as prescribed.

A light diet will then be offered; toast, biscuits and plain crisps are favourites. These sharp foods should be avoided, however, if oral surgery has taken place. Parents will benefit from particular advice on what to eat at home.

## DISCHARGE PLANNING

Planning and organisation enhance the day surgery experience, because at the end of the stay if the family are kept waiting for something, such as a discharge letter, this can cause unnecessary distress for the child and parent. Discharge planning should be initiated at the pre-admission stage in consultation with carers. This will assist the family to plan care and arrange changes to normal activities. Hogg (1994) identifies that attention to detail with discharge planning is paramount, if a quality day care service is to be provided.

Although verbal discharge information is preferable, written information is needed to act as a resource once the family returns home. These instructions cannot cover every eventuality, therefore an outreach service must be offered, providing 24 hour advice from a registered children's nurse. The community paediatric team should be informed of the child's discharge. This service should be promoted in a positive manner, as parents are more likely to seek support if they feel comfortable doing this. They require accessible information and reassurance from a confident, knowledgeable practitioner.

Time spent in hospital will be kept to a minimum, which limits the time parents have to digest information. Concerns for their child's wellbeing during the admission also reduces their ability to comprehend instructions. All information must be clear and should be repeated at appropriate times.

Where possible, parents should be seen by the medical practitioner before the child's discharge to discuss the outcome of the surgery. In many cases, this consultation avoids the need to attend an outpatients clinic.

Before discharge the child should be comfortable, alert, mobile, tolerating small amounts of food and drink and have passed urine. Observations must be assessed as within normal limits. If a wound site is involved, this should be checked to ensure there is no bleeding and that any stitches or dressings are intact.

Teaching and sharing information are time-consuming, but are a vital part of the nurse's role in the day care surgery setting (see Fig. 8.5). Parents are expected to comprehend a considerable amount of information, in a relatively short period of time. Where possible, children should be involved in the discussion concerning postoperative advice. This is necessary, as they may not necessarily remain with the carer who accompanied them into hospital. Armed with this information, they can also take more responsibility for their own recovery.

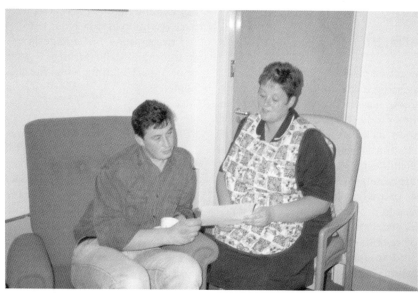

Figure 8.5 Sharing information with a parent.

Driving, riding bicycles, riding horses and operating machinery are not allowed for at least the first 24 hours following a general anaesthetic. Adolescents should be advised to avoid medication that has not been recommended by a pharmacist or medical practitioner, and should be warned to avoid recreational drugs or alcohol within the first 24 hours.

A responsible adult must accompany the child home and be available for at least the first 24 hours. Public transport is not a suitable form of transport home. The journey home should be direct, comfortable and free from interruptions or delays. It is advisable to prepare the vehicle with a pillow, blanket and vomit bowl and tissues. The driver should be prepared to drive slowly and to stop if the child is nauseous. Ideally, another adult will accompany them home to reduce distractions for the driver. Seat belts should not be positioned directly over any operation site.

## ADVICE FOR AFTER DISCHARGE

It is normal practice for a registered children's nurse to telephone the family on the day following surgery, offering advice and reassurance, and generally checking on the child's progress. If possible, this should be someone known to the family. Parents usually appreciate this contact and may ask questions that they would otherwise have felt were trivial and would not have asked in hospital. Details of this call should be recorded in the patient's notes, which will be available for reference. Concerns highlighted during this call must be acted upon, and the nurse should seek further advice from medical staff within the hospital or from the GP or practice nurse. Further telephone links with the family will continue as required. Children's community nurses may be involved after discharge and in some areas they routinely visit children on the first postoperative day. Some parents do not welcome this as they see a visit as time-consuming and an unnecessary invasion of privacy.

## CONCLUSION

The British Paediatric Association's consultation document (1996) predicted a great increase in secondary care outside hospital departments; reduction in overnight admissions was a priority. Children's day care surgery services continue to develop this where possible. However, in some cases the trend for earlier discharge is unsafe or impracticable. This is being addressed within some units where there are plans to introduce 'hotel type' accommodation. This will allow those children prevented from being treated as day case admissions due to social reasons to be discharged but remain nearby overnight. The accommodation would be adjacent to the day care unit/children's ward. A housekeeper would provide hotel type services, such as meals and bed making. Although these plans still remain in their infancy, it is anticipated that when they are introduced the numbers of children treated as day cases will continue to increase.

## References

Audit Commission 1992 All in a day's work: an audit of day surgery in England and Wales. HMSO, London
Audit Commission 1993 Children first: a study of hospital services. HMSO, London
British Paediatric Association 1996 Flexible options for paediatric care. BPA, London
Daborn A, Hatch D, Phillips S 1994 Preoperative fasting for paediatric anaesthesia. British Journal of Anaesthesia 73(4): 529–531
Department of Health 1959 The report of the Platt committee. HMSO, London
Department of Health 1991 Welfare of children and young people in hospital. HMSO, London

Department of Health 1996 The patient's charter: services for children and young people. HMSO, London
Hitchcock M, Ogg T 1993 What is the optimum NPO time prior to day surgery. Journal of One Day Surgery 3(1): 4–5
Hogg C 1994 Setting standards for children undergoing surgery. Action for Sick Children, London
Royal College of Nursing 1996 Annual Congress report. Resolution 10. Royal College of Nursing, Bournemouth
Royal College of Surgeons of England 1992 Commission on the provision of services guidelines for day case surgery. Royal College of Surgeons, London
Thornes R 1991 Just for the day: caring for children in the Health Service. NAWCH, London

# Chapter 9

# Neonatal surgery

## Judith Clegg and Anthony Lander

## INTRODUCTION

This chapter aims to discuss the exciting challenge of surgery in the neonatal period. Advances in antenatal screening, neonatal care and surgery, general and spinal anaesthesia, ventilation techniques and, particularly for the neonatal infant needing surgery, parenteral nutrition have resulted in the increasing survival of neonates born with major congenital malformations. Successful care depends upon the early identification and appropriate treatment of infants with surgical problems. The use of research and evidence-based practice should continue to improve these outcomes.

## HIGH-RISK PREGNANCIES

Identifying at risk neonates is a major component of care. Families with a history of genetic disorders, congenital malformations or premature births are at higher risk. Other indicators of potential neonatal surgical problems are maternal diabetes, infection, low social class, extremes of childbearing age and maternal smoking, alcohol or drug use. Poor nutritional and vitamin intake both prior to and during the pregnancy are associated with malformations, for example folate deficiency and spina bifida. Congenital anomalies are increasingly identified by maternal blood sampling, ultrasound scanning and culturing fetal cells. Maternal blood sampling for raised alpha-fetoprotein levels (AFPs) in relation to gestation can indicate neural tube and abdominal wall defects, whilst low AFP levels are seen in Down syndrome. Routine ultrasound scanning is a non-invasive, well developed procedure for estimating fetal age and amniotic fluid volume, and can identify many malformations.

Amniocentesis is a valuable way of detecting chromosomal abnormalities; fetal cells in the amniotic fluid can be collected via a needle passed through the maternal abdominal wall from 16 weeks gestation. Chorionic villus sampling allows chromosomal analysis from cells removed from the placental surface via the cervix. This test can be carried out earlier now, at 9–12 weeks. Results are available within 10 days but the procedure carries a higher risk of spontaneous abortion.

## ISSUES FOR PARENTS

Early diagnosis often means that parents have difficult decisions to make. Parents have only a short time to make the decision to terminate or continue the pregnancy. They are faced with the dilemma of evaluating their relationship with their unborn child, the potential effect on their family's future welfare and the possibility of caring for a disabled child. Disclosure of the defect needs to be handled sensitively. It is essential that staff who are in contact with the family are well informed of current treatment and prognosis as parents need clear and accurate information to give them realistic expectations and help them make informed decisions.

## FETAL SURGERY

The surgical treatment of fetal abnormalities before birth is ethically and technically complex and is presently concentrated in only a few centres worldwide. Fetal surgery involves opening the uterus, correcting the defect and returning the fetus to the uterus to recover postoperatively and continue gestational development. The following life-threatening problems have been treated: congenital diaphragmatic hernia, cystic adenomatoid malformation of the lung, sacrococcygeal teratoma and posterior urethral valves, although with variable success. Preterm labour, fetal demise and maternal risks remain major obstacles. Less invasive approaches are also developing, including endoscopic fetal surgery, which could have fewer complications. Randomised controlled trials are needed to assess the effectiveness of these approaches.

## TERTIARY CARE

Neonates diagnosed antenatally with major malformations should be delivered as close to a tertiary neonatal surgical unit (NNSU) as possible. Birth is planned in a hospital with a neonatal intensive care unit (NICU) so that prompt and effective care is available at delivery in consultation with the neonatal surgical team. Ideally, parents should visit the NNSU after the diagnosis to gain an insight into the environment and what they can expect once the baby is born and transferred. This is particularly important for mothers who have to stay in hospital and will not be able to accompany their baby. The attitude of staff and the reassurance they give of the high quality of care the baby will receive is vitally important for parents during this first visit.

## NEONATAL CONSIDERATIONS

### BIRTH AND TRANSFER

Infants with congenital abnormalities are commonly born prematurely or by emergency caesarean section. Sometimes delivery occurs unexpectedly, with no antenatal diagnosis, in centres without a neonatal intensive care unit. The unexpected delivery of a compromised, high-risk neonate presents a major challenge, and policies for the initial management, stabilisation and transfer of the newborn baby who requires surgical intervention need to be in place in all maternity units. Maternal blood samples and copies of the mother's and infant's notes and X-rays with details of the labour, delivery and Apgar scores should be provided by the referring hospital. It is important that accurate details of fluid losses, intravenous fluids and drugs administered, particularly vitamin K, and details of any urine or meconium passed since birth are recorded and included in the notes. Consent for surgery will be needed from the parents; this should be from the mother if the parents are unmarried. Ideally, a doctor who is familiar with the procedure to be performed takes consent. This is not always possible when the mother cannot accompany the baby and warrants clear communication between referring and receiving teams. Box 9.1 lists the priorities for transfer of newborn babies requiring surgery.

It is essential that parents are informed and involved, ideally accompanying the baby. Parents need to see their child before transfer and it is useful

**Box 9.1  Priorities for transferring a surgical neonate**

Discussion with accepting centre

Maintenance of airway

Continuous monitoring of oxygenation and cardiovascular status

Gastric decompression using an 8-10 Fg nasogastric tube open to free drainage and aspirated frequently

Maintenance of intravenous access and fluid administration

Temperature support, using a transport incubator and covering exposed defects with an occlusive film

Positioning: to avoid aspiration (e.g. Oesophageal Atresia), pressure on any defect, (e.g. Gastroschisis) and to minimise respiratory compromise (e.g. nurse on affected side with Diaphragmatic Hernia)

to provide Polaroid®/digital photographs, particularly if they will be apart for any length of time. External malformations need to be shown to the parents with sensitivity. This can be difficult for parents as their preconceptions of what defects will look like are often worse than they really are. Handled well, staff can improve parents' understanding of the condition and help them to see positive images of their child, which is vitally important to foster the bonding process.

## ADMISSION TO THE NEONATAL SURGICAL UNIT (NNSU)

A thorough physical assessment is conducted on arrival at the NNSU to evaluate the infant's physiological state and identify any other associated defects. Major difficulties that can occur during transfer are poor oxygenation, acidosis, hypothermia and fluid and electrolyte imbalance. Preterm infants are particularly prone to these problems. In addition, tubes and drips can block or become dislodged, necessitating urgent intervention on arrival.

## PREOPERATIVE CARE

### OXYGENATION

Ventilation can be impaired as a result of prematurity, physical obstruction or metabolic disturbance. Premature babies are at risk from respiratory distress

syndrome (RDS) due to a lack of surfactant and poor lung compliance, and often need mechanical ventilatory support.

All newborns have a limited cough reflex and have an increased risk of aspiration. If they are below 32 weeks gestation or are sick this risk increases, and positioning to maintain and protect their airways is vitally important. Infants with oesophageal atresia (see Ch. 13) require continuous low pressure suction of the upper oesophageal pouch as secretions cannot be swallowed and can easily flow into the trachea. The use of bag and mask oxygenation for babies with tracheoesophageal fistula and those with diaphragmatic hernia can be dangerous, as the resulting gastric distension will impair rather than aid ventilation.

A distended abdomen puts pressure on the diaphragm, the neonate's main respiratory muscle, and can compromise respiratory movements. All neonates with a bowel obstruction or ileus should have an 8–10 Fg nasogastric tube passed and left on free drainage with regular aspiration to reduce abdominal distension, splinting of the diaphragm and the associated risks of vomiting and inhalation of gastric fluids. Lung malformations such as diaphragmatic hernia result in poor inspiratory volume due to hypoplasticity of the lungs. These babies commonly need ventilation or long term supplementation with oxygen to maintain saturations above 92% to avoid hypoxic damage.

Physical obstruction can impede oxygenation as neonates are obligate nose breathers. An oropharyngeal airway maintains patency for infants with choanal atresia. Babies with Pierre Robin syndrome may need nasopharyngeal intubation to maintain their airways due to micrognathia, associated cleft palate, and a tongue that falls into the airway.

Respiratory acidosis occurs when the neonate's ventilation is inadequate and carbon dioxide builds up. Respiratory rate and effort, oxygen saturations and blood gas analysis should be monitored. When self-ventilation is inadequate, mechanical ventilation may be required to correct the acidosis and maintain oxygenation.

### THERMOREGULATION

All newborns have an immature hypothalamus (the temperature regulating mechanism in the brain), a high surface area to body weight ratio and a high metabolic rate. Insulation from subcutaneous fat is small, even at full term, and the premature infant has thin skin, which results in high insensible fluid and heat losses. Heat production from shivering is absent and non-shivering thermogenesis from brown fat is a major means of temperature maintenance. Brown fat is laid down from 26 weeks gestation and provides thermogenesis from the breakdown and reconstitution of triglycerides within the fatty tissue, with heat released directly into the major blood vessels around the heart and neck. The process is dependent upon an adequate supply of glucose and oxygen, which are quickly consumed by the sick neonate. Hypothermia is a major risk to the neonate exposed for extensive examination or the siting of cannulae, with major thermal losses through evaporation and radiation. Any exposed bowel in a gastroschisis leads to serious heat loss from escaping body fluids, and viscera should be covered with clingfilm or the lower body and bowel placed in a bag secured beneath the axillae. A raised respiratory rate also leads to increased insensible losses. A low store of glycogen in the immature liver leads to hypoglycaemia if the neonate is working hard to support temperature maintenance, and it is essential for a neutral thermal environment to be provided where oxygen and glucose consumption are minimised. Initially, the baby should be placed under a radiant heater or incubator at 34–36°C to maintain core temperature at 37°C and the peripheral temperature at 35°C. By monitoring both core (rectal or trunk) temperature and the peripheral temperature (of a foot) a measure of perfusion is obtained, as in shock the small vessels in the peripheral limbs contract to conserve heat as the baby directs blood to essential organs. Normally, the foot is no more than 2°C less than the core temperature. If the toe/core temperature gap increases, it may indicate poor perfusion and impending shock. A widening toe/core temperature gap should therefore be reported to senior staff.

## FLUID BALANCE, HYPOVOLAEMIA AND ACIDOSIS

Haematological and metabolic status are assessed on arrival, with a full blood count, serum urea and electrolyte levels, blood gases and acid-base balance. Metabolic acidosis occurs when the tissues' demand for oxygen exceeds supply, particularly when perfusion is poor. This can occur with large fluid losses or sepsis. Infants with intestinal obstruction can develop 'third-spacing' or capillary leakage, where fluid passes from the vascular into the interstitial compartment, causing hypovolaemia and underperfusion. Hypoglycaemia is an additional major risk as gluconeogenesis is inefficient from limited liver glycogen stores. Glucose levels need to be monitored regularly as demand may exceed supply, which can result in seizures and brain injury. Metabolic acidosis is usually corrected by the replacement of lost fluid with 0.9% saline or a colloid solution such as 4.5% Human Albumin Solution, in addition to maintenance fluids. The infant who is shocked may additionally need a colloid infusion before surgery can take place. One or two volume corrections of 10 mL/kg body weight may be needed; the kidneys can then do the work of correcting the metabolic acidosis.

Normal blood values can be found in Box 9.2. The neonate needs to be haemodynamically stable for optimum tolerance of anaesthesia and surgery, although with continued fluid loss this may not be fully achievable without surgical correction of the defect.

Associated anomalies, particularly heart defects, could affect the infant's ability to withstand surgery. Prior to theatre X-rays, an electrocardiograph (ECG) and an echocardiogram may identify associated cardiac problems. Vitamin K is given prophylactically to prevent major bleeding. Antibiotics are administered for known or suspected sepsis and prophylactically when open lesions are present. Once the infant is stabilised, emergency, urgent or elective surgery is carried out. For many major defects neonates may be ventilated for the first 1–2 days postoperatively, and parents need to be aware of this.

---

**Box 9.2 Normal neonatal blood value**

Potassium (mmol/L) 3.5-5.5
Sodium (mmol/L) 135-146
Urea (mmol/L) 3.4-6.7
pH 7.3-7.4
Bicarbonate ($\mu$mol/L) 18-25
Base excess (mmol/L) −5 to +5
Creatinine ($\mu$mol/L) 37-113
Calcium (mmols/L) 2.1-2.7
Glucose (mmol/L) 2-5.5
Arterial $PO_2$ (kPa) 8.0-12
Arterial $PCO_2$ (kPa) 4.5-6.0
Hb (g/dL) 16.8-18

## POSTOPERATIVE CARE

Following surgery, the neonate will need to be adequately ventilated and cardiovascularly stable to transfer from theatre to the NNSU/ICU. The wound and any drains and stomas should be inspected, and details of analgesia given and postoperative pain relief prescription noted. All intravenous infusions should be assessed for patency and security, with maintenance and replacement fluids titrated. Nasogastric and any drainage tubes should be attached to a drainage bag. When the attending nurse is satisfied with the baby's stability, transfer in a portable incubator can occur. Commonly, oxygen requirements increase after anaesthesia and surgery, and neonates may require oxygen via a headbox/incubator or mechanical ventilation. All oxygen given should be warmed and humidified to avoid cold stress, and analysed to avoid hypoxia/hyperoxia (particularly for preterm babies). On return, core temperature, peripheral temperature, blood pressure, pulse and respiratory rate, oxygen saturation levels and blood sugar levels are recorded, plus arterial blood gas analysis for assisted ventilation/unstable babies. Continuous monitoring of respiratory and cardiovascular status is needed in addition to accurate fluid balance maintenance. Urine output should be measured via a catheter or by weighing nappies to ensure the urine output is >1mL/kg/hour, indicating adequate perfusion and hydration levels. There may be a diuresis after renal surgery, which needs careful fluid balance monitoring to avoid shock. Stomas are covered by petroleum jelly gauze or a clear stoma bag if oozing, and need regular inspection. Parents should be supported and can be actively involved in settling the infant, with all monitoring and support equipment explained. The infant should then be minimally handled and allowed to rest.

## NEONATAL SURGICAL CONDITIONS

### NEONATAL DISORDERS OF THE FACE AND NECK

Visible defects of an infant's face and neck are particularly distressing for parents and may interfere with their ability to bond with their baby. Parents find photographs of postcorrective surgery for other newborns with the same condition comforting in coming to terms with the situation.

### Pierre Robin Syndrome

A baby with this syndrome has a small jaw and a cleft of the palate. The small jaw results in the tongue being too far back in the mouth. The tongue tends to fall back and block the airway, and this happens mainly when the child is tired. Babies can be managed in a number of ways. In the past, babies were supported prone so that the tongue could fall forwards and the airway was safe. However, it can be difficult to nurse babies in this position. A nasopharyngeal airway (an endotracheal (ET) tube measured from the tragus of the ear to the chin in length, split to fix across the cheeks) passed through the nose to the back of the pharynx prevents the tongue obstructing the airway. With careful monitoring of the oxygen saturations, the length of time the airway is needed can be gradually reduced, noting how long the child can manage without running into trouble. Parents may find oxygenation monitoring stressful as the length of time the airway is in place is reduced. Coping with feeds is often the most tiring thing for infants and they need careful supervision. As the child grows, the high cleft palate is repaired. Speech therapy input and orthodontic referral will be needed to develop successful feeding and for the development of language. By the age of 5 years the jaw will usually have grown to near normal size.

### Choanal atresia/stenosis

Choanal atresia is a rare condition when at birth there is little or no patency from the nostrils to the nasopharynx. At delivery, oxygenation is only possible through the mouth as the baby gasps and cries. Diagnosis involves attempting to pass a suction catheter via the nares, which will be unsuccessful. An oropharyngeal tube will maintain the airway adequately until surgery can be carried out. The operation involves boring the bone of the blocked airway and placing firm stent tubes into the nostrils. These are supported in an 'H' shape to avoid pressure on the columella.

The stent tubes need to remain in place for several weeks to avoid natural reclosure of the bone by the neonate's rapid growth and repair ability. Care involves suctioning the tubes before feeds and as necessary to maintain patency. Parents will need to learn how to suction and clean the tubes and will need a portable suction machine for discharge.

## Cystic hygroma

Lymphangiomas are abnormal growths of lymphatic tissue. They consist of multiple cystic elements of variable size. One common site in the newborn is the neck (see Fig. 9.1). At delivery trauma can occur, particularly if the condition is antenatally undiagnosed, causing further swelling and potential bleeding into the tissues. Cystic hygromas can cause difficulty with swallowing and oxygenation due to displacement of the structures within the neck. Excision is important if there is risk of compromise to the airway or major secondary deformation. They can extend into the chest and can be fatal. A tracheostomy may be needed for some infants. Small cystic hygromas can be observed and a few resolve spontaneously or after secondary infection. It may take months for the infant to develop sufficient suck and swallow reflexes to sustain full oral feeding and parents need to be introduced to tube feeding their baby early for successful discharge.

## NEONATAL DISORDERS OF THE CHEST

### Tracheoesophageal fistula and oesophageal atresia

Oesophageal atresia is commonly associated with a tracheoesophageal fistula. The most common arrangement is a blind ending upper oesophageal pouch with the distal oesophagus connected to the trachea. This connection is the fistula (see Fig. 9.2). Antenatally, amniotic fluid is not swallowed into the stomach and polyhydramnios results. The association of polyhydramnios and a small stomach on antenatal scanning suggests the diagnosis, and chromosomal and heart defects are carefully looked for. After birth, an attempt is made to pass a nasogastric tube. This will remain in the upper pouch and on X-ray some gas is seen in the intestine. The gas has entered the intestines via the fistula from the trachea. Sometimes the diagnosis is made after the first feed when the baby coughs and splutters as milk spills over from the upper pouch into the trachea. Preoperative management includes keeping the upper pouch empty to prevent saliva spilling over into the trachea. An ordinary feeding tube on constant low grade suction tends to get blocked with mucosa sucked into its holes. To avoid this, a Replogle tube is used. This tube has a second channel allowing air to break the vacuum at the end of the tube. Regular flushing of the Replogle tube with 1.0–1.5 mL of 0.9% normal saline is needed to maintain patency as the sticky saliva can block suction from the pouch. The surgical repair is carried out through the right chest. The fistula is disconnected from the trachea and joined to the upper pouch. A chest drain may be left for a few days after the operation. A transanastomotic tube allows enteral feeding, bypassing the repair site. Babies

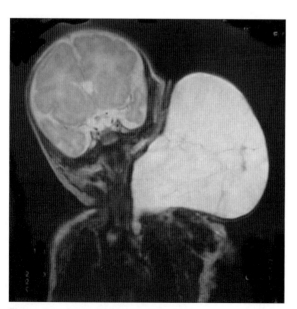

**Figure 9.1** Cystic hygroma on the neck.

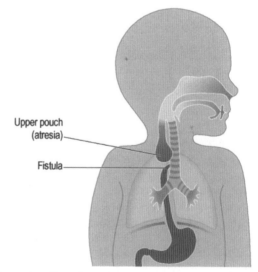

Upper pouch (atresia)

Fistula

**Figure 9.2** Oesophageal atresia with lower pouch fistula (most common type – 85% of cases).

may be fed some days later by mouth, though some surgeons prefer to get a contrast study before oral feeding starts. These babies commonly have reflux and may have associated renal, vertebral, anorectal and cardiac anomalies.

## Diaphragmatic hernia

Diaphragmatic hernias are associated with hypoplastic lungs and consequently problems with ventilation. The defect allowing herniation is usually in the posterolateral aspect of the diaphragm (Bochdalek hernia), most commonly on the left (see Fig. 9.3). Anterior defects (Morgani hernias) are rarer and may present later in life. A wide spectrum of pathology is seen. Many fetuses with diaphragmatic hernias have a trisomy (particularly 18) and/or a major cardiac defect, which is incompatible with life. If this is diagnosed antenatally, a termination is offered. For fetuses surviving to delivery, the prognosis depends on any associated cardiac defects and the respiratory reserve of the lungs. After birth babies are stabilised, sometimes for many days, before surgical repair through the abdomen. Sometimes there is an associated malrotation that needs correction.

A small proportion escape early detection and present with respiratory or gastrointestinal symptoms in infancy and even childhood.

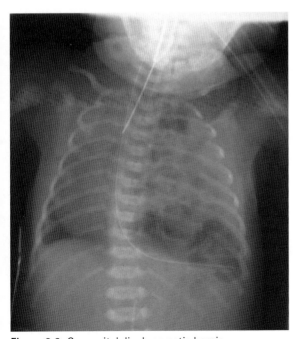

Figure 9.3 Congenital diaphragmatic hernia.

## NEONATAL GASTROINTESTINAL DISORDERS

Gastrointestinal problems can be identified by the history and findings on examination. Box 9.3 shows important features.

### Intestinal atresias and stenoses

In a stenosis there is a narrowing of the gut lumen and in an atresia there is a complete obstruction. Atresias and stenoses are seen in the oesophagus, the duodenum, small bowel, colon, rectum and anus.

### Duodenal atresia and duodenal stenosis (1:10 000 births)

During early development the duodenum used to be thought to go through a brief period of complete occlusion with cells. Failure of this to resolve was thought to result in a stenosis or atresia. We now know the duodenum is normally patent throughout its development. Duodenal atresia is sometimes seen with oesophageal atresia and colonic atresia, and sometimes with both. It is rarely seen with other small bowel atresias. Importantly, about 20% of babies have Down syndrome. Antenatally, a dilated stomach and dilated first part of the duodenum can be detected on ultrasound scans. Chromosomal analysis after amniocentesis is often then performed to look for the trisomy 21 of Down syndrome.

After birth, duodenal atresia presents with dark green bilious vomiting. A plain X-ray shows a dilated stomach and a dilated first part of the duodenum, usually with very little gas in the rest of the bowel. Occasionally, even though there is a complete atresia, some gas enters a y-shaped biliary system, which bridges the atresia, so allowing some gas into the distal bowel.

Preoperative care involves a large bore nasogastric tube (8 or 10 French), regular nasogastric aspiration

### Box 9.3 Common signs of gastrointestinal problems in neonates

- Vomiting
- Green bile vomited or aspirated from a NG tube
- Failure to pass meconium
- An abnormal perineum
- Abdominal distension, erythema or tenderness
- Blood passed per anum

and replacing intravenously any volumes of aspirated fluid with 0.9% NaCl + 0.15% KCl. If the child is suspected to have Down syndrome, a cardiac opinion is usually sought because of the associated heart defects.

The operation consists of joining the duodenum on either side of the atretic segment (duodenostomy). This is performed through a small right upper quadrant transverse incision. A percutaneous silastic long line is usually inserted to give postoperative parenteral nutrition.

Postoperative care involves continued nasogastric suction, initially hourly, together with intravenous replacement. The major postoperative problem is that a hugely dilated duodenum (stretched by antenatally swallowed amniotic fluid blocked by the obstruction) may take time to develop satisfactory peristalsis to empty into the distal bowel. The paediatric surgeon may ask for feeds to be started before the bile has completely cleared from the nasogastric aspirates. This is unusual in normal practice, since children are not fed if there is frank bile in the gastric aspirates. However, with duodenal atresia the pylorus is so stretched that the proximal duodenum is in easy physiological continuity with the stomach and the aspirates are often bilious for a long time. This difference in practice, compared with a child without duodenal atresia, is important to note. Most children with duodenal atresia are on full enteral feeds by 10 days of age, though some children with Down syndrome can be slow to take these feeds by mouth. Surgeons used to use a transanastomic tube but there is no evidence to suggest that this is helpful. When feeds were delivered into the small bowel, they would have been continuous, but bolus feeds into the stomach are appropriate in duodenal atresia. If Down syndrome is diagnosed and had not been suspected antenatally, it is crucial to consider the information that is given to the parents and the support that is to be provided whilst they come to terms with the diagnosis.

Follow-up for the Down syndrome is important, in addition to surgical follow-up. When Down syndrome is present, it is important to remember that, from 3 months of age, special Down's charts are available which show the expected centiles of growth for children with this trisomy. The 50th centile on a Down's chart corresponds approximately to the 3rd centile on a normal growth chart.

## Small bowel atresias

Small bowel atresias can occur anywhere in the jejunum (proximal small bowel) or ileum (distal small bowel). They may be single or multiple. When multiple, the bowel can look like a string of sausages. Sometimes a large section of bowel is missing and the child is left with insufficient intestine to survive without undergoing a lengthy period of intestinal adaptation, which can take many months to accomplish. The bowel upstream of the most proximal atresia is often dilated and has poor function.

Preoperative care is the same as for a child with an obstruction, involving a large nasogastric tube and regular aspiration, together with replacement of gastric losses with normal saline and potassium intravenously.

At operation, intestinal continuity is re-established with one or more anastomoses. If there has been an antenatal perforation and the peritoneal cavity is contaminated, both ends of the bowel may be brought out as temporary stomas, which are subsequently closed. Hugely dilated intestines can be excised or tapered.

There are only rarely other associated non-gastrointestinal abnormalities, and it is thought that these small bowel atresias are caused by vascular problems.

Postoperative care depends on the length of bowel left and the degree of intestinal dysfunction caused by the dilated proximal bowel. Parenteral nutrition is used to support the neonate until nasogastric or oral feeds can be established and increased to a point at which the infant is growing satisfactorily. If the intestine is very short, adaptation can take many months and a degree of malnutrition may be complicated by the problems of intravenous nutrition: sepsis, venous access and liver failure.

## Colonic atresias

Colonic atresias are comparatively rare and present with obstruction, usually with abdominal distension where bilious vomiting may not occur for 1 or more days. Sometimes the dilated colon has been diagnosed antenatally.

## Anorectal malformations

There are a number of different atresias of the anorectal region, most of which present as an imperforate anus. This is why the anus and the genitals should be closely examined in a newborn baby. In girls, there may be a fistula connecting the atretic rectum to the perineum, either immediately behind the vagina or on the perineum, slightly anterior to the external sphincter muscles. In boys, there may be a fistula either onto the skin in the region of the mid line raffe of the scrotum, or into the urethra, or into the prostate, or occasionally into the bladder. Sometimes, therefore, these boys pass meconium from the penis. Depending on the level of the atresia, there will be a variable degree of structural abnormality of the muscles of the pelvic floor. In addition, the muscles that surround the anus and lower rectum are often malformed. The sacrum and innervation of the pararectal tissues and bladder can also be abnormal. When the abnormality is very low, an anoplasty can sometimes be performed in the first few days of life. Low anomalies are not trivial, because many of these babies have long-standing problems with constipation, either because the rest of the bowel is inherently abnormal and sluggish or because of persistent abnormalities in the anorectal region. When the rectum is atretic and a low procedure cannot be performed, most surgeons perform a divided colostomy in the left iliac fossa, in the descending colon. The colostomy is a divided colostomy, so that the stomas are well separated. This means that a bag can be placed over the functioning descending colostomy and stool will not pass into the distal bowel, which may be connected to the urinary tract. Once the stoma has been fashioned the baby is usually able to feed within 24 or 36 hours. Babies are screened for associated anomalies in the urinary tract, vertebrae, limbs and heart, When the baby is thriving, definitive surgery can be planned. A contrast study down the distal stoma demonstrates the level at which the distal bowel is connected to the urinary tract in a boy. Definitive surgery can be done through a posterior mid line incision, when the muscles can be defined and the atretic rectum taken off the urinary tract and brought down to form a new anus within the muscle complex. After the child has recovered from this operation the parents may need to be taught how to dilate the anus, using Hagar dilators (metal rods of various sizes). When the anus is at an appropriate size, the child is readmitted to have the colostomy closed.

In many operated anorectal anomalies, long term problems with constipation and fecal incontinence can occur and are the focus of follow-up.

## Meconium ileus

Some babies present with intestinal obstruction, with a distended abdomen and bilious vomiting, together with failure to pass stool. Plain X-rays may show the baby to be obstructed but with lots of meconium in the bowel. Contrast enemas performed in the radiology department may show an unused distal bowel and contrast eventually gets into the dilated ileum. If gastrograffin is used for the contrast study, the detergent and osmotic effect of this agent helps wash thick sticky meconium from the bowel. Some of these babies need more than one contrast enema to clear the bowel, and others need an operation and a hole to be made in the bowel to clear it out. Many of these babies with thick sticky meconium causing a bowel obstruction are later found to have cystic fibrosis.

## ANTERIOR ABDOMINAL WALL DEFECTS

The two most common anterior abdominal wall defects are gastroschisis and exomphalos. These are two quite different conditions.

## Gastroschisis

In gastroschisis there is a defect to the right of the umbilicus through which intestine, stomach and internal genitalia can prolapse. There is no sac overlying the bowel and the intestine is often thick walled and covered in a peel. The peel is caused by fetal defecatory products in the amniotic fluid affecting the serosa of the bowel. Babies with this problem are often small for dates and have usually been diagnosed antenatally, Antenatal diagnosis allows antenatal counselling for the parents. In gastroschisis there are rarely other associated abnormalities, except those related to the intestine prolapsing through the defect. 10% of these babies have an intestinal atresia probably caused by a vascular accident in the prolapsed bowel.

When these babies are born, their early management is crucial to survival. In the UK these babies are delivered vaginally unless there are other reasons for a caesarean section. Although babies are not allowed to become post mature, they are not deliberately delivered prematurely. When they are born, a large bore nasogastric tube is passed to empty the stomach; an intravenous drip is started to commence intravenous fluids because there can be a lot of fluid lost by evaporation from the open abdomen and the large surface of the intestines that is exposed to the atmosphere. Babies should be wrapped in clingfilm, or the lower part of the body placed into a bowel bag, so that the intestines can be seen but evaporative losses of fluid and heat losses can be minimised. A bolus of intravenous fluid is usually given, together with intravenous antibiotics. A postnatal volvulus of prolapsed intestine can be a catastrophe. The bowel, therefore, has to be watched closely, noting its colour. Dusky or blue intestine should initiate a prompt examination of the bowel. Usually, it is best to nurse the baby on the right hand side with the intestine also lying on the right hand side. A baby lying on the right with the intestine lifted over onto the left is one in whom the bowel is likely to have severe compromise to its circulation. There are three ways in which these babies are managed:

1. Traditionally, under a general anaesthetic, the bowel is cleaned and reduced into the abdominal cavity with or without rectal washouts. Sometimes the defect in the abdomen is enlarged to allow the intestines to return.
2. If the intestines will not fit in the abdominal cavity easily, a synthetic silo or chimney can be created. This allows the intestines to be reduced gradually over a period of a few days whilst the child is ventilated on the ICU.
3. More recently, in selected infants, it is possible to return the intestinal contents to the abdomen without a general anaesthetic and without the child suffering any significant discomfort. A silo may be used in some babies. This can avoid a lengthy period of ventilation on intensive care.

Babies with gastroschisis can take 3–6 weeks or more for intestinal function to fully return. Parents need to be aware of the potential time their baby will need to be in hospital for the bowel to develop effective function. Some of these babies develop necrotising enterocolitis, but overall the survival rate is 90%.

## Exomphalos

In exomphalos, the intestines are prolapsed in the mid line into a sac covered with peritoneum and amnion (see Fig. 9.4). At one end of the spectrum there may be a small defect and a few loops of small intestine in the base of the umbilical cord. At the other end of the spectrum, there can be a large defect in a small baby and the sac can contain the liver and a large quantity of small intestine. When the liver is

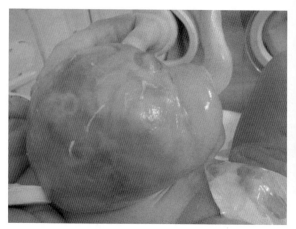

**Figure 9.4** Exomphalos.

in the sac the condition is known as exomphalos major. Antenatal diagnosis is common and because these babies have a high incidence of associated chromosomal abnormalities and cardiac defects, amniocentesis and terminations are common. Those babies who survive are transferred to neonatal surgical units. There is less of an emergency in managing exomphalos compared with gastroschisis. The sac that covers the intestines will keep them warm and heat and fluid loss are reduced. The clinical approach in exomphalos will depend on the size of the defect and its contents. A small defect can be repaired at a single procedure, obtaining skin and muscle cover. In larger defects skin coverage is sometimes obtained at a first procedure, and later on the anterior abdominal wall is repaired. Treatment options include putting on a mesh, or again a silo can be constructed with gradual reduction of the intestines. Alternatively, a very large exomphalos can be managed conservatively. The sac will dry out and a skin-like membrane will grow over the sac, and delayed surgery can be planned. Intestinal function usually returns much more quickly with exomphalos than with gastroschisis, because the intestine has not been exposed to amniotic fluid.

## Necrotising enterocolitis

Premature and intrauterine growth retarded neonates, especially those with cardiac abnormalities, are at risk of developing necrotising enterocolitis. The immature gut is not ready to receive enteral feeds or cope with intestinal bacteria. An immature gut that in addition has a degree of impairment of its blood supply is at great risk of developing patches of localised gangrene and perforation. This is what is called necrotising enterocolitis. The baby may pass blood in the stool and on X-ray abnormal loops of bowel and gas in the bowel wall or biliary tree may be seen. When the intestine is rested and antibiotics are given, the condition may settle down and completely resolve. However, sometimes the intestine perforates and a potentially fatal peritonitis can develop. Intestinal perforation is usually an indication for surgical intervention. These babies can be very sick and often need close monitoring in the ICU. They can become acidotic and have problems with their coagulation. They are often septic. Once stablised, the baby may require an urgent laparotomy. At laparotomy, necrotic intestine is removed and either an anastomosis is made between two healthy ends of bowel, or one or both ends of the intestine are brought out onto the anterior abdominal wall as intestinal stomas (see Fig. 9.5).

Postoperative care involves stoma management and the resolving of sepsis in the child. Sometimes necrotising enterocolitis resolves without the need for surgical intervention; however, sometimes the piece of damaged bowel scars down forming a stricture, often in the colon. This can cause distension when the baby is fed and may require an elective operation to resect the obstructing region.

## Hirschsprung's disease

New born babies usually pass meconium in the first 24 hours of life. Hirschsprung's disease usually presents with failure to pass meconium in the first 24 hours of life, abdominal distension and vomiting. It is seen at any gestational age, but premature babies may be slower than normal to pass meconium without them having aganglionosis. A rectal biopsy can be performed on the ward. In Hirschsprung's disease it shows thickened cholinergic nerve trunks and absent ganglion cells in the submucosal nerve plexus and myenteric nerve plexus. The affected intestine fails to relax, so causing a functional obstruction. The aganglionic region runs proximally for a variable distance from the internal sphincter. The ganglionic bowel further upstream dilates, and if left untreated leads to a megacolon. About 75% are aganglionic up to the sigmoid colon, 10% have a longer segment of colon involved, and a further 10% have total colonic and some small bowel involvement (male:female 4:1, 1 per 5000 live births).

Babies may need intravenous fluids for resuscitation. Rectal washouts help decompress the intestine. When the baby is well, a temporary stoma in the ganglionic bowel is performed. Later, definitive surgery involves a pull through of ganglionic bowel to the level of the anus. Alternatively, a primary pull through can be done using microscopic examination of frozen sections at the time of surgery to determine the level of the upper limit of the pathology.

Hirschsprung's disease sometimes presents later in childhood (see Ch. 13) or, rarely, in adult life, with constipation without soiling, but there is often a neonatal history of delay in passage of meconium or problems with constipation from early on.

## Malrotation and volvulus neonatorum

A baby with dark green bilious vomiting may have malrotation with a volvulus (twisting) of the intestine, causing obstruction (see also Ch. 13). An upper gastrointestinal contrast study is used to assess intestinal rotation. Sometimes there are signs of vascular compromise, in which case an urgent laparotomy is indicated.

Sometimes the small bowel mesentery is not fixed at the duodeno–jejunal (DJ) flexure (in the left paravertebral gutter) or in the ileocaecal region (in the right paravertebral gutter). This means that the base of the mesentery is short and unstable, predisposing to volvulus. It is thought that the DJ flexure failed to rotate adequately to the left (anticlockwise from the front) around the superior mesenteric vessels. Sometimes, the caecum fails to rotate and descend on the right (anticlockwise from the front).

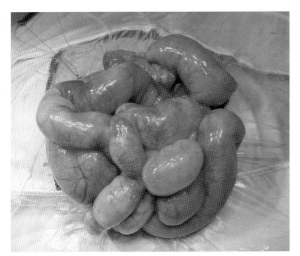

Figure 9.5 Appearance of necrotising enterocolitis at laparotomy.

Normal DJ rotation is illustrated in Figure 9.6, whilst a volvulus of the small intestine is seen in Figure 9.7. Sometimes bands (Ladd's bands) cross the duodenum and contribute to the obstruction. The baby may present with simple obstruction or obstruction with a compromised blood supply. If there is infarction of the bowel, there may be blood in the gastric aspirates or in the stools. Obstruction with bilious vomiting usually presents in the first few days of life but can be seen later. At operation, the volvulus is untwisted (see Fig. 9.8), the duodenum is mobilised and the bowel placed in the non-rotated position with the DJ flexure on the right and the caecum and appendix on the left. The malrotation is not 'corrected' but the mesentery is broadened. The appendix may be removed to avoid later diagnostic confusion in the event of appendicitis.

## Biliary atresia

Biliary atresia presents as a gradual onset obstructive jaundice, which is due to an extrahepatic atresia that obstructs biliary drainage. It is to be considered in any jaundiced neonate in whom the conjugated bilirubin is raised. Tests demonstrate typical hepatic histology on biopsy and an absence

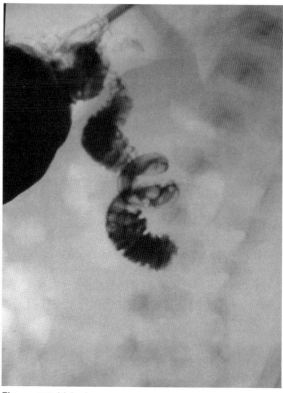

Figure 9.7 Volvulus.

of biliary drainage. Early operation (Kasai procedure) is performed at 8 weeks, bringing a loop of intestine up to the porta hepatis, which is aggressively dissected until biliary drainage is witnessed. If this procedure fails, liver transplantation is considered. Early detection and operation is essential for optimum outcome.

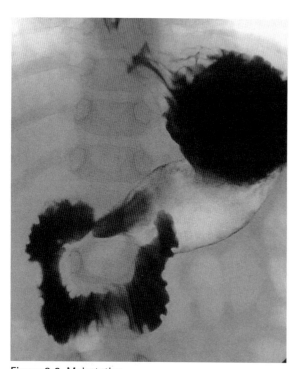

Figure 9.6 Malrotation.

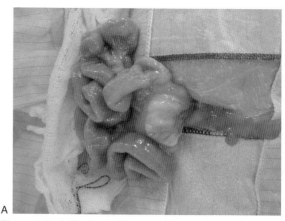

A

Figure 9.8 A. The bowel is twisted with some creamy chyle collected in the mesentery from obstructed lymphatic vessels.

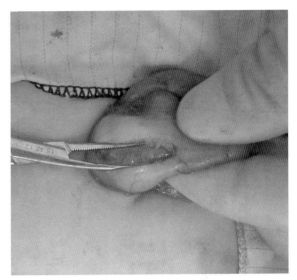

Figure 9.9 Pyloromyotomy.

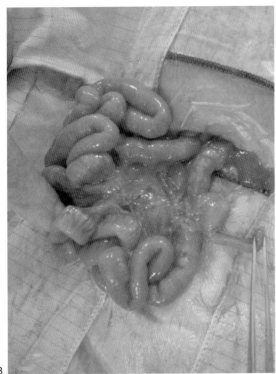

B

**Figure 9.8—cont'd** B. The bowel is untwisted with the caecum and appendix on the left and the duodenum on the right.

## Pyloric stenosis

Vomiting is common in babies in the first weeks of life; bilious vomiting is the most serious and needs urgent referral and assessment. The commonest cause of non-bilious vomiting is reflux, which is often present from birth and is not particularly forceful. Pyloric stenosis, however, presents after the first few weeks of life with increasingly frequent and ever more forceful non-bilious vomiting in a hungry baby (see also Ch. 13).

Pyloric stenosis is more common in boys than girls and there may be an associated family history. Protracted loss of gastric fluid results in a hypochloraemic metabolic alkalosis. This needs correction with normal saline intravenously before operation, and the stomach should be kept empty with aspiration on a large bore (10 Fg) nasogastric tube. The operation can be performed through a right upper quadrant muscle cutting incision or through an umbilical incision. At operation, the pyloric muscle is cut (pyloromyotomy), taking the compression off the pyloric channel (see Fig. 9.9). Only rarely is the mucosa breached, needing a repair, and postoperative feeding is then delayed. There is always a degree of gastric ileus after the operation and feeds can be restarted the following morning. There is no need to keep the nasogastric tube in after the operation and no need to have complex feeding regimens. These babies have been vomiting for many days preoperatively and will often have a few vomits in the first 24 hours after starting feeds. Parents need to be told that this is to be expected.

## Stoma management (see also Ch. 13)

Stomas are formed for the management of Hirschsprung's disease, necrotising enterocolitis, high imperforate anus and to rest infected or damaged bowel. Commonly, infants with colostomies are discharged home prior to closure. Neonates have their ileostomies closed as soon as possible as fluid loss and poor feed absorption are major difficulties. Two stomas are usually formed. The proximal stoma is functional and the distal is non-functioning as a mucous fistula of the lower bowel.

Preoperatively, it is useful for the proposed site to be marked for optimum positioning. Siting the stoma in the centre of the abdomen or close to the groin causes problems with bag adhesion and leaking, which can cause serious damage to the surrounding skin. Postoperatively, the new stomas may be slightly dusky and oedematous but should develop a shiny reddish pink appearance within the first hour. A clear stoma bag allows visibility of the stoma and output.

It is vital for the flange to fit snugly and using a template of the stoma size ensures the flange is cut accurately. This is important as ileostomy fluid is particularly corrosive, with an enzyme content that can cause considerable breakdown of the surrounding tissue. The opening of the drainage bag should be directed towards the side for ease of emptying. Once established, the stoma bag can remain in place for 3–4 days. Cotton wool and warm water are adequate to clean stomas and some superficial bleeding is normal. All stoma output should be measured and recorded and loose stool tested for faecal sugar to determine feed absorption.

Parents should be encouraged to participate in their baby's stoma care as early as possible. Their confidence and competence should be carefully assessed prior to the baby's discharge to avoid difficulties at home.

## NEONATAL DISORDERS OF THE RENAL AND REPRODUCTIVE SYSTEMS

### Pelviureteric junction obstruction

Pelviureteric junction (PUJ) obstruction is intermittent and incomplete and is caused by a stenosis, a kink, a lower pole vessel or a functional problem in the region where the renal pelvis joins the ureter.

A PUJ obstruction can present with antenatal dilatation, with infantile urinary tract infections or with episodic loin pain in childhood. Mild degrees of dilatation in an asymptomatic child may be observed to resolve spontaneously. Only rarely is surgery needed in the neonatal period.

### Posterior urethral valves

The most common cause of urinary obstruction in boys is a membrane or valves in the posterior urethra. This can be fatal. The valves are prominent flaps of tissue near the lowest limits of the verumontanum. The obstruction is often diagnosed antenatally when there is a big bladder and hydronephrosis. The back pressure can damage the kidneys. Sometimes part of the urinary tract, for example the pelvis of the kidney, perforates and decompresses the system, thus preventing damage but causing urinary ascites. These boys can be quite sick with renal failure that is relieved by the passage of a urinary catheter. There may be a profound diuresis, which needs close monitoring and intravenous fluid replacement. Surgical management involves destruction of the valves.

### Hypospadias/epispadias/bladder exstrophy (see also Ch. 13)

Hypospadias occurs in about 1 in 300 boys. The urinary meatus is found on the ventral surface of the penis anywhere from the corona (the groove below the glans) to the scrotum. Religious circumcision is contraindicated as the foreskin may be needed in the repair. Repair is usually done at about 1 year and may be staged.

Epispadias is very rare and describes a urinary meatus on the dorsal surface of the penis. It is seen with bladder exstrophy. In bladder exstrophy the bladder is open on the lower abdominal wall and needs neonatal closure. In the UK there are only 3 centres doing this type of closure.

### Ambiguous genitalia

Occasionally it is not clear what the sex of a baby is. This is a major problem because the sex and name of a new born baby are the first thing that family and friends wish to know and they are usually told promptly. This pressure sometimes tempts staff to guess the sex. This is a disaster if the guess is wrong. It is a mistake to give the baby an ambiguous name, like Charlie or Leslie, which might do for either sex. It is wrong to refer to the baby as 'it' but also care should be taken to avoid 'he' or 'she' and staff should use 'baby' instead. Parents need a lot of support and should be informed of all investigations and their results as they happen. The management is urgent and multidisciplinary.

## DISCHARGE PLANNING

Discharge from the NNSU can equal the stress of admission for parents. Taking their baby home after what can be months of hospital care causes great anxiety. It is common for parents to distance themselves from their child in the early stages of diagnosis and surgery as they try to protect themselves from the potential pain of losing the child. Consequently, facing the thought of taking over the responsibility for care can be daunting as they never envisaged the possibility of the child surviving and coming home with them. For others, discharge is the final achievement from a challenging experience, and finally they can be a family. It is common for these families to feel more ready than they really are when faced with 24-hour care at home, often at some distance from the regional unit and the staff they have come to depend upon for advice and support.

## PREPARATION FOR DISCHARGE

From the time of admission, planning for discharge can occur. The family's health visitor and GP need to be informed of the admission and subsequent progress of the baby. It is useful if the health visitor or community paediatric nurse can visit the family in the unit to develop a rapport with them prior to discharge.

## ASSESSING READINESS FOR DISCHARGE

Certain criteria, involving both physical and emotional considerations, need to be met for discharge to be successful. The new born baby needs to be able to maintain his temperature and to have a regime that is achievable for parents. Feeding should be no more frequent than 3 hourly, with a pattern of weight gain at 150–200 g per week. For infants who need nasogastric continuous/intermittent feeds, or feeding using special equipment, parental teaching and competence are essential.

Babies can also be nursed at home when receiving parenteral nutrition via a central venous line, although this involves considerable skills, understanding and facilities within the home to support aseptic line management.

Elimination also needs to be manageable. Commonly, after intestinal surgery babies may have a temporary colostomy. Parents need to be competent in emptying and changing stoma bags and caring for peristomal skin. They will also need a week's supply of stoma equipment and details of where to obtain further supplies as the local nursing and GP service may not be able to offer specific advice.

In addition to their competence to manage the baby's physical needs, the NNSU staff need to assess the family's emotional readiness to take on the full care of the baby at home. If such an assessment is not made, the likelihood of readmission is increased when the family find they cannot cope. It is important that staff indicate that after a long hospital stay the baby may be initially unsettled in a home environment. Carpets, soft furnishings and relative quiet are unfamiliar to the infant and initially may affect behaviour, feeding and sleeping patterns. It often helps if the family have 'home visits' prior to discharge, particularly if special equipment will be used in the home.

It is useful for families to be assured that they can contact the unit for advice following discharge, and accurate notes of any concerns and postdischarge advice given needs to be recorded by unit staff. The receiving team of health visitor, community paediatric nurse and GP should also be welcomed to contact the unit for any clarification of the baby's needs and treatment. Written information is very useful for both parents and community teams to refer to following discharge. Outpatient appointment dates or a readmission date for further surgery need to be given to the family and community team.

## CONCLUSION

This chapter outlines the surgical management and intensive nursing care of infants who require surgery in the neonatal period. In the past many babies with the problems discussed would not have survived, yet now the majority are able to recover and live full lives. The care of neonates pre- and postoperatively poses a challenge to surgical teams and gives exciting and ongoing opportunities to be involved in research and developments in care to make further improvements for this special group of surgical patients.

## References

Martin V (ed) 2004 The TOF child. TOFS, Nottingham

## Further reading

Bilodeau JA 1995 A home parenteral nutrition program for infants. Journal of Obstetric, Gynaecological and Neonatal Nursing 24(1): 72–76
Cuckle H 1998 Antenatal screening today and in the future. RCM Midwives Journal 1(6): 177–179

Fisk N, Moise K (eds) 1997 Fetal therapy. Cambridge University Press, Cambridge
Hancock J 2000 Nursing the preterm surgical neonate. Journal of Child Health Care 4(1): 12–18

Howell LJ 1994 The unborn surgical patient: a nursing frontier. Nursing Clinics of North America 29(4): 681–694

Kenner C, Wright Lott J, Flandomeyer J 1998 (eds) Comprehensive neonatal nursing: a physiologic perspective, 2nd edn. WB Saunders, London

Leslie A 1997 Transferring sick babies. The new practicalities. Journal of Neonatal Nursing 3(2): 6–12

Mollohan J 1999 Extrophy of the bladder. Neonatal Network: Journal of Neonatal Nursing 18(2): 17–26, 49–52

Parry A 1998 Stoma care in neonates: improving practice. Journal of Neonatal Nursing 4(1): 8–11

Prem Puri (ed) 1996 Newborn surgery. Butterworth Heinemann, Oxford

Prows CA, Bender PL 1999 Beyond Pierre Robin sequence. Neonatal Network: Journal of Neonatal Nursing 18(5): 41–44

Sadler TW 1990 Langman's medical embryology, 6th edn. Williams & Wilkins, Baltimore

Shannon L, Quinn D 1996 Neonatal radiology. Congenital abnormalities. Neonatal Network: Journal of Neonatal Nursing 14(8): 25–28, 15(1): 63–66

# Chapter 10

# Neurosurgery

## Lindy May

## INTRODUCTION

The knowledge and experience acquired by skilled children's nurses will help them in anticipating the needs of their patients and their families. However, to understand the needs of the child with a neurological deficit, nurses must also be able to assess the child's neurological status, understand the implications, and act accordingly. Communication with all disciplines and clinicians is essential, and since families understand their children far better than any professionals, their involvement in the assessment and treatment of their children throughout their care, is paramount.

## NEUROLOGICAL ASSESSMENT

Nurses are in a unique position to detect subtle changes in a child's neurological status as they are usually the most consistent carers on the multidisciplinary team; where appropriate, they should also use the mother's unique understanding of her child in their assessment. Attention should be given to children's activities and surroundings during this assessment, along with their response to their mothers. Formal neurological assessment should always take place in conjunction with, and not instead of, general observation of the child.

Many coma charts have been devised in an attempt to standardise clinical assessment of consciousness. The Glasgow coma chart (GCS) is used worldwide, and adaptations for its use in paediatrics have been many. The scales are divided into three categories comprising eye opening, best verbal response and best motor response; each category is further divided and the resulting graph gives a visual recording of the patient's neurological improvement or deterioration. The resulting numerical score is used in conjunction with the child's vital signs in identifying the patient's status and any necessary interventions. A chart, however, is only as good as the person using it and consistent assessment between observers has been shown at times to be unreliable. Consequently, whatever chart is used, appropriate education is essential to minimise this variation and maximise reliability in scoring, and local policies should be put in place to ensure this. Figure 10.1 shows a typical paediatric coma chart.

Further information regarding coma scoring and education in children can be found in papers by Simpson & Reilly (1982), Raimondi & Hirschner (1984) and Moray et al (1984).

## CHANGES IN VITAL SIGNS

Cushing's response describes the changes in vital signs that occur due to raised intracranial pressure. This includes a drop in pulse, rise in blood pressure and a variation in respiratory pattern. However, in the young child, blood pressure and pulse remain relatively stable in the early stages of raised intracranial pressure, and Cushing's response is considered a late indication of raised pressure in this age group. In contrast, changes in respiratory pattern in the infant, commencing with apnoea attacks and leading to respiratory arrest, are far more common than in the adult patient. It is therefore essential that assessment of the child includes a neurological assessment, observation of vital signs, observation of headache, irritability and vomiting, and that all this is performed, where appropriate, in conjunction

with the mother's account of her child's symptoms and behaviour.

## NEUROLOGICAL IMAGING

X-rays remain an invaluable tool in the diagnosis of skull and spinal fractures, and abnormal skull formations. Computerised tomography (CT) scanning is now widely available, although cranial ultrasound may be adequate in diagnosing hydrocephalus in the neonate. Magnetic resonance imaging (MRI) scanning is becoming increasingly available and provides more detailed views to those obtained from CT. However, scanning young children often requires sedation or anaesthesia, and so becomes more of an undertaking than in the older and more cooperative child. Preparation in the form of explanation, photographs and relaxation techniques may help reduce anxiety and increase compliance, and can be undertaken by the nurse or play specialist in conjunction with the parent or carer.

## HYDROCEPHALUS

Hydrocephalus is a clinical symptom rather than a disease and is characterised by an increase in cerebrospinal fluid (CSF) volume and enlarged ventricles.

Hydrocephalus occurs when the production of CSF exceeds its absorption. CSF is produced continuously at a rate of approximately 22 mL per hour in the adult (smaller amounts are produced in children but the amount is undetermined). CSF is produced by the vascular choroid plexus of the third ventricle and in smaller amounts in the third and fourth ventricles and brain parenchyma. CSF moves from the lateral ventricles to the third and fourth ventricles and then into the subarachnoid space; here it is reabsorbed via the arachnoid villi into the venous system. CSF also flows down the spinal cord. It is a clear, colourless fluid and provides buoyancy for the brain and also helps maintain brain homeostasis.

Hydrocephalus can be described as communicating or non-communicating. In communicating hydrocephalus, the arachnoid villi are unable to absorb CSF in the normal manner, resulting in a 'backlog' of CSF and, consequently, enlarged ventricles. In non-communicating hydrocephalus, there is an obstruction to the flow of CSF within the ventricles, which results in enlarged ventricles.

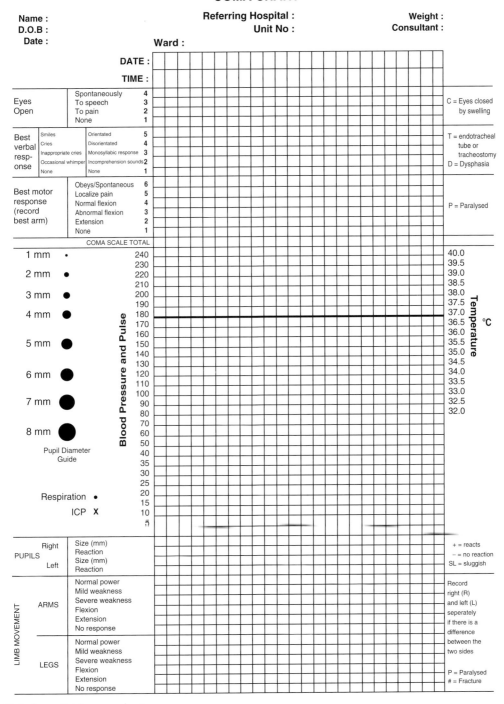

Figure 10.1  A paediatric coma chart.

There are many causes of hydrocephalus, including congenital abnormalities, intraventricular haemorrhage (for example in the premature infant), cerebral tumours, trauma and post meningitis.

The outcome for children with hydrocephalus is variable and is associated with the degree and duration of raised intracranial pressure, and the underlying primary brain pathology.

## PRESENTATION

The typical appearance of a baby with hydrocephalus includes increased head circumference and bulging fontanelle, sunsetting eyes and dilated scalp veins; poor feeding, vomiting, irritability and drowsiness will also occur. The older child will display symptoms of vomiting and headache, lethargy, possible developmental delay and poor school performance.

## DIAGNOSIS

An initial diagnosis of hydrocephalus can be made in the infant using cranial ultrasound through the anterior fontanelle. It is of particular benefit for the clinically unstable, premature, ventilated infant, and in addition avoids radiation to the young brain.

For the vast majority of children, however, a CT scan will provide a definitive diagnosis of hydrocephalus. Although performing a CT head scan is now a rapid procedure, infants and toddlers will often require sedation or occasionally a general anaesthetic.

## TREATMENT

A ventricular peritoneal shunt is the most common form of treatment for hydrocephalus: a short proximal catheter is inserted into the lateral ventricle, connected to a reservoir and then to a one way valve which controls the flow rate of CSF passing through it; the distal catheter leading downwards from the valve enters the abdominal cavity, and CSF is reabsorbed into the venous system. A ventricular atrial shunt is used when the peritoneal cavity is unsuitable, for example if the child has peritoneal adhesions due to previous infections.

A shunt is intended to stay in place for life, although alterations and revisions may well be required. The incidence of mechanical shunt malfunction is approximately 30% over 1 year and peaks in the first few months after shunt insertion.

Shunt blockage is the most common shunt complication in paediatrics and constitutes 50% of all shunt complications (Detwiller et al 1999).

Neuroendoscopic ventriculostomy is becoming a popular alternative for the treatment of obstructive hydrocephalus such as idiopathic aqueduct stenosis, or secondary to a cerebral tumour (Drake 1993). During this procedure, an endoscope is passed into the lateral ventricle, through the foramen into the third ventricle. The floor of the ventricle is then fenestrated and the resulting hole dilated with a balloon catheter, which is then withdrawn. CSF draining through the fenestration is absorbed via the basal cisterns back into the venous system. Successful ventriculostomy and fenestration avoids the need for a shunt and is consequently highly desirable.

## PREOPERATIVE CARE FOR THE CHILD WITH HYDROCEPHALUS

Treatment begins on admission and this includes the family's participation in the care of their child, and their involvement in discussions regarding treatment plans and options. Once diagnosis has been established with a CT scan, the parents should be provided with written and verbal information regarding hydrocephalus, and given time to discuss their anxieties and concerns.

The age and cognitive ability of the child will determine the extent of preparation and explanation required. A play specialist can assist with the child's psychological preparation, using dolls, drawings and discussions as appropriate.

A blood profile and cross match will be required; this may be the child's first experience of venepuncture, and particular care should be taken to minimise trauma, using explanation and an anaesthetic cream.

## POSTOPERATIVE CARE

In addition to the usual postoperative requirements, the child's neurological status should be regularly assessed using a paediatric coma scale, and any deterioration promptly reported. An open fontanelle is a good indication of a baby's intracranial pressure, and should be used in conjunction with the coma scale. Following insertion of a ventricular peritoneal shunt, the child should initially be nursed flat in accordance with local policy, and slowly elevated over the following days. The breast feeding mother may be anxious and lacking in confidence, and can be assisted in feeding her infant by placing the baby on a pillow and thus maintaining the desired position. Winding can be a problem whilst the baby is nursed flat, and placing the baby on his stomach during winding will usually relieve this.

Following a ventriculostomy, the child will often be nursed in a semi-upright position, to aid flow of CSF through the newly formed fenestration.

Following either of the above procedures, intravenous fluids may be necessary until oral feeding is re-established. Regular analgesia is required, particularly following a shunt procedure, where the neck and abdomen may cause particular discomfort due to the passing of the peritoneal catheter. Codeine phosphate in addition to paracetamol and diclofenac should be used where required and appropriate. Local hospital policy with regard to wound care and dressings should be followed.

Family involvement is essential throughout the child's care, and the nurse and parent should work in partnership in assisting the child's recovery.

## COMPLICATIONS OF TREATMENT

### Following ventriculostomy

Patient selection is an important factor in the success of fenestration (Buenolz 1991). The probability of success includes the diagnosis of idiopathic aqueduct stenosis in a baby over 3 months of age and the absence of meningitis or subarachnoid haemorrhage (Koch & Wagner 2004). With appropriate patient selection, 56–87% of patients will achieve shunt independence, with adults having a better outcome than children (Grunert et al 1994). Surgical complications following ventriculostomy are rare, but include infection and haemorrhage.

### Following shunt insertion

1. Shunt blockage can occur at any time and at any age. This constitutes a neurosurgical emergency and requires a revision of part or all of the shunt system. Prolonged delay in treatment can result in neurological deterioration, coma and eventually death. To educate a family in the dangers of shunt blockage, whilst encouraging them to allow their child a degree of independence, takes skill and understanding from the team and courage from the family.

2. Shunt infection is usually due to contamination at the time of surgery and is most likely to occur within 2–3 months of shunt insertion (Scheinblum & Hammond 1990). Signs and symptoms of shunt infection include pyrexia, sepsis and probable shunt blockage. Should a shunt infection occur, the child will require to have the existing shunt removed and an external ventricular drain inserted. The nursing care required is very specific and should only be undertaken by those trained to do so (Birdsall & Greif 1990). Following a period of intravenous and intrathecal antibiotics, a new shunt will be inserted.

3. Overdrainage can also occur following shunt insertion and although this usually resolves as the child adjusts to the new intracranial pressure in the following postoperative weeks, further surgery may occasionally be required. This involves changing the valve in the shunt system, utilisation of a 'programmable' shunt or insertion of an anti-siphoning system. In very extreme cases, a decompression temporal craniectomy may be performed, which acts as a false fontanelle and allows fluctuations in intracranial pressure.

## DISCHARGE PLANNING

By the time the child has recovered sufficiently from surgery to be discharged from the neurosurgical unit, the parents need to feel educated and confident in the care of their child. The ward should produce written information regarding the child's care and this should be used in conjunction with verbal discussion and education. In the light of growing litigation today, many units will require the parents' signatures to confirm that they have read and understood the literature provided.

Following ventriculostomy, the family should be advised to contact the neurosurgical unit if the child does not recover from the presenting symptoms, or if these symptoms reoccur in the future. Again, written information should be provided in addition to verbal discussion.

For those children who have required a shunt, it is often initially difficult to distinguish between shunt blockage and common children's illnesses. Headaches and vomiting are common childhood ailments, but are also classic signs of shunt blockage, particularly in association with increasing drowsiness. Parents must therefore be encouraged to contact their GP, local hospital or neurosurgical unit should their child become unwell. The neurosurgical unit has a responsibility to ensure that the community carers (GP, health visitor, community nurse) are fully informed about the child's discharge and care needs. Written information regarding hydrocephalus is often appreciated by community teams, who may not be familiar with the diagnosis.

The Association of Spina Bifida and Hydrocephalus (ASBAH) (see useful addresses, below) offers support to many families, including local fieldwork services, and study days for professionals, parents and people with hydrocephalus; it also provides a wide range of information sheets.

## LONG TERM OUTLOOK FOR CHILDREN WITH HYDROCEPHALUS

The long term outlook for children with hydrocephalus is very variable, and is dependent on aetiology, complications such as infection, and the degree of any underlying neurological damage. Many children with hydrocephalus have normal cognitive abilities and IQ: however, subtle difficulties such as problems with visual and spatial awareness can be difficult to recognise. Additional difficulties may include problems with sequencing and an inability to organise tasks in the correct order; there may also be difficulties with recognising patterns, shapes and words. In a study by Hoppe-Hirshe and colleagues (1998) 60% of children with hydrocephalus entered mainstream school, although a significant number were 1 or 2 years behind their age group.

Each child is unique and the level of skills attained depends on many factors (May & Carter 1995). However, the attitude of the child's family and the surrounding environment will greatly influence the child's overall development and adaptation to the world. Confident and informed parents are therefore very important, and the process of educating and supporting them should be commenced by the ward nurse and multidisciplinary team, and continued into the community setting.

## SPINA BIFIDA

When spina bifida was first recognised 2000 years ago, most children died from secondary infection or hydrocephalus. Today, the expectation is to facilitate a long life span, with optimum quality of life.

Neural tube closure is completed by the 28th day of conception; in the case of spina bifida, a section of the neural tube fails to develop in the normal fashion and the surrounding bone and muscle cannot form around the spinal cord.

Geographical, racial and environmental factors are all associated with spina bifida, but the maternal use of folic acid and vitamin B, when commenced at least 1 month before conception, has been shown to reduce the incidence dramatically (May 2001).

Myelomeningocele occurs in 1 in 2000 births (Tulipan & Bruner 1997) and is the most devastating form of spina bifida. The lesion is usually exposed and leaking CSF; occasionally it may be covered by a thin membrane. Meningocele is a less common abnormality, consisting of a skin sac enclosing normal meninges; since neural tissue is not exposed, the neurological outlook for the child is more optimistic than in the case of myelomeningocele. Spina bifida occulta describes a collection of other congenital spinal abnormalities which include tethering and splitting of the lower end of the cord; these rare conditions may benefit from corrective surgery and are not described below.

Spina bifida can be identified in utero, and in the Western world ultrasound is routinely available for all pregnant women. Amniocentesis can also be performed, which measures the amount of alpha-fetoprotein in the amniotic fluid; this is known to be raised in cases of open spina bifida. Termination of the pregnancy may be an option for certain families.

Spina bifida will be apparent at birth. The baby's leg movement will be assessed, bowel and bladder function considered and any signs of hydrocephalus noted. An open lesion should be kept moist until surgically closed, and saline soaked gauze or paraffin gauze should be applied. Babies should be nursed prone or on their sides to protect the lesion.

Despite any antenatal knowledge of the presence of spina bifida, most parents will be distressed following delivery of their baby. A frank discussion should take place involving the doctor, nurse and parents with regard to the possible long term implications for the baby and the whole family. Presuming that the level of dysfunction is not so devastating as to consider withholding treatment, treatment should commence immediately in the hope of reducing the risk of complications. This would include early surgical closure of the lesion to reduce the risk of infection, and to assist the bonding process between mother and infant by making the baby easier to handle, and perhaps more aesthetically pleasing. A ventricular peritoneal shunt is often required for the treatment of secondary hydrocephalus which may become more evident following closure of the back lesion. Urethral catheterisation may be required, and assistance with defecation in the form of laxatives and suppositories may be necessary.

## PREOPERATIVE CARE

In addition to the above, the normal neonatal requirements such as warmth, establishing feeding, and hygiene are necessary, and the nurse should encourage and assist the mother with the care of her baby. The psychological needs of the family also need addressing, and whilst recognising their grief and sadness, the nurse should adopt a realistic but positive approach with the family and encourage them to bond with, and care for their child.

## POSTOPERATIVE CARE

Alongside the routine postoperative requirements of any neonate, neurological observations must be performed to assess any increase in intracranial pressure, and also to assess limb movement, which may have altered following surgery. It is routine practice to nurse these babies flat and off their backs for a few days following surgery, in an attempt to promote wound healing by avoiding local pressure. Intravenous fluids may be required, but oral feeding should be established as early as possible. The mother may need assistance from the nurse when feeding her baby, and this can be a time for discussion and psychological support.

Analgesia should be given as required, and particularly prior to any interventions such as moving the baby and physiotherapy treatment. The parents should be encouraged by the physiotherapist to perform passive limb movements and correct positioning, so that they can continue this necessary treatment themselves in the future.

Contamination of the wound from feces and urine is highly likely and should be attended to promptly to avoid infection. Assessment of bladder and bowel function will continue, and appropriate actions should be taken.

Involvement of the family in the baby's care is essential in the bonding process, and also helps address difficulties they may face in the future. Many of these difficulties may not yet be apparent

to the family, but early involvement from a social worker can mean that potential needs and requirements are anticipated and met. Practical advice can be given with regard to potential future needs such as wheelchairs and seating, early financial support in the form of Disability Living Allowance (DLA) can be encouraged.

## DISCHARGE PLANNING

The urodynamics team and general paediatrician will continue to work with the family with regard to urinary and fecal incontinence. Parents will initially be taught to catheterise the baby intermittently if necessary, and to give regular glycerine suppositories as required.

Head circumference will need measuring by the community team as hydrocephalus can occur if the baby is not already shunted.

Physiotherapy will be a long term requirement. Most children will achieve their maximum level of ambulation at around 4 years of age (McLone & Ito 1998), and parents should therefore be encouraged to assist with physiotherapy treatment from when the child is at an early age.

The immediate needs of the baby on discharge may be relatively simple, and only as time progresses will longer term requirements become evident. The hospital team will liaise with the community team with regard to the baby's condition on discharge, and good communication should be continued. Any signs of hydrocephalus or problems with an existing shunt should prompt a referral back to the neurosurgeon. Physiotherapy is essential, and an occupational therapist, if available, will become a good resource for the family. ASBAH provide invaluable support to these children and their families, and should be contacted at an early stage.

## LONG TERM OUTLOOK FOR THE CHILD WITH SPINA BIFIDA

The prognosis is extremely variable and is directly related to the degree of neurological damage. Regular hospital visits will disrupt the child's schooling and the family's lifestyle. Many difficulties will be faced during infancy, and will become more evident during puberty, adolescence and adulthood. Mobility and continence are major factors in the child's self-image, and life quality, and a supportive family environment can do much to assist with this. It is therefore essential that early bonding and caring is established within the family and this should be encouraged immediately following birth. The hospital multidisciplinary team can have an important impact on the long term outcome for these children, and must ensure they are appropriately educated in the relevant care needs.

## HEAD INJURY

Approximately 40 000 children a year are admitted to hospital in the UK following a head injury; head injury is now the most common cause of death in children, accounting for 10% of all deaths in the 0–15 age group (Appleton 1994). Head injuries in children vary according to the age of the child, a significant number occurring in children under 1 year of age; this includes birth injury and non-accidental injury. The disproportionately larger and heavier heads of young children make them more prone to head injury, for example by falling against furniture and down stairs as they become more mobile. Between 4 and 8 years of age, head injury is more likely to occur due to accidents in playgrounds, road traffic accidents and bicycle accidents. During the warmer summer months when windows are left open, the incidence of head injury increases. Incidence decreases until the mid teens when there is a rapid increase in head injury associated with motor vehicles and alcohol intoxication (May 2001).

Mild head injury is presented in over half the children seen in the Accident and Emergency department. Memory impairment, sleep disturbance and reduced concentration can occur even following mild head injury, and the Medical Disability Society recommends that all children should routinely be followed up following all head injuries.

Primary head injury describes the initial injury, and can be focal or diffuse. Approximately two thirds of deaths occur at the scene of the accident; for those who survive, the outcome is unpredictable, although the severity of the injury gives some indication of the long term outcome. Secondary injury describes the cascade of events which follow the primary injury and which may lead to ischaemia and infarction.

### EMERGENCY MANAGEMENT

Initial resuscitation and stabilisation at the scene of the accident and en route to the hospital will have a profound effect on the outcome for the child. Adequate oxygenation and maintenance of blood pressure are essential in providing brain perfusion, whilst also maintaining haemodynamic stability throughout the body. Early liaison between relevant teams such as neurosurgeons and intensivists is important in ensuring optimum treatment for the child.

Assessing and monitoring the neurological status of a young, distressed child can be immensely difficult, and yet level of consciousness is a good indicator of neurological change.

Whilst a team approach is always adopted in the management of these children, it is often the nurse who is the most consistent assessor of the child, and it is therefore important that nurses are appropriately educated and competent in such assessments. Nurses must be able to utilise an appropriate coma scale and act upon the findings. Michaud et al (1992) found that the Glasgow coma scale (GCS) was a better predictor of morbidity 72 hours following head injury, as opposed to immediately following the trauma. Clearly, many other factors will be involved in the outcome, including severity of total injuries and pupillary responses in the emergency room. However, Michaud's study does indicate the importance of ongoing neurological assessment following head injury. Nurses are responsible for ensuring their own competence in this process.

The family must be kept informed and updated of the child's progress. Although it may be impractical for them to remain at the bedside the entire time, they may wish to assist in their child's care where appropriate, for example by performing mouth care and washing their child. Parents are often reassured to hear what treatment and care their child is receiving, because they interpret this to mean that the situation is not hopeless (Hazinski 1992). Families will watch staff and interpret their behaviour and interventions as clues about their child's condition; a competent and experienced nurse will help reassure and support them. The nurse must also provide information, correct misconceptions and validate concerns. Additional support should be provided for family members as appropriate, for example from the social worker or hospital chaplain (Plowfield 1999).

### THE INTENSIVE TREATMENT UNIT (ITU)

Traumatic head injury is a series of pathophysiological events that vary in severity, and over time.

Oxygenation and haemodynamic stability remain in the forefront of management protocols. Avoidance and active treatment of intracranial hypertension is essential: surgical mass lesions should be removed as soon after injury as possible; raised intracranial pressure will occur in 75% of all children with severe head injuries and medical management should be instigated immediately in an attempt to reduce or control this.

Ventilation will be required in children with severe head injuries. Hyperventilation may be used to reduce cerebral blood flow and intracranial pressure, although the period of hyperventilation and its effectiveness remain controversial.

Patient positioning has an effect on intracranial pressure: elevating the head of the bed by 30 degrees and maintaining the head of the child in the neutral position, avoiding neck flexion, both help facilitate venous return from the brain. Intrathoracic and intraabdominal pressure can also interfere with venous return and intracranial pressure, so the nurse should avoid placing the child prone, or with extreme hip flexion. These are simple measures which can assist with improved patient outcomes, and it is the nurse's responsibility to provide good positioning and pressure area care as soon as the child's condition allows.

Intracranial pressure monitoring may be undertaken and treatment strategies planned accordingly. Hyperventilation, external ventricular drainage and the use of diuretics are among the strategies commonly utilised to control or reduce raised intracranial pressure; sedation and neuromuscular blocks alongside analgesia are routine practice in assisting this treatment aim. The control of hyperthermia and seizures and consequent cerebral metabolism is essential. Fluid management consists of maintaining blood pressure and organ perfusion; current thinking is that restricting fluid input has minimal effect on cerebral oedema and may cause hypotension (Hickey 1997).

Nutrition should be implemented in the form of parenteral nutrition or enteral feeding, according to the child's condition. Early neurological recovery has been found to occur more rapidly when early nutrition has been established, although it is recognised that this may take several days (Gardener 1986).

Chest physiotherapy should be given where indicated, and concerns about transient increases in intracranial pressure due to treatment should not deter from good positioning, oxygenation and treatment of chest consolidation and collapse.

Rehabilitation of the child with head injuries begins on admission to the unit, and the physiotherapist can explain to the nurse and parents the importance of good positioning and movement; parents often wish to feel useful and this can be one way they can help with their child's care in conjunction with the nurse.

Greater detail concerning the child's care on the ITU can be obtained from Hazinski (1992).

## REHABILITATION

As ventilation is withdrawn, an early picture of the child's neurological status becomes evident. There is often a stage of extreme agitation, due to pain, fear, withdrawal of medications (in particular morphine), cerebral irritation or raised intracranial pressure. Parents will often feel a sense of immense relief that their child has survived, alongside a growing fear of what the future may hold. This unpredictability can result in stress and frustration. Parents will usually be utterly exhausted. Parental involvement is an essential part of the child's care but each situation should be assessed individually: sleep and support may be appropriate for some families at this stage, whereas others may need to be involved in all stages of their child's care. The experienced nurse will treat each family individually and advise accordingly.

Protecting the child from self harm may be an important part of the nurse's role during this early stage of recovery from severe head injury, and constant supervision and the use of cot sides on the bed are essential. The child may display aggressive behaviour and have violent and abusive outbursts; this status is usually temporary, but in the case of extreme brain damage this may be a permanent state. Once again, the unpredictability of outcome, and the feeling of helplessness that the parents experience (and embarrassment at their child's language) need to be recognised and addressed. If the family feel understood and supported, they will be able to provide a higher level of support for their child (Addison & Shah 1999).

Families feel more in control when nurses ask for their assistance in caring for their children, for example by giving medications, or helping decrease children's agitation by holding their hands or reading to them (Plowfield 1999). It is often difficult for the family to see their child distressed by necessary treatment such as physiotherapy; explanation of the importance of such treatment and encouraging their participation will help dissipate this distress. Teaching parents how to perform stretching and positioning, application of splints and so forth has a dual purpose: the child receives more physiotherapy than the therapist alone can offer, and the parents feel useful and that they are contributing to the rehabilitation of their child.

The nurse must involve the family members in assisting in meeting the child's needs and implementing the stages of rehabilitation, and this includes safety, hygiene, nutrition, physiotherapy, stimulation, play and forward planning. Early intervention usually involves the child's physical needs and the emphasis gradually changes to encourage functional and intellectual recovery.

Play is an important rehabilitation tool for the young child; the role of the play specialist is recognised as being distinct from nursing, but the two team members should work together to provide a continual catalyst for play. Behaviour such as self-injury can arise through frustration and lack of stimulation and children with restricted mobility and communication should be provided with appropriate play opportunities. Activities designed to promote sensory stimulation can be both educational and enjoyable. Basic play activities that involve physical contact and holding may give pleasure to the child and family, although this may not apply to all children, particularly in the early stages of recovery, when the child may resist such contact.

Speech and language therapy may be required and will often be used in conjunction with the dietitian with regard to feeding, and with the clinical psychologist if there are problems with communication.

Nurses are usually pivotal in coordinating the child's complex care and integrating all the disciplines to provide the optimum mixture of treatment, rest, play and sleep on a 24 hour basis. Weekends are usually times when many other professionals on the team are absent, and the nurse and family need to continue the child's treatment programmes to the best of their abilities.

## DISCHARGE PLANS

Children may be transferred to a local hospital, a rehabilitation unit, or directly home, depending on their condition and the availability of local services.

The aim of the occupational therapist – resources permitting – is to attempt to rehabilitate the child in terms of play, feeding, washing and other activities of daily living. Occupational therapists will often work in conjunction with social services and local teams to assess the finances and resources available with regard to wheelchairs, seating and the home environment.

Realistic and achievable goals must be set in conjunction with community teams and early communication regarding the child's condition is essential for forward planning.

Returning to school is a goal for the child and family, although cognitive problems may necessitate a change in schools. Reassessment of the child will involve many professionals, including the occupational therapist, educational psychologist and school teacher. Aggressive or antisocial behaviour may be present, and add further complication to schooling.

The expectation for this group of children is that their recovery progresses and that the goals set in conjunction with the family are realistic and achievable. From the early stages of recovery and rehabilitation it is essential that nurses teach parents to be involved in their child's care, and that the family's needs are met. Self-care and independence are promoted as they would be in normal childhood development, but many families need encouragement to achieve this (Greenwood 1994). Empowering families will lead to improved outcomes for the child and family.

## LONG TERM OUTCOME

Mortality rates following severe head injury in children remain high, particularly when associated with a low GCS score, multiple trauma, shock and hypoxia. Whilst mortality rates vary, Scott-Jupp et al (1992) found that 35% of children in their study required special schooling following severe head injury, and 42% had persistent neurological impairment; long and short term memory is often affected with serious consequences. Following minor head injuries, families will often describe the child as 'just not the same'.

Normal patterns of family behaviour are disrupted and the family structure and functioning may change. Up to 50% of families with a child with severe head injury suffer high levels of stress and disrupted family dynamics (Rivara et al 1992). Hospital and community teams must continue their support of these families in the long term.

## THE FUTURE

National guidelines for the treatment of children with head injury remain difficult to establish due to the lack of clinical trials. However, treatment should be based on studies of recovery rather than mortality.

The aim of care should be prevention. Cycle accidents are the most common cause of head injury: government policy, motoring associations, parental cooperation, education and school involvement should all be involved in helping to reduce the incidence of cycle accidents.

## NON-ACCIDENTAL INJURY (NAI)

Brain injury caused by NAI can be caused by blows to the head, being thrown against a hard surface, strangulation or, most frequently, violent shaking. Any child under 2 years of age with a head injury should be evaluated with regard to having suffered an NAI, and it should be considered that this injury may have been caused by a parent or carer. All staff should be familiar with the Trust's child protection policies and procedures so that appropriate action and treatment are instigated. This may include immediate involvement of social services and the police to ensure the safety of other family members, particularly other children.

In the absence of any external injury, children may be brought to the Accident and Emergency department with a history of vomiting, irritability and seizures. Alternatively, children may arrive by ambulance, with parents or carers reporting that they found the child cyanosed and had attempted to revive the child by shaking.

The child's immediate needs may be resuscitation, seizure control and blood transfusion. Once the child is stabilised, a CT scan may provide the diagnosis of subdural haematoma. This may occasionally require 'tapping' (withdrawal of subdural blood via the anterior fontanelle). The child should be examined for signs of retinal haemorrhage and fractures to other areas of the body, rib fractures of differing ages being a common occurrence in association with NAI.

Children who are not ventilated may be extremely irritable and dislike handling. Analgesia does little to soothe the child at this stage and caring for these young children can be very distressing. Nursing staff are particularly vulnerable emotionally, since they are the most consistent carers of these children, and discussion, support and an open approach from the team are helpful.

When NAI is suspected, communication between parents and professionals must be maintained. Investigations and discussions must be conducted fairly and openly, despite the emotions that may be aroused by the professionals now caring for the child. Professionals may initially be reluctant to be involved in a process that might bring about the separation of children from their families, or cause disruption of the entire family unit. The social worker can help guide colleagues, and provide a support network should this become necessary.

Mortality and morbidity are variable, depending on the degree of neurological damage. Should the child survive, blindness, seizures and developmental delay are among the common complications of severe NAI involving the brain. Occasionally, a subdural peritoneal shunt will be required on a short term basis, but will do little to improve the longer term morbidity.

## BRAIN TUMOURS

Brain tumours are the most common solid tumour of childhood and the second most common neoplasm (Shiminski–Mayer & Shields 1995). Brain tumours in children account for 20% of childhood cancers, 400–500 new brain tumours being diagnosed annually in the UK. Brain tumours in children differ from those found in the adult population with regard to their position and histology (Tobias & Hayward 1989).

50–60% of childhood brain tumours originate in the posterior fossa and these include medulloblastomas, ependymomas and astrocytomas. The remaining 40–50% are supratentorial and include craniopharyngiomas, optic pathway tumours, hypothalamic tumours and astrocytomas. Primitive neuroectodermal tumours (PNETs) can occur in any position.

Medulloblastoma is the most common malignant brain tumour in children and accounts for 20% of all childhood brain tumours. It originates in the cerebellum and often invades the fourth ventricle and brain stem; dissemination down the spinal cord is not uncommon. The prognosis remains poor, particularly for the infant; the presence of metastatic disease at diagnosis and an incomplete surgical resection are also indicative of a poor outlook.

Survival is estimated at 50–60% overall, following treatment with radiotherapy and/or chemotherapy.

Astrocytomas comprise 33–40% of childhood brain tumours and can occur anywhere within the brain, although they are more commonly found in the posterior fossa and brain stem. Prognosis depends on histology (20% are malignant) and surgical accessibility. Complete removal of a benign astrocytoma offers a long term cure, whereas incomplete removal of a malignant astrocytoma offers a poor prognosis.

Ependymomas originate from the ependymal cells of the ventricular lining, commonly in the fourth ventricle; hydrocephalus is common and spinal metastases sometimes occur (less than 10% at diagnosis). Surgical excision of this posterior fossa lesion remains the initial treatment, followed by chemotherapy in the infant, and radiotherapy and/or chemotherapy in the older child, depending on the degree of surgical resection. A total surgical excision offers the best prognosis; recurrence following surgery and radiotherapy offers a poor prognosis long term.

Further details regarding specific childhood brain tumours can be obtained from more detailed literature (e.g. May 2001).

The presenting signs and symptoms of the child with a brain tumour depend on the position of the tumour, related cerebral oedema and the presence of hydrocephalus. Since many of the presenting signs and symptoms mimic those of common childhood illnesses (lethargy, vomiting, irritability and headache), diagnosis is often difficult to establish. A delay in diagnosis may lead to anger and guilt on the part of the parents, and lack of trust in the medical team. Reassurance must be given that an earlier diagnosis would have been unlikely to alter the long term prognosis.

Signs and symptoms may vary depending on the age of the child and the position of the tumour. Most children will present with headaches and those with posterior fossa lesions will suffer from vomiting and ataxia; visual disturbance and cranial nerve involvement may also be present. Seizures and hemiparesis, intellectual deterioration and endocrine disturbance may occur in supratentorial lesions, depending on the structures involved. The child may have visited the GP on several occasions before the presence of raised intracranial pressure, and particularly hydrocephalus, may tip the balance and render the child acutely ill. Retrospectively, it may be seen that other symptoms may have been present over the previous weeks/months.

The diagnosis of a brain tumour as established by CT or MRI scanning is totally devastating to the family. The immediate concerns are for their child's survival, but as the diagnosis sinks in, thoughts of physical and intellectual disability arise, and the medical team can offer no definite outcomes at this preliminary stage.

The anxiety and uncertainty following diagnosis of a brain tumour will cause enormous distress to the family, and an anxious family will result in an anxious child. The nursing team in particular can offer support, information and explanation to the family and, where appropriate, to the child.

## PREOPERATIVE CARE

In the majority of cases, surgical excision will be attempted. The use of steroids, in particular dexamethasone, will reduce oedema around the tumour and improve the child's symptoms temporarily. Explanations need to be simple and repeated, both to the family and to the child. Information should be consistent, which requires good communication between professionals.

In addition to CT and MRI scanning, investigations are minimal: a blood profile and cross match will be required and a physiotherapy assessment may be appropriate; a thorough baseline assessment of the child by a paediatrician is required. Consent for surgery should be taken by the surgeon performing the operation, and the potential complications explained. The presence of a nurse during the consent process will enable the parents to question points they are unclear about, and to receive a consistent explanation.

Preparation of older children begins by discovering what they perceive as their illness and what they think is going to happen. All preparation should be undertaken with parents' consent, and assessed on the individual child's needs and comprehension, answers being given as fully and honestly as appropriate. Preparation can be given by the play specialist if available, or the ward nurses. Parents will also need preparing, and in addition to discussion with the doctor, time for discussion with a nurse usually proves invaluable.

## POSTOPERATIVE CARE

In addition to the routine management of the child's airway and haemodynamic state, the following care is required postoperatively: regular neurological assessment and early recognition, reporting and treatment of raised intracranial pressure; fluid management, including blood replacement as required; recognition and treatment of complications such as seizures; administration of analgesia; safety of the child (visual disturbance, ataxia and confusion may render the child more vulnerable to self-harm and cot sides and supervision may be required); comfort and support to both child and family.

The care required by these children should ideally be undertaken within a paediatric neurosurgical unit, where all team members are skilled in this speciality. Deterioration can be rapid, particularly in the baby and infant, and nurses, who will usually be the frontline carers, must therefore ensure that they have adequate knowledge and skills to deal with such situations quickly and efficiently.

Nausea and vomiting can persist in the days following surgery, and the child will need supporting with intravenous fluids and antiemetics; plasma electrolytes will need to be checked. Feeding should be re-established as soon as tolerated, although nasogastric feeding may be required for those children who remain reluctant to feed, or who have difficulty in swallowing. Visual disturbance can be difficult to assess in the young, non verbal child and the parents' understanding of their child should be used in conjunction with professional assessment. Diplopia is usually temporary and can be relieved to a certain extent by eye patching (if tolerated); visual field defects can occur due to surgical trauma or increased intracranial pressure, and placing toys or books on the side of the bed where the child's vision is intact may help reduce frustration.

Motor and sensory deficits will relate to the surgical site. Young children adapt remarkably well to changes in mobility and with the help of physiotherapy, occupational therapy and a positive approach from parents, most children will mobilise to the best of their ability.

Any member of the team should be available to advise and support the child and family; resources permitting, this should include a clinical and educational psychologist, both in the immediate and longer term. A social worker and hospital chaplain also form an important part of this support system, and it usually falls to the nurse to coordinate such links.

The implications of complications following treatment for a brain tumour can be profound. Long term concerns include changes in body image, cognitive changes, the presence of hydrocephalus, quality of life, changes in family dynamics, endocrine disturbances, personality changes and long term prognosis. Clearly these children need an individual who coordinates their care and this is, when available, a clinical nurse specialist, who can also guide the parents through the next stage of treatment, whether that be chemotherapy, radiotherapy, a watch and wait policy or palliative care.

Discharge planning can be complex. The damaging effect of a brain tumour on the developing brain is highly significant but not always immediately apparent. Survivors of central nervous system (CNS) disease are identified as having special educational needs and requiring physical and psychological support after treatment (Glaser et al 1997). Families must be able to recognise and access available sources for support and advice and this should be facilitated by healthcare professionals. With such assistance, the family will become more confident and independent, and reintegration back into society is made easier.

Adjuvant therapy is required for the majority of children with brain surgery since surgery alone is rarely curative with malignant CNS tumours. External beam radiation is generally used to treat CNS tumours and this can include craniospinal radiation, radiation to the whole brain or localised radiation. Treatment is given daily over a period of 5–6 weeks, and toddlers may require sedation or general anaesthesia for each treatment. In addition to the consequences from this, other short term effects can include cerebral oedema, drowsiness, apathy and irritability. Radiation results in damage to the cell nucleus and although many cells survive the initial onslaught of radiotherapy, they are rendered unable to divide at mitosis. Demyelination and white matter necrosis occur and the long term consequences include cognitive and educational deterioration, pubertal disturbance, a reduction in growth hormone production and a disturbance in thyroid production

Chemotherapy alone is not curative in intent for the majority of children with CNS tumours. It has been used to delay or avoid the use of cranial radiation, particularly in the young child, and is currently utilised as part of an integrated treatment plan which comprises surgery, radiation and chemotherapy. The blood–brain barrier is a physiological constraint impeding drug delivery to the brain and, consequently, high doses of chemotherapy are required. This can result in severe immunosuppression and further complications and hospitalisation for the child. Long term effects include neurodevelopmental decline, endocrine disturbance, hearing loss, renal impairment and infertility.

As survival following surgery, radiotherapy and chemotherapy improves, so the spectrum of late effects becomes more evident. Specific definitions of morbidity must be identified, if the consequences of cure are to be reduced.

## TUMOURS OF THE SPINE AND SPINAL CORD

Primary spinal tumours are rare. Surgical removal of the tumour is not always possible or desirable (as in the case of a diffuse intrinsic tumour). However, surgery for acute spinal decompression may be necessary and a spinal jacket may be required for support following extensive laminectomy. Torticollis, kyphosis, limitation of movement and pain are all consequences following extensive laminectomy and long term follow-up throughout childhood should be undertaken.

Despite chemotherapy and radiotherapy, the prognosis is variable and dependent on the extent of the tumour and its histology.

Metastases from primary infratentorial tumours can seed into the spinal cord causing localised pain, bladder and sphincter disturbance and motor impairment. Surgical excision is rarely possible and treatment is by localised radiotherapy and occasionally chemotherapy can be beneficial in the short term.

## CONGENITAL MALFORMATIONS

### ANENCEPHALY

Anencephaly describes a rare congenital abnormality where the neural groove has failed to develop in utero, and has not formed a covering of mesoderm or ectoderm. The exposed brain is represented by a dysfunctional mass of nervous tissue including the brain stem and a few cranial nerves. Most fetuses are stillborn, but may occasionally survive for a few hours.

### ENCEPHALOCELES

Encephaloceles are very rare and occur most frequently in the occipital position, although anterior encephaloceles do occur. The aetiology of encephaloceles is unknown.

Posterior encephaloceles are obvious at birth and if diagnosed antenatally will be a tremendous shock to the family. The soft swelling protrudes through the underlying bone defect and may contain meninges alone, or meninges and cerebral tissue. The head is small and there are often abnormalities within, such as hydrocephalus, and Chiari type malformations (the latter involves a spectrum of abnormalities involving the hind brain). Neurological examination may be normal at birth due to the immaturity of the brain, with defects such as seizures, focal weakness, spasticity, visual impairments and cranial nerve involvement becoming more obvious as the child develops.

In addition to the normal requirements of the newborn baby, these babies require careful handling of the encephalocele. Ulceration, weeping and infection can occur and, in the presence of hydrocephalus, the sac may increase rapidly in size. The head should be turned regularly and particular attention given to skin integrity. With caution paraffin gauze can be gently applied to a weeping or ulcerated area (see Ch. 4). A hat can be applied over the encephalocele if the parents find this more aesthetically pleasing, particularly in front of other parents. The mother may need advice and encouragement from the nurses when handling her baby. The uncertainty of long term outcome may cause additional problems with bonding between baby and parent; race, religion and cultural background may affect the family's attitude to the baby and various members of the multidisciplinary team, including the social worker and hospital chaplain, should be involved.

Attention must be given to temperature control because of excessive heat loss from the head. Nasogastric feeding may be necessary if the baby is reluctant to feed orally, and the mother may wish to express her own milk and then participate in her baby's feeding.

Discussions with the family concerning the ethics of surgery are important. Encephaloceles may become necrotic and rupture, and surgical excision is recommended except where the child's condition is clearly not compatible with life. The risks of mortality and morbidity should be discussed, and there must be a clear understanding that although surgery is aimed at preserving existing neurology, it is unlikely to improve it.

Surgery involves preserving normal cerebral tissue where possible, and excision of dysplastic tissue; the sac will be removed and a watertight repair performed; treatment for hydrocephalus may be necessary at this time or at a later date.

The postoperative needs involve the normal requirements of a neonate: warmth, comfort and nutrition are all essential and the mother should be encouraged to participate in her baby's care. She should feel more confident in handling her baby following removal of the encephalocele, and perhaps find her baby more 'acceptable' to other parents on the ward. Nurses must be aware of the complex emotions felt by the parents and in addition to offering their own support, they should facilitate support from other team members.

The baby's immediate needs on discharge are not complex, although the family may need much support from the community team in coming to terms with what the future holds, and coping with disabilities as they arise. There is a 9–47% mortality rate during the first few years of life (Date et al 1993), and the quality of that life is variable and unpredictable.

Anterior encephaloceles are apparent at birth with a skin covered midline swelling and a degree of hypertelorism. The majority of frontal encephaloceles contain non-functional cerebral tissue which can be surgically removed and a cosmetic repair performed. Hypertelorism may need to be corrected at a later date. The majority of these children will have normal motor skills and normal intelligence and once the shock of the abnormality has been addressed, bonding between parent and baby is usually good.

## ARACHNOID CYSTS

Arachnoid cysts can occur following trauma or cerebral atrophy, but a congenital arachnoid cyst can occur due to abnormal development of the arachnoid membrane. Arachnoid cysts causing mass effect or hydrocephalus require surgery either by removal of the cyst, fenestration, or insertion of a shunt. A Dandy Walker cyst describes a cystic malformation of the fourth ventricle and is associated with developmental delay.

Arnold Chiari malformations are a spectrum of abnormalities involving the hindbrain. The most common is Chiari type 2 and is found in most children with spina bifida. Compression of the brainstem can result in abnormalities affecting all associated functions, and obstruction to the flow of CSF from the fourth ventricle is responsible for hydrocephalus. In the majority of cases, insertion of a shunt is required and, very occasionally, surgery will be undertaken to provide more space for the hindbrain in the form of a foramen magnum decompression.

## SURGERY FOR EPILEPSY

Epilepsy is a chronic condition characterised by seizures; seizures can be defined as malfunctions of the brain's electrical system resulting from cortical neuronal discharge. The type of seizure is determined by the site of origin and may include involuntary movements, changes in perception, sensation and posture, and loss of or altered consciousness. Seizures can be induced by various acute neurological or medical conditions, including hypoxia, hypoglycaemia, pyrexia, drugs or infection. The term epilepsy can only be applied when seizures occur over a prolonged timescale. The aetiology of epilepsy is variable but it can be due to trauma, infection, prenatal (such as toxoplasmosis), congenital, vascular or idiopathic causes.

Epilepsy occurs in 1 in 200 of the population (0.5%), 75–90% commencing before the age of 20 (Austin & McDermott 1988). 80% of people with chronic epilepsy become seizure free on anticonvulsant therapy (Shorvon et al 1987), but the adverse effects of these drugs must be considered. Ideally, drugs should be introduced alone and adjusted until seizure control is achieved, or until the side effects of therapy become intolerable; only then should a second drug be introduced. Of the 20–25% of children in whom epilepsy therapy is ineffective, a small portion will be selected for surgery. Improvements in patient selection and operative techniques have now made epilepsy surgery a viable and reasonably safe alternative for this small group of children.

There are two types of surgery for epilepsy. The first type is functional, aimed at modifying seizure spread and thus defined as a palliative procedure; this includes corpus callosotomy (incision of the corpus callosum) and multiple subpial transection (transections are made horizontally in the superior cortex at 5 cm intervals). The second type is resective, aimed at removing the epileptogenic process, and this includes lobectomy, hemispherectomy (removing part or all of one cerebral hemisphere) and lesionectomy.

Seizures are thought to interfere with brain maturation, resulting in delay or arrest of developmental milestones; in addition, antiepileptic drugs may interfere with cortical maturation. The aim of epilepsy surgery is to stop/reduce the number of seizures and thus allow the child to develop. Many hopes and fears surround the family during the time of investigation and potential selection for surgery. The possibility of a real improvement in the quality of their child's life, and that of the whole family, can be overwhelming. Investigations can be traumatic and invasive, and with an uncertain outcome good communication between professionals and the family is essential in ensuring understanding and compliance.

## PRESURGICAL INVESTIGATIONS

The goal of investigations is to localise the epileptogenic focus and to assess the functional and structural normality of tissue beyond resection. Investigations are many. An initial electroencephalogram (EEG) will be performed, to identify and analyse seizure activity. Telemetry will then follow, during which continuous EEG recording will be performed alongside video monitoring. Invasive telemetry monitoring may be undertaken, during which intracranial electrodes will be used for EEG recording; the latter should only be undertaken in specialised units where both medical and nursing staff are appropriately trained. An MRI scan will be performed to detect abnormal lesions, cerebral atrophy or abnormal signal activity. Functional imaging may be performed, including single photon emission tomography (SPECT) scanning, where cerebral blood perfusion is measured and, more rarely, positive emission tomography (PET) scanning, where glucose, oxygen and metabolic activity are measured. Neuropsychological assessment forms an essential part of the investigation process in determining the location and extent of brain dysfunction. It further assists in identifying cognitive function, memory, language, visual–spatial function, processing and attention, and school attainment. Much of this assessment can be applied to underlying focal pathology or lesions, and to atypical cerebral disorganisation. The psychologist will also act as a source of guidance and advice for the family, who may be dealing with a child with multiple psychosocial difficulties, with behaviour and language that is unacceptable to society.

A multidisciplinary approach is required, with a key team member coordinating the very complex requirements of this family; this may be a liaison nurse or clinical nurse specialist if available.

Anticonvulsants will normally be withdrawn during this period of assessment, to ensure enough seizures occur for identification. This may render the child's behaviour and activity unpredictable, and this can be frightening for the child and family; skilled and understanding nursing is required, ensuring the child's safety alongside parental cooperation. Anxiety will be high with so much at stake, and support should be provided by all team members, including the social worker and hospital chaplain. Should the child be selected for surgery, a discussion should be undertaken between the parents and doctors about the realistic expectations and potential outcomes for their individual child. Surgery does not guarantee freedom from seizures, and the decision to proceed with surgery is difficult for many parents, when faced with a major surgical procedure with an uncertain outcome.

It is customary for the child to be discharged following these investigations and readmitted from the waiting list; this can be a long and difficult wait for many families, and the liaison nurse should remain in contact with the family, offering support and advice during this time.

## PREOPERATIVE CARE

Further discussion is often required with the parents at the time of surgery, and reassurance that they are allowing their child a chance for an improved quality of life.

The preoperative care is similar to that required for any craniotomy; in addition to the normal blood profile and cross match, clotting studies must be undertaken as anticonvulsant medication may have altered the normal clotting status. Anticonvulsants should be taken as prescribed to coincide with the last oral fluids taken prior to theatre; extra supervision may be required during the starvation time as some children may not be compliant with this, or understand what is explained. Preparing the child psychologically for theatre should be undertaken in conjunction with the parents, who have a unique understanding of their child's comprehension and coping mechanisms.

## POSTOPERATIVE CARE

Maintenance of a patent airway is of paramount importance, particularly if seizures occur; these fits, whilst of great concern to the family, are rarely of any significance and are related to handling of the brain rather than being an indication that surgery has failed. Protocols for control of postoperative seizures should be in place, and instigated when required. The child's normal anticonvulsant drugs must be continued postoperatively (orally, rectally or intravenously). Neurological assessment of the child must be undertaken as appropriate and possible: pupil reaction may be difficult to assess in the non-compliant child, and for those children with severe behavioural disturbances, experience and common sense are required by nurses when assessing the child's level of consciousness. Parents can be very helpful in recognising what is normal behaviour and verbalisation for their child, and they may be the only ones who can settle the child during this period. Analgesia should be given regularly, remembering that children may be unable to communicate their pain verbally. Monitoring of vital signs will be undertaken in line with local policy and used in conjunction with the coma scale to observe for relevant changes. Constant supervision of the child is essential, to ensure safety during the giving of intravenous fluids and blood products, and to ensure any Redivac bottles stay in place. Head bandages may be used, but compliance may once again be an issue.

Once sufficiently recovered and released from Redivac bottles and intravenous lines, these children usually become rapidly active and mobile. It is tempting to allow early discharge from hospital, but a period of lethargy and exhaustion often follows this period of hyperactivity, and each child and family must be assessed individually. Visual field defects may be present postoperatively, but this is usually best assessed at a later date.

Recovery is significantly slower following hemispherectomy, with lethargy, sleepiness and vomiting often occurring. Pyrexia is not uncommon and an infective cause is rarely found for this. Hemiparesis will be apparent to varying degrees following surgery, although this will not be a new symptom for many children. Physiotherapy and occupational therapy will enable the majority of children to regain acceptable mobility – young children are very adaptable and versatile.

In the days and months following surgery, it will become evident whether surgery has been successful or not. An absence or reduction in seizure activity and an improvement in their child's behaviour will provide a very different lifestyle for the families of those in whom surgery has been successful; if unsuccessful, there may be issues the family members wish to address, and much support will be required to help them deal with their disappointment and sadness.

# References

Addison C, Shah S 1999 Neurosurgery. In: Guerrero D (ed) Neuro-oncology for nurses. Whurr, London

Appleton R 1994 Head injury rehabilitation for children. Nursing Times 90(22): 29–30

Austin J, McDermott N 1988 Parental attitude of coping behaviour in families of children with epilepsy. Journal of Neuroscience Nursing 20(3): 174–178

Birdsall C, Greif I 1990 How do you manage external ventricular drainage? American Journal of Nursing Nov: 47–49

Buenolz RD 1991 Endoscopic coagulation of choroid plexus using the wand. Neurosurgery 28(3): 421–427

Date L, Yagyu Y, Assari S, Ohmoto T 1993 Long term outcome in surgically treated encephaloceles. Surgical Neurology 40:125–130

Detwiller PW, Porter RW, Rekate HL 1999 Hydrocephalus – clinical features and management. In: Choux M, Di Rocco C, Hockley A et al (eds) Paediatric Neurosurgery. Churchill Livingstone, London, p 263–264

Drake JM 1993 Ventriculostomy for treatment of hydrocephalus. Neurosurgical clinics of America AM 4: 657–666

Gardener D 1986 Acute management of the head injured adult. Nursing Clinics of North America 21: 555–561

Glaser AW, Abdul Rashid NF, Walker DA 1997 School behaviour and health status after central nervous system tumours in childhood. British Journal of Cancer 76(5): 643–650

Greenwood I 1994 The aims of paediatric rehabilitaion. Paediatric Nursing 6(9): 21–23

Grunert P, Perneczky A, Resch K 1994 Endoscopic procedures through the foramen intraventriculare of Munro under stereotactic conditions. Minim Invasive Neurosurgery 37: 42–47

Hazinski M 1992 Nursing care of the critically ill child. Mosby, St Louis, MO

Hickey JV 1997 The clinical practice of neurological and neurosurgical nursing. Lippincott, Philadelphia, PA

Hoppe-Hirshe E, Laroussinie F, Brunet L et al 1998 Late outcome of the surgical treatment of hydrocephalus. Child's Nervous System 14: 97–99

Koch D, Wagner W 2004 Endoscopic third ventriculostomy in infants less than 1 year of age: which factors influence outcome? Child's Nervous System 20: 405–411

May L 2001 Paediatric head injury. In: May L (ed) Neurosurgery – a handbook for the multidisciplinary team. Whurr, London

May L, Carter B 1995 Nursing support and care: meeting the needs of the child and family with altered cerebral function. In: Carter B, Dearmun AK (eds) Child health care nursing, concepts, theory and practice. Blackwell Science, Oxford, p 363–390

McLone D, Ito J 1998 An introduction to spina bifida. Children's Memorial Spina Bifida Team, Chicago IL

Michaud LJ, Rivara FP, Gradys MS et al 1992 Predictors of survival and severity of disablement after severe brain injury. Neurosurgery Aug 31(2): 254–256

Moray JP, Tyler DC, Jones TK et al 1984 Coma scale used for brain injured children. Critical Care Medicine 12: 1018–1020

Plowfield L 1999 Waiting following neurological crisis. Journal of Neuroscience Nursing Aug 31(4): 231–238

Raimondi AJ, Hirschner J 1984 Head injury in the infant and toddler. Coma scoring and outcome scale. Child's Brain 11: 12–35

Rivara JB, Fay JC, Jaffe KM et al 1992 Predictors of family functioning one year following head injury in children. Archives of Physical Medical Rehabilitation 73(10): 899–910

Scheinblum S, Hammond M 1990 The treatment of children with shunt infections: external ventricular drainage system care. Pediatric Nursing March/April 16(6): 2

Scott-Jupp R, Marlow N, Seddon N et al 1992 Rehabilitation and outcome following severe head injury. Archives of Disability in Childhood 62(2): 222–226

Shiminski–Mayer T, Shields M 1995 Pediatric brain tumours: diagnosis and management. Journal of Pediatric Oncology Nursing 12(4): 188–198

Shorvon SD, Chadwick D, Galbraith A et al 1987 One drug for epilepsy. British Medical Journal 1: 474

Simpson D, Reilly P 1982 Paediatric coma scale. Lancet August 450

Tobias JS, Hayward RD 1989 Brain and spinal cord tumours in children. In: Thomas DAF (ed) Neurooncology. Edward Arnold, London

Tulipan N, Bruner J 1997 Myelomeningocoele repair in utero, a report of three cases. Child's Nervous System 15: 435–443

## Useful Addresses

ASBAH (Association of Spina Bifida and Hydrocephalus)
ASBAH House,
42 Park Road,
Peterborough,
PE1 2UQ

# Chapter 11

# The child requiring cardiac surgery

## Caroline Haines and Sandra Pedley

## INTRODUCTION

With the development of cardiopulmonary bypass techniques, the increased technological advances in healthcare, and expansion in the knowledge and expertise of health personnel, cardiac surgical techniques have developed rapidly. Today, intricate and complex paediatric cardiac surgery has become the norm. The identification and recognition of specialist paediatric centres providing intensive, high dependency and continued care, the early detection of children with congenital heart disease (CHD) and high quality pre-, intra- and postoperative care have led to improved survival and ensured a better quality of life for these children.

To manage the care of children who require cardiac surgery holistically, it is important to understand normal anatomy, physiology and haemodynamic principles before applying them to children with CHD. This chapter therefore initially focuses on the above principles, prior to reviewing the most commonly presenting defects, their altered physiology, and the care provided for these children both pre- and postoperatively.

## CARDIAC ANATOMY AND PHYSIOLOGY

### BLOOD FLOW THROUGH THE HEART
(see Fig. 11.1)

- Venous blood enters the right atrium via the superior vena cava (SVC) from the head and upper body, and the inferior vena cava (IVC), from the lower body.

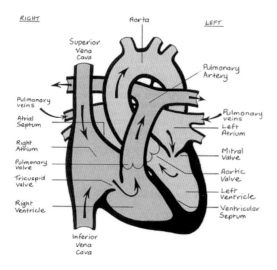

NORMAL CIRCULATION

**Figure 11.1** Diagram of the heart showing blood flow (Reproduced from *The Heart Children Book* with kind permission from HeartLine Association).

- Blood flows from the right atrium through the tricuspid valve into the right ventricle.
- The right ventricle pumps blood through the pulmonary valve into the pulmonary artery and then to the lungs, where it will be oxygenated. The main trunk of the pulmonary artery divides into two, the right and left pulmonary arteries, supplying blood to each lung.
- From the lungs the oxygenated blood flows via the pulmonary veins to the left atrium.
- From the left atrium the blood flows through the mitral valve into the left ventricle.
- The left ventricle pumps the oxygenated blood through the aortic valve into the ascending aorta and from there to the systemic circulation.

## INTRACARDIAC PRESSURES AND OXYGEN SATURATIONS

The heart receives systemic venous blood and ejects it to the lungs and then receives pulmonary venous blood and ejects it into the body. This serial circulation occurs due to the sequential relaxation and contraction of the atria, followed by the sequential relaxation and contraction of the ventricles (Hazinski 1992). Normally, circulation to the right and left sides of the heart is separate.

As blood flows through the heart (see Fig. 11.1), the oxygen saturation of this blood alters, depending on whether it is pre or post the lungs (see Fig. 11.2), and

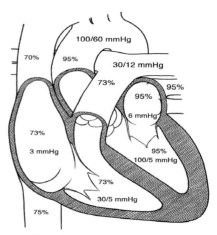

**Figure 11.2** Normal intracardiac pressures and oxygen saturations.

the pressures generated within each chamber of the heart relate to the sequential relaxation and contraction (diastole and systole) of the heart (see Fig. 11.2). Figure 11.3 shows the blood supply to the heart.

## THE CONDUCTING SYSTEM OF THE HEART

A network of specialised muscle fibres generates and distributes electrical impulses which stimulate the cardiac muscle to contract:

- The sinoatrial node (SA node/pacemaker) in the right atrium initiates the contraction or depolarisation and sets the pace for the heart (see Fig. 11.4).

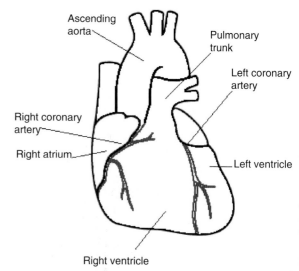

**Figure 11.3** Blood supply to the heart through left and right coronary arteries.

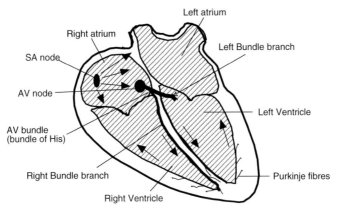

**Figure 11.4** The conducting system.

• The impulse spreads over both atria causing them to contract together, until it reaches the atrioventricular node (AV node). Conduction is fractionally delayed to allow the atria to finish contracting. From the AV node the impulse passes rapidly down the single atrioventricular bundle (bundle of His), then this divides in the septum between the ventricles into the left and right bundle branches. Conduction spreads though the ventricular muscle due to specialised fibres called purkinje fibres (see Fig. 11.4).
    • Repolarisation then occurs.

### Electrocardiogram (ECG)

An ECG measures the electrical activity of the heart and if recorded on graph paper allows the sequence and magnitude of the electrical impulses generated by the heart to be analysed and evaluated.
    The ECG provides information on:

• Heart rate and rhythm
• Abnormalities in conduction pathways
• Muscular damage (ischaemia)
• Hypertrophy
• Effects of electrolyte imbalance
• Effects of drugs
• Pericardial disease.

Figure 11.5 shows a normal sinus rhythm, with the following features marked:

• P wave – represents the contraction and depolarisation of the atria.
• PR interval – represents the time taken for the impulse to spread from the SA node through the atrial muscle and the AV node, down the bundle of His and into the ventricular muscle.

• QRS complex – represents ventricular depolarisation. As the ventricles are large, there is a large deflection of the ECG when they contract.
• T wave – represents the return of the ventricular mass to the resting electrical state, or depolarisation.

## CLASSIFICATION OF CONGENITAL HEART DISEASE

CHD may be classified in many differing ways and Figure 11.6 demonstrates just one of these.

## CLINICAL PRESENTATION OF CONGESTIVE HEART FAILURE

Box 11.1 illustrates the clinical presentation of congestive heart failure.

## PREOPERATIVE MANAGEMENT

As with any operation, preoperative preparation of the child who needs cardiac surgery is imperative to ensure a safe procedure with minimum complications. There is no doubt that the families of these children experience overwhelming stress, fear, anxiety and a desire to protect their child, and these concerns and feelings must neither be underestimated nor ignored. Appropriate support networks, from psychologists, social workers, cardiac liaison nurses, unit nurses and medical or allied health professionals, must be offered and accessible to these families.
    Box 11.2 focuses on the specific medical investigations, information and management that should

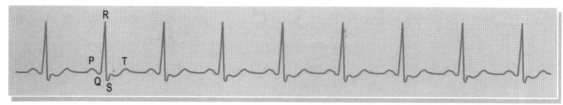

**Figure 11.5** Normal sinus rhythm.

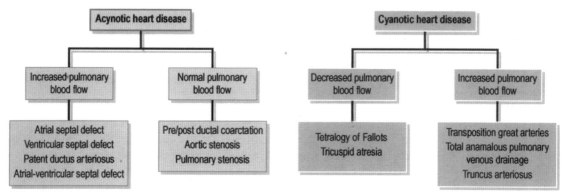

**Figure 11.6** Classification of congenital heart disease.

---

**Box 11.1 Clinical presentation of congestive heart failure**

| Impaired cardiac function | Pulmonary congestion | Systemic venous congestion |
|---|---|---|
| • Tachycardia | • Tachypnoea | • Weight gain |
| • Altered blood pressure | • Dyspnoea | • Peripheral oedema |
| • Pale, cool, mottled peripheries | • Recession | • Ascites |
| • Weak peripheral pulses | • Nasal flaring | • Hepatomegaly |
| • Oliguria | • Cough | • Splenomegaly |
| • Sweaty | • Wheezing | |
| • Fatigue | • Grunting | |
| • Weakness | • Cyanosis | |
| • Agitation | • Clubbing | |
| • Anorexia/failure to thrive | • Pulmonary oedema | |
| • Weight loss | • Exercise intolerance | |
| • Dysrhythmias | | |
| • Cardiomegaly | | |

---

be undertaken or obtained prior to a child receiving cardiac surgery.

## IMMEDIATE POSTOPERATIVE CARE

### AIRWAY AND BREATHING

- The child will be intubated and ventilated in the immediate postoperative period.

- The child will be extubated when
  — cardiovascularly stable
  — making good respiratory effort with good gas exchange on minimal ventilatory support.
- Continuous monitoring and hourly recordings of the following observations are essential in the immediate postoperative period
  — respiratory rate (set ventilator rate and child's overall respiratory rate)
  — chest expansion

— chest auscultation
— appropriate ventilator observations.
- The nurse will also regularly assess
  - chest expansion
  - chest auscultation
  - respiratory effort.

## Potential complications

These may be detected by:

- unequal chest expansion
- unequal air entry
- a decrease in the child's saturations
- increased respiratory effort in the self-ventilating child.

Potential complications are as follows:

1. Pneumothorax: Air within the pleural space has caused part, or all of the lung to collapse. This may occur if the pleura are opened during surgery and the air is not adequately removed, or by damage to the lung tissue causing an air leak.

It can be treated by insertion of a pleural drain which will bubble on inspiration and 'swing' in time with respiration.

2. Haemothorax: Blood within the pleural space has caused part of the lung to collapse. This may occur if there is bleeding within the thorax.

It can be treated by insertion of a pleural drain which will drain blood-stained fluid.

3. Chylothorax: Lymph fluid, or chyle, has collected within the pleural space. This may occur if the lymph vessels are damaged or bruised during surgery or if the child has a high central venous pressure postoperatively.

It can be treated by insertion of a pleural drain which will drain milky coloured fluid, and a medium-chain triglyceride diet to reduce thoracic lymph flow.

4. Pleural effusion: Fluid within the pleural space has caused part of the lung to collapse. Congestive heart failure may contribute to the accumulation of this fluid.

It can be treated by insertion of a pleural drain which will drain the accumulated fluid, and treatment of congestive heart failure.

5. Consolidation: There is a build up of secretions within the airways, usually within the small bronchioles and alveoli.

It can be treated by chest physiotherapy and postural drainage.

## CIRCULATION

- Continuous monitoring and hourly recordings of the following observations are essential in the immediate postoperative period
  - heart rate and rhythm
  - blood pressure
  - central venous pressure
  - core and peripheral temperature
  - drainage loss, volume and quality
  - urine output.

- In addition, children who are prone to pulmonary hypertension will also have continuous observation and hourly recording of
  - left atrial pressure
  - pulmonary artery pressure.

## Potential complications

**Dysrhythmias**    These may be caused by:

- inflammation and oedema around atrial or ventricular incisions or around the sinoatrial or atrioventricular nodes

- surgical damage to the SA node, AV node or the conduction pathways
- hypoxia of the SA node, AV node or the conduction pathways
- acidosis
- electrolyte disturbance.

They may be treated by:

- correcting any hypoxia
- correcting any acidosis
- correcting any electrolyte disturbances
- use of anti-dysrhythmics e.g. adenosine, amiodarone, flecanide
- cardioversion
- pacing.

Nursing issues when caring for a child being paced include:

- atrial wires exit to the right of the child's sternum
- ventricular wires exit to the left of the child's sternum
- entry site must be kept clean and dry to minimise risk of infection
- 12 lead ECG and clotting profile must be checked prior to removal of pacing wires
- tamponade is a risk post pacing wire removal
- permanent damage to the SA node, AV node or the conduction pathways may necessitate permanent pacing via an implanted pacing system.

**Bleeding**   This may be caused by:

- failure to fully reverse the anti-coagulation given whilst on cardiopulmonary bypass
- an open vessel.

Nursing observations will reflect:

- tachycardia
- hypotension
- low central venous pressure
- excess, bloody drainage
- poor peripheral perfusion.

Treatment involves the following:

- Check clotting profile, if clotting is extended administer the appropriate clotting factor.
- If clotting is normal, call the surgeon and the theatre team, re-open the chest and seal the bleeding point.
- Volume, e.g. blood, may need to be given to support the child's circulation until the above measures have been instigated.

**Cardiac Tamponade**   There is a collection of excess fluid in the pericardium. As the pericardium is a fibrous sac it is unable to expand. Excess fluid in the pericardium will therefore 'compress' the heart, restricting its function, and lead rapidly to cardiac arrest. In the postoperative cardiac patient, cardiac tamponade is usually caused by bleeding into the pericardium. This may be due to:

- poor drainage of the pericardial area by the existing chest drains
- blockage of an existing chest drain resulting in blood collecting in the pericardium.

Nursing observations will reflect:

- tachycardia – due to bleeding
- hypotension – due to bleeding and reduced stroke volume
- increased central venous pressure due to increased right atrial pressure as the heart is 'compressed'
- unusually faint heart sounds
- poor peripheral perfusion
- distended neck veins.

Chest drain output may be:

- excessive, the child may have a generalised bleed which is evident by excess loss from the drains as well as bleeding into the pericardium
- minimal, if the drain is blocked or the tip of the drain is not near the bleeding point.

Treatment is as follows:

- children who are tamponading will usually develop dysrhythmias and lose cardiac output very quickly. Full resuscitation must be instigated. The surgeon and theatre team must be called immediately to re-open the child's chest and evacuate the excess blood from the pericardium.

**Reduced Cardiac Output/Hypotension**   This is caused either by hypovolaemia or decreased cardiac function.

*Hypovolaemia*   Nursing observations will reflect:

- tachycardia
- hypotension
- low central venous pressure
- poor peripheral perfusion
- reduced urine output.

Treatment is:

- 10 mL/kg colloid, review effect and repeat bolus if necessary.
- human albumin solution (4.5%) is readily available and is the colloid of choice for acute incidents of hypovolaemia
- blood or fresh frozen plasma should be considered if the child has a low haemoglobin or deranged clotting.

Colloid is the optimum fluid for resuscitation in this situation. The large molecular structure of colloids ensures that they stay within the circulation longer than crystalloid, thus restoring the child's blood pressure quickly and effectively.

*Decreased Cardiac Function*  Nursing observations will reflect:

- tachycardia
- hypotension
- normal, high or low central venous pressure
- poor peripheral perfusion
- reduced urine output.

Treatment is:

- continuous inotrope infusion to improve contractility
- afterload reduction
- optimise preload.

Inotropes are drugs that increase heart rate and contractility (force of contraction), thereby increasing the child's blood pressure. They work by stimulating receptors that are located within the heart and the blood vessels. There are several types of receptors, each having a different effect (see Table 11.1). Inotropes may stimulate one or several receptors (see Table 11.2).

Afterload reduction may be achieved by using phosphodiesterase inhibitors, e.g. milrinone or enoximone. These drugs improve cardiac output by causing an increase in contractility and also arterial dilation, i.e. the myocardial contractions are stronger and there is less resistance to forward flow into the arterial circulation. The overall effect of these actions is to improve the child's cardiac output.

Preload may be optimised by the administration of volume and/or the use of selective vasoconstrictors, e.g. noradrenaline (norepinephrine).

**Pulmonary Hypertensive Crisis**  Children who have a large left to right shunt, e.g. those with an

**Table 11.1** Receptor sites and the cardiovascular effect when stimulated

| Receptor | Action |
| --- | --- |
| Alpha receptor | Vasoconstriction |
| Beta$_1$ receptor | Increase heart rate and contractility |
| Beta$_2$ receptor | Vasodilation |
| Dopamine receptor | Renal, coronary, cerebral and mesenteric vasodilation |

**Table 11.2** Commonly used inotropes and their receptor sites

| Inotrope | Receptors stimulated | Action |
| --- | --- | --- |
| Adrenaline (epinephrine) | Alpha and beta$_1$ receptors | Vasoconstriction, increase in heart rate and contractility |
| Noradrenaline (norepinephrine) | Alpha | Vasoconstriction |
| Dobutamine | Beta$_1$ | Increase in heart rate and contractility |
| Dopamine | 2–5 mcg/kg/min – dopamine | Renal, coronary, cerebral and mesenteric vasodilation |
| | 5–10 mcg/kg/min – dopamine and beta$_1$ | Renal, coronary, cerebral and mesenteric vasodilation |
| | >10 mcg/kg/min – alpha | Vasoconstriction |

atrioventricular septal defect (AVSD), also have a large increase in pulmonary blood flow – they have hyperdynamic pulmonary hypertension. During the immediate postoperative period, these children are prone to acute increases in pulmonary pressures, which can cause a pulmonary hypertensive crisis. This acute reaction is exacerbated by endothelial damage and an increase in circulating vasoactive substances following cardiopulmonary bypass.

Pulmonary hypertensive crisis may be precipitated by:

- hypoxia
- hypercarbia
- pyrexia
- pain/anxiety.

The stimulus, e.g. hypoxia, causes a chain reaction as depicted in the flow diagram in Figure 11.7.

The optimum management is to reduce the risk of a pulmonary hypertensive incident actually occurring. This can be achieved by:

- maintaining a high pO$_2$ (>90 mmHg)
- maintaining a low normal pCO$_2$ (35–40 mmHg)
- maintaining normothermia (use cooling blanket if necessary)
- maintaining optimum analgesia, sedation and muscle relaxation for at least 24 hours postoperatively (use of fentanyl/vecuronium infusion)
- use of vasodilator e.g. phenoxybenzamine
- minimal handling.

If pulmonary artery (PA) pressures remain high or unstable then the use of nitric oxide may be considered.

Treatment is:

- hand ventilate on 100% oxygen
- administer a bolus of intravenous (IV) fentanyl.

Care such as physiotherapy, which may precipitate a pulmonary hypertensive episode, is managed by prophylactically administering a bolus of intravenous (IV) fentanyl and preoxygenating the child.

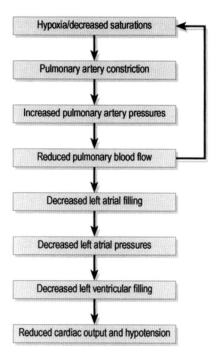

**Figure 11.7** Physiology of a pulmonary hypertensive crisis.

## NEUROLOGICAL

Cerebal insult may occur due to:

- hypoxia
- hypotension
- cerebral bleed (related to anticoagulation for bypass)
- air embolism (related to bypass procedure)
- thrombus (related to bypass procedure).

It is therefore important to perform an early neurological assessment on children following cardiac surgery.

Nursing observations will assess:

- pupil reaction
- posture and muscle tone
- seizure activity
- consciousness level.

Any abnormality or change in the child's neurological status must be referred to the medical staff for further investigation and management.

## RENAL

Renal insult may occur due to:

- hypoxia
- hypotension.

Nursing observation will assess:

- hourly urine output
- hourly fluid balance
- serum creatinine, urea and electrolytes.

Regular frusemide may be given to maintain a good urine output (>1 mL/kg/h) and to optimise cardiac function.

Acute renal failure can be detected by:

- decreased urine output (less than 0.5 mL/kg/h)
- raised serum urea and creatinine
- electrolyte disorders
- metabolic acidosis.

It can be treated by:

- peritoneal dialysis
- haemofiltration.

## FLUIDS AND NUTRITION

Fluids are strictly restricted to 50% of normal maintenance requirements following open heart surgery.

This is because the children may become quite oedematous as a result of the capillary leak associated with cardiopulmonary bypass. The child's fluid balance should be calculated hourly and the electrolytes and blood sugar level should be checked regularly.

Nutrition is also an extremely important aspect of the child's recovery following cardiac surgery. A nasogastric tube should be passed and enteral nutrition should be commenced, ideally within 3–4 hours of the child returning from theatre. Due to the severe fluid restriction post cardiac surgery, it may be advisable to liaise with the dietitian regarding optimisation of the child's calorific intake.

## CONGENITAL HEART DEFECTS, SURGERY AND CARE

### ACYANOTIC DEFECTS WITH INCREASED PULMONARY BLOOD FLOW

In these defects there is an abnormal connection between the right and left sides of the heart. As pressure is higher in the left, systemic side of the heart, blood shunts from left to right and pulmonary blood flow is increased.

### Atrial Septal Defect (ASD) (see also Fig. 11.8)

#### Altered Anatomy and Haemodynamics

- *Ostium secundum* – located high in the septal wall.
- *Ostium primum* – located low in the septal wall close to the endocardial cushion.
- *Sinus venosus* – located close to the opening of the superior vena cava.

Blood will shunt left to right, from the high pressure left atrium to the low pressure right atrium.

#### Signs and Symptoms

- Murmur
- Chest X-ray
  — increased pulmonary vascular markings
  — enlarged right atrium, right ventricle and pulmonary artery
- ECG – right ventricular hypertrophy.

#### Surgical Technique

- Open heart
- Sternotomy

- Stitch closure or patch repair
- Small ASDs may be closed with a septal occlusion device at cardiac catheter.

#### Postoperative complications related to specific defect

- Atrial dysrhythmias.

### Ventricular Septal Defect (VSD) (see Fig. 11.9)

#### Altered Anatomy and Haemodynamics

- *Perimembranous* – located below the aortic valve, high in the left ventricular outflow tract
- *Muscular* – located lower down at the apex of the septum.

Blood shunts left to right from the high pressure left ventricle to the low pressure right ventricle.

#### Signs and Symptoms

- Murmur
- Increased respiratory effort
- Chest X-ray
  —cardiomegaly
  —increased pulmonary vascular markings
- ECG – right ventricular hypertrophy.

#### Surgical Technique

- Open heart
- Sternotomy
- Stitch closure or patch repair.

#### Postoperative complications related to specific defect

- Ventricular dysrhythmias
- Pulmonary hypertension if large VSD.

### Patent Ductus Arteriosus (PDA) (see Fig. 11.10)

#### Altered Anatomy and Haemodynamics    The ductus arteriosus connects the pulmonary artery and the aorta and is a normal part of fetal circulation. However, it should close within 10–15 days of birth; failure to do so results in a persistent patent ductus arteriosus.

Blood shunts left to right from the high pressure aorta to the low pressure pulmonary artery.

#### Signs and Symptoms

- Murmur
- Increased respiratory effort

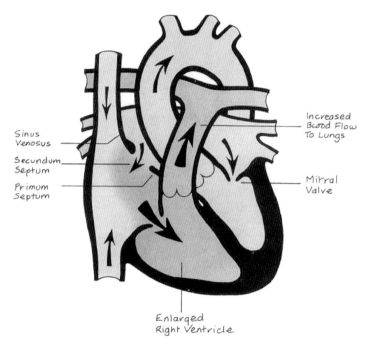

Sinus
Venosus

Secundum
Septum

Primum
Septum

Increased
Blood Flow
To Lungs

Mitral
Valve

Enlarged
Right Ventricle

**Figure 11.8** Atrial septal defect (Reproduced from *The Heart Children Book* with kind permission from HeartLine Association).

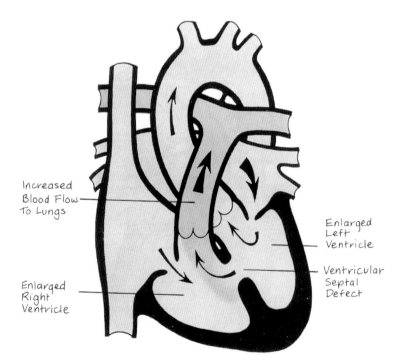

Increased
Blood Flow
To Lungs

Enlarged
Left
Ventricle

Ventricular
Septal
Defect

Enlarged
Right
Ventricle

VENTRICULAR SEPTAL DEFECT

**Figure 11.9** Ventricular septal defect (Reproduced from *The Heart Children Book* with kind permission from HeartLine Association).

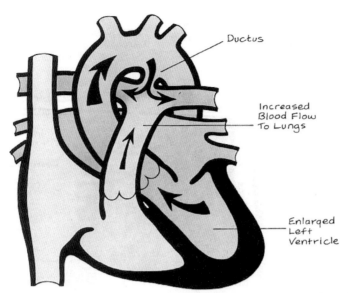

**Figure 11.10** Patent ductus arteriosus (Reproduced from *The Heart Children Book* with kind permission from HeartLine Association).

- Chest X-ray – increased pulmonary vascular markings
- ECG – left ventricular hypertrophy.

**Medical Treatment**

- Indometacin (a prostaglandin synthesis inhibitor), administered intravenously, may cause constriction of the duct
- Insertion of a ductal occlusion device at cardiac catheter.

**Surgical Technique**

- Closed heart
- Thoracotomy
- Ligation or division of duct.

**Postoperative complications related to specific defect**

- Laryngeal nerve palsy.

## Atrioventricular Septal Defect (AVSD)
(see Fig. 11.11)

**Altered Anatomy and Haemodynamics**   This defect is caused by abnormal development of the endocardial cushion. This can result in either a partial or complete AVSD.

- *Partial* – there is a defect of the mitral valve and either an ostium primum ASD, or a VSD. Blood will regurgitate through the incompetent mitral valve

and will also shunt left to right through the septal defect.

- *Complete* – there is a common atrioventricular valve, an ostium primum ASD and a VSD. Blood will shunt left to right through the septal defect and through the incompetent valve.

**Signs and Symptoms**

- Increased respiratory effort
- Congestive heart failure
- Chest X-ray – right ventricular hypertrophy or cardiomegaly
- ECG – biventricular hypertrophy.

**Surgical Technique**

- Open heart
- Sternotomy
- Patch closure of septal defect.

  In addition:

- Partial – repair of mitral valve
- Complete – division of common AV valve and creation of two competent valves.

**Postoperative complications related to specific defect**

- Residual mitral/tricuspid valve regurgitation
- Pulmonary hypertension
- Dysrhythmias/complete heart block.

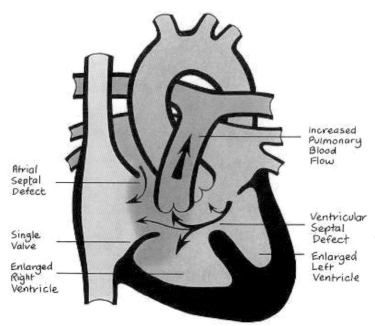

**Figure 11.11** Atrioventricular septal defect (Reproduced from *The Heart Children Book* with kind permission from HeartLine Association).

## ACYANOTIC DEFECTS WITH NORMAL PULMONARY BLOOD FLOW

In these defects there are no abnormal connections between the right and left sides of the heart; therefore pulmonary blood flow is not increased.

### Preductal coarctation of the aorta, where the narrowing is before the patent ductus arteriosus (see Fig. 11.12)

**Altered Anatomy and Haemodynamics**  Oxygenated blood from the left ventricle perfuses the head and upper body as the carotid, innominate and brachiocephalic arteries arise from before the narrowed segment of aorta. There is minimal flow from the ascending to the descending aorta through the narrowing. As the ductus arteriosus is after the narrowing, unoxygenated blood will shunt from the pulmonary artery into the descending aorta to perfuse the lower body. This is possible because pressure in the descending aorta is low due to the minimal blood flow through the narrowed segment.

### Signs and Symptoms

- Congestive heart failure
- Relative hypertension i.e. blood pressure (BP) in upper limbs at least 20 mmHg higher than in lower limbs

- Femoral pulses weak and delayed
- Lower limb cyanosis
- Chest X-ray – cardiomegaly
- ECG – right ventricular hypertrophy.

### Specific preoperative care

- Prostin infusion to maintain ductal patency.

### Surgical Technique

- Closed heart
- Thoracotomy
- Left subclavian artery mobilised and used to enlarge narrowed area of aorta.

### Postoperative complications related to specific defect

- Residual obstruction
- Hypertension
- Mesenteric ischaemia
- Spinal cord damage.

### Postductal Coarctation of the aorta, where the narrowing is after the patent ductus arteriosus (see Fig. 11.12)

**Altered Anatomy and Haemodynamics**  Oxygenated blood from the left ventricle perfuses the head and upper body as the carotid, innominate and

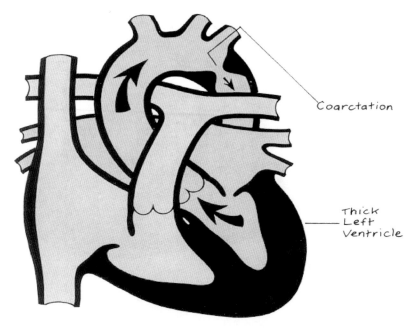

## COARCTATION OF AORTA

**Figure 11.12** Coarctation of the aorta (Reproduced from *The Heart Children Book* with kind permission from HeartLine Association).

brachiocephalic arteries arise from before the narrowed segment of aorta. There is minimal flow from the ascending to the descending aorta through the narrowing. The ductus arteriosus is before the narrowing so blood cannot shunt via this to perfuse the lower body, as happens with a preductal coarctation. Instead, collateral circulation will have developed in utero. These vessels will branch off the aorta before the narrowing, and connect distal to the narrowing. Lower body perfusion is dependent on flow through these collateral vessels.

### Signs and Symptoms

- Congestive heart failure detected in first few months or at routine medical
- Frequent headaches and nosebleeds
- Poor peripheral perfusion – 'cool feet'
- Hypertension
- Weak femoral pulses
- Chest X-ray
  — enlarged left atrium and ventricle
  — dilated ascending aorta
  — collateral circulation
  — rib notching in older children (caused by collateral circulation)

- ECG – left ventricular hypertrophy.

### Surgical Technique

- Closed heart
- Thoracotomy
- Resection and end-to-end anastomosis or patch repair.

### Postoperative complications related to specific defect

- Residual obstruction
- Hypertension
- Mesenteric ischaemia
- Spinal cord damage.

## Aortic valve stenosis (see Fig. 11.13)

### Altered Anatomy and Haemodynamics

- *Valvular* – the cusps of the aortic valve remain fused and this, combined with stenotic muscle around the valve, causes obstruction and turbulent flow. This results in left ventricular hypertrophy and aortic dilation.
- *Subvalvular* – a fibrous ring below the valve causes obstruction to flow. The increased stress on

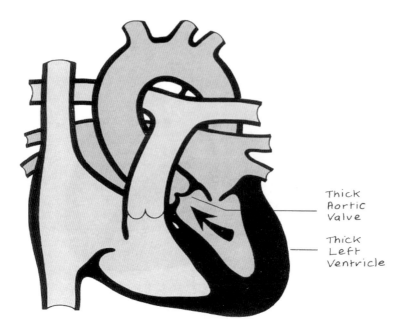

AORTIC VALVE STENOSIS

**Figure 11.13** Aortic valve stenosis (Reproduced from *The Heart Children Book* with kind permission from HeartLine Association).

the left ventricle will lead to left ventricular hypertrophy.

• *Supravalvular* – the obstruction is caused either by a fibrous membrane situated above the valve or by a hypoplastic aorta. This results in left ventricular hypertrophy.

• *Idiopathic hypertrophic subaortic stenosis (IHSS)* – the valve is normal but obstruction is caused by hypertrophy of the left side of the ventricular septum. The obstruction becomes progressively worse as the septum continues to grow and left ventricular hypertrophy develops.

Blood flow from the left ventricle is obstructed by the stenosis. Neonates may also have a patent ductus arteriosus.

### Signs and Symptoms

• Murmur
• Chest X-ray – left ventricular hypertrophy
• ECG – left ventricular hypertrophy.

### Surgical Technique

• Open heart
• Sternotomy.

• *Valvular* – The valve is dilated and the commisures incised. Valve replacement is avoided in childhood as the implanted valve will not grow with the child. In adolescents a Ross procedure may be performed.
• *Subvalvular* – The fibrous membrane is excised and any residual narrowing is dilated or enlarged with a patch.
• *Supravalvular* – The fibrous membrane is excised and any residual narrowing is dilated or enlarged with a patch.
• *IHSS* – The hypertrophied muscle is resected.

### Postoperative complications related to specific defect

• Aortic insufficiency
• Poor ventricular function
• Persistent stenosis.

### Pulmonary valve stenosis (see Fig. 11.14)

### Altered Anatomy and Haemodynamics

• *Valvular* – the cusps of the valve remain fused and may also be thickened. The valve may also consist of two, rather than three cusps. The increased stress on the right ventricle will lead to right ventricular hypertrophy.

- *Subvalvular* – due to hypertrophied muscle in the right ventricular infundibulum (outflow tract). The increased stress on the right ventricle will lead to right ventricular hypertrophy.
- *Supravalvular* – due to narrowing of the pulmonary artery or its branches in either one or several places. The increased stress on the right ventricle will lead to right ventricular hypertrophy.

If the stenosis is severe, right-sided pressures may exceed pressures on the left and blood may shunt right to left through a patent foramen ovale. This will cause cyanosis.

### Signs and Symptoms

- Murmur
- Chest X-ray – right ventricular hypertrophy
- ECG – right ventricular hypertrophy.

### Medical Treatment

- If the stenosis is mild, the narrowing may be dilated with a balloon tipped cardiac catheter.

### Surgical Technique

- Open heart
- Sternotomy
- *Valvular* – the valve is dilated and the commisures incised
- *Subvalvular* – surgical resection of infundibulum; patch enlargement of outflow tract.

### Postoperative complications related to specific defect

- Poor right ventricular function
- Residual pulmonary stenosis.

## CYANOTIC DEFECTS WITH DECREASED PULMONARY BLOOD FLOW

In these defects there is some obstruction to pulmonary blood flow on the right side of the heart and an abnormal communication between the right and left sides of the heart. The obstruction causes pressure in the right side of the heart to be abnormally high and blood therefore shunts from right to left through the abnormal communication. This results in oxygenated blood perfusing the systemic circulation and causes cyanosis.

## Tetralogy of Fallot (see Fig. 11.15)

**Altered Anatomy and Haemodynamics**    The altered haemodynamics are as a result of the four defects associated with tetralogy of Fallot. These are:

- Pulmonary stenosis (usually subvalvular)
- Right ventricular hypertrophy
- Ventricular septal defect
- Overriding aorta.

The pulmonary stenosis causes reduced pulmonary blood flow and an increase in workload for the right ventricle, resulting in the right ventricular hypertrophy. Pressure in the right ventricle is increased due to the pulmonary stenosis and right ventricular hypertrophy and so blood shunts right to left through the ventricular septal defect.

The degree of pulmonary stenosis determines the degree by which the pulmonary blood flow is reduced, the volume of right to left shunt and consequently the severity of the child's cyanosis. Children with very mild pulmonary stenosis may be relatively asymptomatic, simply requiring definitive surgery when they have reached suitable size. However, a child with severe pulmonary stenosis will present as a neonate and will require a shunt to increase pulmonary blood flow, prior to definitive repair at a later date.

### Signs and Symptoms

- Murmur
- Cyanosis
- Chest X-ray – 'boot' shaped heart due to the small pulmonary arteries and right ventricular hypertrophy
- ECG – right ventricular hypertrophy
- 'Tet' spells – periods of severe cyanosis and loss of consciousness caused by infundibular spasm.

The more severe the pulmonary stenosis, the earlier the child will present.

### Surgical Technique
*Severe pulmonary stenosis*

- Closed heart
- Thoracotomy
- Modified Blalock Taussig shunt as neonate, followed by definitive repair. This involves:
  — Dacron® or Gore-Tex® conduit from right or left subclavian artery to corresponding pulmonary artery
  — blood flow from the subclavian artery will therefore flow to the pulmonary system and increase pulmonary blood flow and oxygenation.

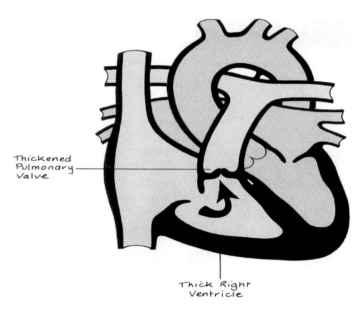

PULMONARY VALVE STENOSIS

**Figure 11.14** Pulmonary valve stenosis (Reproduced from *The Heart Children Book* with kind permission from HeartLine Association).

*Definitive Repair*

- Open heart
- Sternotomy
- Closure of VSD so that the aorta arises from left side of septum
- Resection of infundibular stenosis
- Patch enlargement of right ventricular outflow tract.

**Postoperative complications related to specific defect**

- Residual shunt
- Residual right ventricular outflow obstruction
- Poor ventricular function
- Dysrhythmias.

## Tricuspid atresia (see Fig. 11.16)

### Altered Anatomy and Haemodynamics

- The tricuspid valve is absent resulting in congestion and high pressure in the right atrium.
- High right atrial pressure results in blood shunting right to left through a persisting patent foramen ovale.
- Blood will shunt left to right, from the high pressure aorta to the low pressure pulmonary artery via the ductus arteriosus. The ductus arteriosus

remains patent primarily due to the neonate's low oxygen levels.
- Pulmonary blood flow is dependent on the left to right shunt through the ductus arteriosus.
- The right ventricle, pulmonary valve and pulmonary artery will be hypoplastic.

### Signs and Symptoms

- Murmur
- Cyanosis
- Increased respiratory effort
- Metabolic acidosis
- Chest X-ray
  — decreased pulmonary vascular markings
  — left ventricular, right ventricular and right atrial hypertrophy
- ECG – left ventricular, right ventricular and right atrial hypertrophy.

### Surgical Technique

- Open heart
- Sternotomy
- Modified Blalock Taussig shunt as neonate. This involves:
  — Dacron® or Gore-Tex® conduit from right or left subclavian artery to corresponding pulmonary artery

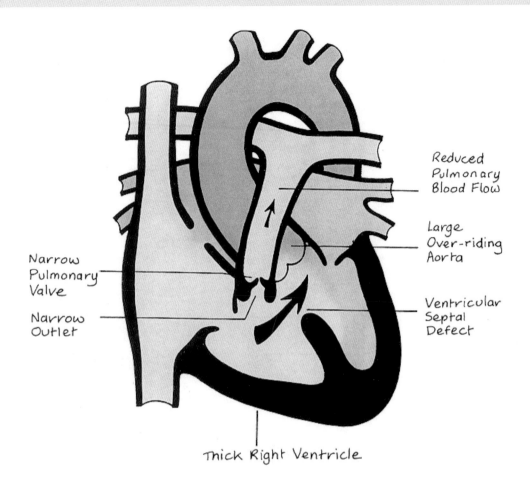

Reduced
Pulmonary
Blood Flow

Large
Over-riding
Aorta

Ventricular
Septal
Defect

Narrow
Pulmonary
Valve

Narrow
Outlet

Thick Right Ventricle

## TETRALOGY OF FALLOT

**Figure 11.15** Tetralogy of Fallot (Reproduced from *The Heart Children Book* with kind permission from HeartLine Association).

— blood flow from the subclavian artery will therefore flow to the pulmonary system and increase pulmonary blood flow and oxygenation

- Glenn shunt at 12–18 months. This constitutes:
  — right pulmonary artery separated from main pulmonary artery and 'pulmonary' end ligated
  — SVC separated from right atrium and hole oversewn
  — open end of SVC joined to open end of right pulmonary artery
  — venous return from the SVC will therefore flow directly to the right pulmonary artery and increase pulmonary blood flow and oxygenation
- Total caval pulmonary connection (TCPC) at 2–3 years. This involves:

—right pulmonary artery separated from main pulmonary artery and 'pulmonary' end ligated
—SVC and IVC separated from right atrium and holes oversewn
—open ends of SVC and IVC joined to open end of right pulmonary artery
—venous return from the SVC and IVC will therefore flow directly to the right pulmonary artery and increase pulmonary blood flow and oxygenation.

**Postoperative complications related to specific defect**

- Poor ventricular function
- Atrial dysrhythmias

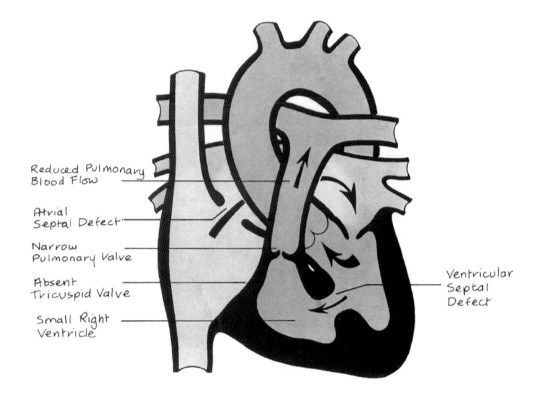

Reduced Pulmonary Blood Flow

Atrial Septal Defect

Narrow Pulmonary Valve

Absent Tricuspid Valve

Small Right Ventricle

Ventricular Septal Defect

## TRUCUSPID ATRESIA

**Figure 11.16** Tricuspid atresia (Reproduced from *The Heart Children Book* with kind permission from HeartLine Association).

- Increased venous pressure which may cause pleural effusions or chylothoraces.

## CYANOTIC DEFECTS WITH INCREASED PULMONARY BLOOD FLOW

In these defects there is no obstruction to pulmonary blood flow but there is an abnormal communication between the right and left sides of the heart.

### Transposition of the Great Arteries (TGA)
(see Fig. 11.17)

#### Altered Anatomy and Haemodynamics

- The pulmonary artery arises from the left ventricle and the aorta arises from the right ventricle.
- Unoxygenated, venous blood from the body returns to the right atrium, as normal. It enters the right ventricle and is pumped into the aorta

from where it perfuses the body. There is cyanosis as unoxygenated blood is perfusing the systemic circulation.

- Oxygenated blood from the lungs returns to the left atrium, as normal. It enters the left ventricle and is pumped into the pulmonary artery from where it perfuses the lungs.
- Essentially there are two parallel circulations, with oxygenated blood circulating around the pulmonary system and unoxygenated blood circulating around the systemic system.
- The ductus arteriosus remains patent due to the low systemic oxygen levels.
- The pulmonary artery pressure is high as it arises from the left ventricle, and the aortic pressure is low as it arises from the right ventricle. Oxygenated blood, therefore, shunts from the pulmonary artery to the aorta via the ductus arteriosus.
- Systemic oxygenation is dependent on the left to right ductal shunt.

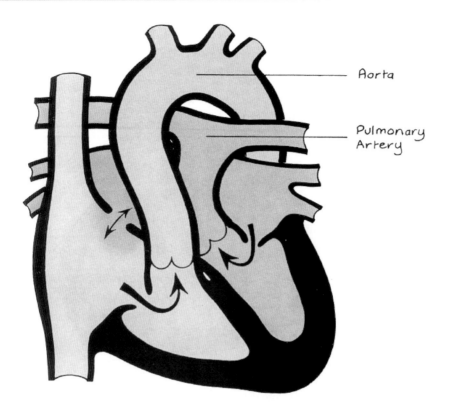

Aorta

Pulmonary Artery

## SIMPLE TRANSPOSITION

**Figure 11.17** Transposition of the great arteries (Reproduced from *The Heart Children Book* with kind permission from HeartLine Association).

### Signs and Symptoms

- Murmur
- Cyanosis
- Increased respiratory effort
- Congestive heart failure
- Chest X-ray
  — cardiomegaly
  — increased pulmonary vascular markings
- ECG – right ventricular and right atrial hypertrophy.

### Specific preoperative care

- Prostin infusion to maintain ductal patency.
- Atrial septostomy (Rashkind's procedure). Under X-ray supervision, a balloon-tipped catheter is inserted in the femoral vein and guided through the right atrium and the foramen ovale to the left atrium. The balloon is then inflated with saline and the catheter is pulled back to the right atrium. This results in a 'man-made' atrial septal defect through which oxygenated blood will shunt from left to right, so increasing systemic oxygenation.

**Surgical Technique**   Arterial switch is the operation of choice. The patient needs to have good left ventricular function and coronary arteries suitable for resection and re-anastomosis. Surgery is performed within the first few weeks of life, before the right ventricle becomes hypertrophied and the left ventricular function decreases. The arterial switch procedure involves the following:

- Open heart
- Sternotomy
- The aorta and the pulmonary artery are excised above the respective valves and anastomosed in the correct position.
- The coronary arteries are removed on a 'button' of tissue from the right sided aortic root and reim-

planted at the root of the original, left sided pulmonary artery.

### Postoperative complications related to specific defect

- Spasm or kinking of the reimplanted coronary arteries resulting in myocardial ischaemia and raised S–T segments on the ECG
- Left ventricular failure
- Pulmonary hypertension
- Aortic regurgitation
- Dysrhythmias.

## Total anomalous pulmonary venous drainage (TAPVD) (see Fig. 11.18)

### Altered Anatomy and Haemodynamics

- *Supracardiac* – the four pulmonary veins drain, via a common pulmonary vein, into the superior vena cava or directly into the right atrium.
- *Cardiac* – the four pulmonary veins drain, via a common pulmonary vein, into the right atrium via the coronary sinus.
- *Infradiaphragmatic* – the four pulmonary veins drain, via a common pulmonary vein, into the ductus venosus or portal vein.
- *Mixed* – the four pulmonary veins drain to a combination of sites.
- There is always a coexisting ASD.
- The pulmonary veins may be obstructed. This is most likely with infradiaphragmatic TAPVD when the diaphragm constricts the pulmonary veins. The obstruction means that blood flow to the right side of the heart is only slightly increased. However, the obstruction causes back-pressure in the pulmonary veins, which will lead to congestion in the pulmonary arteries and pulmonary hypertension.
- If the pulmonary veins are not obstructed the increased blood flow to the right side of the heart results in raised pressures and right atrial and ventricular hypertrophy. The raised right sided pressures cause blood to shunt right to left through the ASD.

### Signs and Symptoms

- Congestive heart failure
- Cyanosis
- Increased respiratory effort
- Chest X-ray – increased pulmonary vascular markings

- ECG – right ventricular hypertrophy.

Presents earlier if there is obstruction of pulmonary venous flow.

### Surgical Technique

- Open heart
- Sternotomy
- Pulmonary veins redirected to left atrium either directly or through the construction of conduits.

### Postoperative complications related to specific defect

- Residual pulmonary vein obstruction
- Pulmonary hypertension
- Dysrhythmias.

## Truncus arteriosus (see Fig. 11.19)

**Altered Anatomy and Haemodynamics**    One common vessel, with a common or truncal valve, arises from the right and left ventricles. There is a VSD high in the ventricular septum. The 'truncus' acts as the aorta and the pulmonary artery branches from it in one of the following ways:

- *Type I* – the main pulmonary artery branches from the truncus arteriosus just above the truncal valve.
- *Type II* – the right and left pulmonary arteries branch individually from the posterior of the truncus arteriosus.
- *Type III* – the right and left pulmonary arteries branch individually from the anterior of the truncus arteriosus.

Pulmonary blood flow is increased due to the high pressure within the truncus arteriosus. The child will be cyanosed as unoxygenated blood from the right ventricle perfuses the truncus arteriosus and so the aorta and systemic circulation.

If the pulmonary vessels are dilated (e.g. due to high oxygen levels and/or low carbon dioxide levels), pulmonary blood flow and oxygenation will be good. However, as a consequence of the good pulmonary blood flow, systemic flow is compromised and the systemic blood pressure will be low. Conversely, if the pulmonary vessels are constricted (e.g. due to low oxygen levels or high carbon dioxide levels), pulmonary blood flow and oxygenation will be poor. However, as a consequence of the poor pulmonary blood flow, systemic flow is strong producing good systemic blood pressures. This is referred to as a 'balanced circulation'.

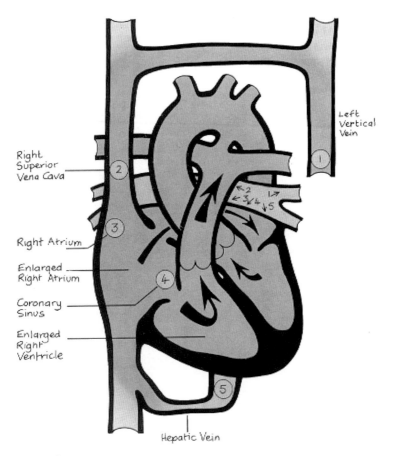

## TOTAL ANOMALOUS PULMONARY VENOUS DRAINAGE

**Figure 11.18** Total anomalous pulmonary venous drainage (Reproduced from *The Heart Children Book* with kind permission from HeartLine Association).

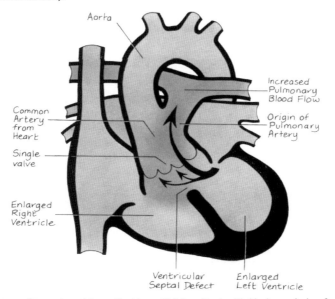

**Figure 11.19** Truncus arteriosus (Reproduced from *The Heart Children Book* with kind permission from HeartLine Association).

## Signs and Symptoms

- Murmur
- Cyanosis
- Congestive heart failure
- Chest X-ray – increased pulmonary vascular markings
- ECG – right and left ventricular hypertrophy.

## Surgical Technique

- Open heart
- Sternotomy
- VSD closed to establish flow from left ventricle to aorta
- Pulmonary arteries excised from the common vessel and anastomosed to a valved conduit, which is joined to the right ventricle.

## Postoperative complications related to specific defect

- Pulmonary hypertension
- Dysrhythmias.

## DISCHARGE PLANNING AND CONTINUED CARE

Discharge planning should ideally commence on admission of the child to hospital. It should include an assessment of the parents' ability to acknowledge and accept the child's altered health status and the role they will need to play in managing their child's care. The family may need assistance in recognising both their child's improved health status and the need to allow the child more independence.

Both verbal and written instructions on medications, nutrition, activity restrictions, a return to school, wound care, signs and symptoms of infections and potential complications will all need to be provided. Organisation of referrals to community support may be required to assist families in the transition from hospital to home and to help rein-force the management of care, and these should be planned well in advance of discharge.

Families will need clear instructions on when and where to seek medical advice if concerned with their child's condition and a follow-up outpatients appointment should be made prior to discharge. Additionally, appropriate identification, such as a medical alert device, should be organised for those children receiving anticoagulation or antidysrhythmic therapy.

The nurse will also need to discuss with families the possibility of sleep disturbance, overdependence and separation anxiety following cardiac surgery, and should provide consistent advice and reassurance.

Despite the advancement in cardiac surgical techniques, many children will require repeated surgery to replace conduits, grafts or valves as they grow and develop. Consequently, the long term prognosis for some children is uncertain and a full recovery is not always possible. Families therefore need continuing emotional and psychological support, together with encouragement and understanding by all health professionals involved, and nursing staff caring for these children are in an ideal position to take the lead in this.

## SUPPORT GROUPS FOR PARENTS AND CHILDREN (See Box 11.2)

| Box 11.2    Support groups |
|---|
| • Cardiomyopathy Association<br>• Children's Heart Federation<br>• Contact a Family<br>• Down's Syndrome Association<br>• GUCH association (Grown-up congenital heart)<br>• Heartline Association<br>• Marfan Association<br>• The British Heart Foundation |

## GLOSSARY

*Afterload*  The resistance to ejection from a ventricle. Ventricular afterload is the sum of all the forces that oppose ventricular emptying. A decreased afterload is often associated with an improvement in ventricular function.

*Cardiac Index*  Cardiac output ÷ body surface area $m^2$. Normal range = 3.5–5.5 $L/min/m^2$ body surface area.

*Cardiac Output*  The amount of blood ejected by the ventricle per minute, measured in mL/L.

Cardiac output = stroke volume × heart rate. Normal cardiac output is higher per kg of body weight in the child than in the adult. Hazinski (1992) gives the following values:

- At birth      400 mL/kg/min
- Infancy      200 mL/kg/min
- Childhood   150 mL/kg/min
- Adulthood   100 mL/kg/min.

**Chronotropic** Refers to drugs that affect heart rate.

**Contractility** Refers to the strength and efficiency of contraction. It is the force generated by the myocardium, independent of preload and afterload. Contractility is reduced by many factors, including hypoxia, acidosis, excessive preload or afterload, hypocalcaemia and nutritional deficiencies.

**Depolarisation** The contraction of any muscle is associated with electrical changes called depolarisation.

**Diastole** The resting stage of the heart muscle during which the chamber fills with blood.

**Hypertrophy** Excessive thickening of a part, or organ by increasing of its own tissue.

**Inotropic** Refers to drugs that increase myocardial contractility due to the movement of intracellular calcium.

**Preload** The amount of myocardial fibre stretch that is present before contraction and is related to the volume of blood in the ventricles prior to contraction, the central venous pressure and the left atrial pressure. Factors that affect preload include ventricular compliance and tachycardia.

**Repolarisation** The return of the ventricular fibres to the resting electrical state.

**Stroke Volume** The quantity of blood ejected from the ventricles during each contraction. It increases as the child grows from 5 mL at birth to 84 mL at 15 years. The preload, afterload and contractility determine stroke volume.

**Systemic Vascular Resistance (SVR)** (Mean arterial pressure (MAP) – central venous pressure (CVP)) ÷ cardiac output (CO).

**Systole** The contraction of the ventricle.

## Reference

Rees P, Tunstill A, Pope T et al 2002 Heart children – a practical handbook for parents of children with congenital heart problems. DK Creative Services, Surrey, UK

## Further reading

Alderman LM 2000 At risk: adolescents and adults with congenital heart disease. Dimensions of Critical Care Nursing 19(1): 2–14

Beck JR, Mongero LB, Kroslowitz RM et al 1999 Inhaled nitric oxide improves hemodynamics in patients with acute pulmonary hypertension after high-risk cardiac surgery. Perfusion 14(1): 37–42

Boyle J, Rost MK 2000 Present status of cardiac pacing: a nursing perspective. Critical Care Nursing Quarterly 23(1): 1–19

Chan D 1998 Critical care nursing series: pulmonary hypertension and inhaled nitric oxide therapy. Hong Kong Nursing Journal 34(2): 14–19

Curely MAQ, Bloedel-Smith J, Moloney-Harmon PA 1996 Critical care nursing of infants and children. WB Saunders, Philadelphia

Dalton HJ, Heulitt MJ 1998 Extracorporeal life support in pediatric respiratory failure: past, present, and future. Respiratory Care 43(11): 966–977

Davoric GO 1995 Haemodynamic monitoring: invasive and non-invasive clinical application. WB Saunders, Philadelphia

Dwyer D 2000 Device safety. Pacing your patients. Nursing 30(3): 82

Gaskin K 1998 The implications of pulmonary vascular resistance on the nursing care of an infant with hypoplastic left heart syndrome. Nursing in Critical Care 3(6): 296–300

Hazinski MF 1992 Nursing care of the critically ill child. Mosby, St Louis

Hazinski M 1999 Care of the critically ill child. Mosby, St Louis

Hess DR 1999 Adverse effects and toxicity of inhaled nitric oxide. Respiratory Care 44(3): 315–330

Jordan SC, Scott O 1989 Heart disease in paediatrics, 3rd edn. Butterworth, London

Nichols D, Cameron D, Greenley W et al 1995 Critical heart disease in infants and children. Mosby, St Louis

Levine DM, Farrell HC 1999 Clinical perspectives. Pediatric mechanical ventilation with nitric oxide. American Association of Respiratory Care Times 23(10): 53–56

Macnab A, Macrae D, Henning R 1999 Care of the critically ill child. Churchill Livingstone, London

Park MK 1997 The pediatric cardiology handbook, 2nd edn. Mosby, St Louis

Prasad SA, Hussey J 1995 Paediatric respiratory care: a guide for physiotherapists and health professionals. Chapman & Hall, London

Qureshi SA 1997 Practical interventional paediatric cardiology. In: Grech DE, Ramsdale DR (eds) Practical interventional cardiology. Martin Dunitz, London

Royal College of Paediatrics and Child Health 1999 Medicines for Children. Royal College of Paediatrics and Child Health Publications Ltd, London

Sokol J, Jacobs SE, Bohn D 2000 Inhaled nitric oxide for acute hypoxemic respiratory failure in children and adults. The Cochrane Library, Oxford p 17

Stark J, De Leval M 1994 Surgery for congenital heart defects, 2nd edn. WB Saunders, Philadelphia

Thompson J, Bateman ST, Betit P 1999 Pediatric applications of inhaled nitric oxide. Proceedings of the 1998 Respiratory Care Journal Conference. Respiratory Care 44(2): 177–183

Weiland AP, Walker WE 1996 Physiological principles and clinical sequelae of cardio-pulmonary bypass. Heart and Lung 15(1): 34–39

Williams C, Asquith J 2000 Paediatric intensive care nursing. Churchill Livingstone, Edinburgh

# Chapter 12

# Ear, nose and throat

## Christine English and Ann Macfadyen

## CHAPTER CONTENTS

## INTRODUCTION

This chapter will consider care of children undergoing ear, nose and throat surgery. The care required by children undergoing the most common surgical procedures will be explained. This includes tonsillectomy, adenoidectomy, myringotomy, insertion of grommets/T-tubes, mastoidectomy, pinning back of prominent ears, nasal surgery, dental surgery and tracheostomy.

The general pre- and postoperative care of children is detailed elsewhere in this book, therefore only specific nursing care for each procedure will be given in this chapter.

## BACKGROUND

Historically children undergoing surgery to their ear, nose or throat have been cared for in specialist ear, nose and throat (ENT) and plastic surgery areas rather than on paediatric surgical units. The Audit Commission (1993) suggested several possible reasons for this situation: the surgeons' preference for children to be cared for in adult ENT wards instead of children's wards, stemming from their perceived lack of control of beds in children's wards; the need for the nurses to be skilled in the surgical speciality; and the need to maintain the viability of their speciality (Audit Commission 1993). Elsewhere in the Audit Commission report (1993) there are recommendations that children should be cared for in separate facilities from adults, and that children's nurses should undertake specific in-house training to gain the skills and knowledge required to care for these children.

The need for children to be cared for in designated children's areas, including theatre, recovery and outpatient departments, by appropriately trained staff has been well documented (Caring for Children in the Health Services 1987, 1991, Department of Health 1991, 1997, 2001, Audit Commission 1993, Action for Sick Children 1996). Most recent guidance in the National Service Framework for Children, Young People and Maternity Services further reinforces these requirements (Department of Health 2003a, 2004).

Many of the procedures discussed in this chapter are undertaken as day case surgery. This method of care delivery became increasingly popular in the late 1990s because of the advances in surgery and anaesthetics as well as the political demands on the National Health Service (NHS). Day surgery has many benefits; however, to ensure quality services are offered there must be appropriate facilities, staffing and care packages (which include pre-admission preparation and follow up care). Quality standards for children undergoing day case surgery have been developed (Caring for Children in the Health Services 1991) (see also Ch. 2).

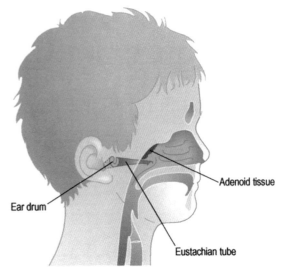

Figure 12.1 Position of adenoids in relation to eustachian tube.

## TONSILLECTOMY

Tonsillectomy is one of the most commonly performed surgical procedures in the UK and approximately 100 000 tonsillectomies are performed in Britain annually over half of which are in children under 15 years.

The tonsils are masses of lymphoid tissue and their main function is protection of the gastrointestinal tract and respiratory system from pathogens. They are situated one on either side of the pharyngeal cavity, and tend to be larger in children than in adults, so inflammation can cause them particular difficulty with eating or breathing.

## ADENOIDECTOMY

If the adenoids are enlarged, they can impede the passage of air to the throat from the nose (see Fig. 12.1). This can interfere with speech, impair taste and smell and cause mouth breathing, with potential for mouth odour. If they are very large, they may obstruct the eustachian tube, with resulting recurrent otitis media.

There is some controversy over the necessity of many tonsillectomies and adenoidectomies, however both continue to be carried out routinely in the UK, primarily for the reasons mentioned above, although, in a small number of cases, it may be necessary because of malignancy. Contraindications to the surgery include cleft palate (since both tonsils help minimise escape of air during speech) and acute infection at the time of the surgery.

In January 2001 the Department of Health recommended the use of single use instruments during tonsillectomy and adenoidectomy procedures. This change in procedure was to counteract the theoretical risk of transferring variant Creutzfeldt–Jakob disease (vCJD) from a patient incubating the disease to other patients. In the pre-clinical stages of vCJD it was recognised that high concentrations of abnormal prion protein in lymphoid tissue existed and conventional sterilisation techniques did not eliminate this prion protein from surgical instruments.

In December 2001 surgeons were advised (Department of Health 2001) to return to using reusable instruments, following an increase in reports of primary and secondary haemorrhage during surgery. Current guidelines address action to be taken in the case of high or medium infectivity on a possible CJD or vCJD patient (Department of Health 2003b).

## PREOPERATIVE CARE

Although often seen as common, routine operations, tonsillectomy or adenoidectomy can be painful and frightening experiences for a child. Children are admitted for surgery at a time when they are well but pain is often suffered afterwards and so effective psychological preoperative preparation is particularly important. Pain assessment and management should be discussed with the child and family at this time.

The child and family should be reassured that they might see some old blood, which is dark brown in colour, in the child's secretions postoperatively.

## POSTOPERATIVE CARE

The child's comfort and safety are key aspects of the postoperative nursing care. Safe positioning of the child in the immediate postoperative period is especially important to allow secretions to drain. These secretions will probably be bloodstained from surgery, but observation for fresh bleeding from the throat is vitally important. Frequent swallowing or clearing of the throat may indicate bleeding. The child's pulse, respiratory rate and colour will be monitored regularly to detect signs of postoperative complications such as haemorrhage or respiratory difficulty. A decrease in blood pressure may not be apparent until the child's condition has seriously deteriorated.

Primary haemorrhage (where bleeding occurs within the first 12 hours following surgery) may necessitate a return to theatre for ligation of a bleeding vessel, and therefore the surgeon should be informed if bleeding is continuous.

Children have often reported that this surgery is very painful and therefore effective pain prevention strategies should be used to minimise the pain experience for the child. Perioperative administration of rectal analgesics can be used to prevent pain on awakening following surgery. This needs to be discussed with the child and family preoperatively. Analgesia should be given regularly, with pain assessment being carried out before and after administration.

Once awake, the child may find cool fluids comforting. It should be noted that citrus juices and milky drinks could cause children to cough or clear their throats more often, which could lead to bleeding. Normally children will be discharged home the day following their surgery provided that they have made a full recovery from the anaesthetic, there are no signs of surgical complications and they are tolerating food and drinks. A sore throat and slight earache may persist for a few days and parents should be advised to administer simple analgesics regularly. It may be particularly helpful to administer analgesia prior to meal times to ease swallowing.

In recent years there has been some controversy regarding recommendations for post-tonsillectomy diet. At one time it was thought that soft diet was preferable, then rougher foods were advocated as it was thought that they helped in promoting healing and preventing infection. Current recommendations tend to advocate that the child eats normally and does not avoid rougher foods. Chewing and swallowing are viewed as important, and increased fluid intake and the chewing of gum may, therefore, also be helpful. Normal brushing of teeth is generally recommended to maintain good oral hygiene. Poor diet and infection may be associated with secondary bleeding (bleeding occurring several days following surgery) which requires immediate medical attention. Strategies to prevent infection include avoidance of people with coughs and colds, crowded places or smoky atmospheres. Parents should be warned that their child will need some time off school but should be able to resume normal activities within 1–2 weeks post surgery.

Before discharging the child and family the nurse should ensure that any verbal advice given is also provided in clear, understandable, written format. Parents should be provided with a contact number in case they have any concerns about their child's recovery at home. Some units have found that a follow-up visit or telephone call the following day is reassuring to parents.

## ACUTE OTITIS MEDIA WITH EFFUSION ('GLUE EAR')

The presence of fluid in the middle ear commonly follows upper respiratory tract infection in children. Obstruction of the eustachian tube by mucus and oedema causes pressure build up in the middle ear and the air which is normally present is replaced by inflammatory or mucous fluid. This may become infected by viral or bacterial pathogens resulting in acute otitis media with effusion, better known as 'glue ear'.

Language development can be affected and there is evidence that this condition can affect cognitive ability and behaviour because the child is not hearing information.

There is some contention about the need for surgical treatment; however, it continues to be one of the most common reasons for ENT surgical intervention in children. These procedures are normally carried out as day case surgery and children may be discharged a few hours after surgery.

A variety of surgical procedures are carried out for the treatment of 'glue ear' including myringotomy (surgical incision of the tympanic membrane to relieve pressure and allow drainage), insertion of grommets or T-tubes and adenoidectomy. There is some debate as to the benefits of surgical intervention, but any improvements in hearing are often immediate.

## MYRINGOTOMY

This involves surgical incision of the tympanic membrane to relieve pressure and allow drainage.

## INSERTION OF GROMMETS

Grommets are tiny plastic tubes, which are inserted into the middle ear through myringotomy incision to promote drainage and prevent build up of pressure in the middle ear (see Fig. 12.2).

Grommets usually remain in situ for up to a year and fall out spontaneously. If the drainage needs to be maintained over a longer period of time the surgeon may elect to insert T-tubes instead of grommets.

## INSERTION OF T-TUBES

T-tubes are similar to grommets and inserted in the same manner but are more secure, usually being removed under general anaesthesia after 2–4 years.

## POSTOPERATIVE CARE

Recovery is generally rapid because of the short anaesthetic and the small incision required in this relatively avascular area. However, postoperatively the child's general condition should be observed to detect any complications and to assess pain and distress.

Simple analgesics (e.g. paracetemol or ibuprofen) should be given in combination with comfort

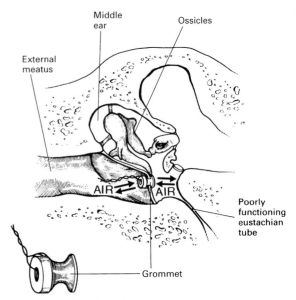

**Figure 12.2** Position of grommet.

(e.g. heat or cold pads) and distraction appropriate to the child's age and stage of development. Diet and fluids can be given when the child is awake.

Small amounts of discharge or bleeding, which may continue for a day or two, should be cleaned away but no attempts should be made to clean inside the ear canal. If discharge increases or begins to smell, medical advice should be sought. Generally, advice to parents indicates that care should be taken when washing hair. Parents are generally advised not to take their child swimming for 2 weeks and to prevent bath water from going in the child's ear whilst the grommets/T-tubes are in place. Diving under water should be avoided.

Longer term complications include early expulsion of the grommets from the ears, recurrence of otitis media, blockage of grommets by wax or exudate and sclerosis of the tympanic membrane.

## MASTOIDECTOMY

One potentially dangerous consequence of otitis media with effusion is the formation of a cholesteatoma in the middle ear space. This can grow and erode bony structures, causing hearing loss. It is important that the whole growth is removed.

## Preoperative care

The child may have been admitted with acute mastoiditis, which is very painful and normally results in a high temperature. Intravenous antibiotics may have been administered in the days prior to surgery; however, if the inflammation does not respond to these a mastoidectomy may be required.

An audiogram should be performed prior to surgery to assess hearing ability.

## Postoperative care

Postoperatively, nausea and sickness are not uncommon, and children should lie flat on return from theatre and be encouraged to sit up gradually as they awake from the anaesthetic, because their balance may have been temporarily affected.

The suture line will be behind the ear, and children will often have soluble sutures. Medical staff should be informed if bleeding is more than an ooze. Damage to the facial nerve is a potential complication, and this can be detected if the child cannot smile or grimace.

An antibiotic wick may be inserted into the ear in theatre and left in situ until follow up in the outpatient department (normally 2 weeks later) when the surgeon may wish to remove it personally. A pressure bandage may be applied in theatre and left on overnight.

## PINNING BACK OF PROMINENT EARS

This procedure is normally undertaken for cosmetic reasons by plastic surgeons. The main reason for the surgery is because of teasing by other children, and it is often performed at a young age – before starting school, or in the early school years. At one time the surgery was usually at the request of the parents although many surgeons will not carry out the procedure unless the child wishes to have it done.

The surgery is normally carried out under a general anaesthetic, and children return from theatre with a head bandage. Observations for bleeding are important, and an additional bandage may be applied to apply pressure if bleeding is slight. Length of stay in hospital varies, depending on local preferences. The bandage should remain on for 1–2 weeks, with hair washing discouraged. If the bandage falls off (a not uncommon problem), some centres will replace it, while others do not.

## NASAL SURGERY

This includes a variety of procedures:

- Nasal polypectomy (removal of polyps)
- Nasal cautery
- Submucosal resection
- Rhinoplasty
- Correction of deviated septum (which may be congenital or due to injury).

Principles of specific care in the immediate postoperative period focus on monitoring of the airway and detection of bleeding.

Bleeding will often be controlled by application of cold pack (or ice) to the bridge of the nose and gentle pinching of the soft part of the nose. The child should be positioned with the head tilted forward. Uncontrolled, continuous bleeding may require further surgical intervention.

Nasal packing may be used and is often left in situ for several days. Removal of packing is an uncomfortable experience for which the child should be well prepared. Moistening of the packing around the nose prior to removal may lessen some of the discomfort.

In the days following surgery the child's nose will feel blocked due to inflammation and dried blood. Some centres advise that children are discouraged from blowing their noses but that they may sniff if necessary. Others advocate regular steam inhalation followed by firm blowing to dislodge mucus or clots.

## DENTAL SURGERY

Dental extractions under general anaesthetic are a common procedure, despite recommendations that they should be avoided (Department of Health 1990). It has been recognised that for some groups of children, anaesthesia may be required if essential treatment is to be carried out. These include children who are extremely anxious, some who have physical disabilities, some children with learning difficulties, and those who require extensive treatment. An example of this is when children require total clearance of first teeth because of dental decay.

Since 1st January 2002 general anaesthesia for dental treatment has been undertaken in hospitals, in order to ensure the availability of emergency facilities should they be required (Department of Health 2000).

## PREOPERATIVE CARE

Children generally find the presence and taste of blood in their mouths a frightening and unpleasant experience, and it is important that this is discussed with them preoperatively. Some children wish to keep any teeth that are removed and they should be asked about this before their surgery.

## POSTOPERATIVE CARE

Effective pain management is a key consideration postoperatively as, if this is not provided, children may be reluctant to resume eating and drinking. The majority of children may prefer to start with a soft diet initially, particularly where several teeth have been removed at one time.

Nurses should be aware that a health promotion target was set by the Department of Health with regard to children's teeth to be achieved by the end of 2003: '5 year old children should have, on average, no more than one decayed, missing or filled primary tooth: and 70% of 5 year olds should have no experience of tooth decay' (Department of Health 2000, p. 42). Although progress was made towards this target, it was not fully achieved (National Statistics 2003).

Nurses should be able to advise parents on the benefits of brushing children's teeth from infancy, using toothpaste that contains fluoride, and reducing sugar intake in their diet.

## TRACHEOSTOMY

A tracheostomy is where a surgical incision is made into the trachea (tracheostomy) and a temporary or permanent opening is developed (see Fig. 12.3). Normally this would be performed in an operating theatre but rarely, and in extreme emergency situations, this procedure may be carried out elsewhere.

A tracheostomy is most commonly undertaken if the baby or child's upper airway is obstructed, or if there are problems with respiratory function and airway access for long term ventilation is required.

## UPPER AIRWAY OBSTRUCTION

There may be a range of causes for the upper airway obstruction which include:

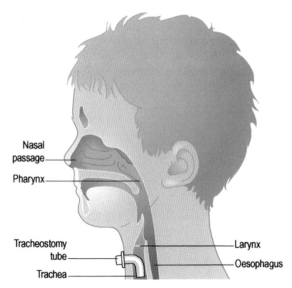

**Figure 12.3** Position of tracheostomy tube in trachea.

- Foreign bodies
- Trauma
- Acute infection – acute epiglottitis, croup, diphtheria
- Glottic oedema
- Bilateral abductor paralysis of the vocal cords
- Tumour of the larynx such as cystic hygroma
- Congenital web or atresia
- Laryngectomy
- Airway or facial burns.

A tracheostomy is kept patent by the insertion of a tube, which can be metal, but is more commonly plastic or silastic. It is important to ensure that this does not become blocked with secretions that may become crusted. This is less likely to happen with the more modern tubes, but metal tubes will have both an outer tube (which remains secured) and an inner tube that can be removed for cleaning. All of the tubes should be secured, usually with tapes that are attached to the side of the tracheostomy tube (see Fig. 12.4). When these tapes are changed, it is important to ensure that the new tapes are secured before the old ones are removed. Methods used to tie tapes are illustrated in Figure 12.5. Figure 12.4 shows a tied tracheostomy tube in situ and its proximity to the trachea and smaller airways. A small non-adhesive dressing is often placed beneath the flanges of the tube and this should be changed regularly to prevent infection around the tracheostomy opening.

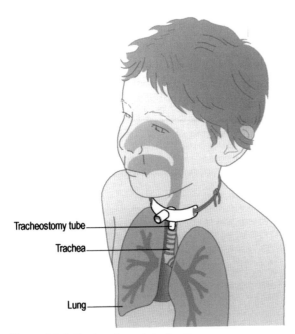

Figure 12.4 Tracheostomy tube in situ.

## POSTOPERATIVE CARE

Maintenance of the airway is of vital importance, and the child should be constantly observed for the first few days. Frequent suctioning to remove secretions is normally required, and indications for this include the sound or appearance of mucus in the airway or signs of respiratory difficulty (increased respiratory rate, sternal or intercostal recessions, nasal flaring, change in colour [to pale or dusky] and restlessness). Aseptic technique should be used to prevent the introduction of infection to the lower respiratory tract and the length of the suction tubing should be determined by estimating the length of the tracheostomy tube, as it should not be inserted further than half a centimetre beyond the end of this. If there is an inner tube, this can be removed and cleaned in normal saline after each suctioning and any crusting can be removed with pipecleaners of specially made brushes.

If the tube does become blocked or displaced, another one should be inserted immediately, and in order to ensure that the airway is not compromised, the following equipment must be readily available at the bedside:

- tracheal dilators
- a spare tracheostomy tube (which is ready to use with ties attached)

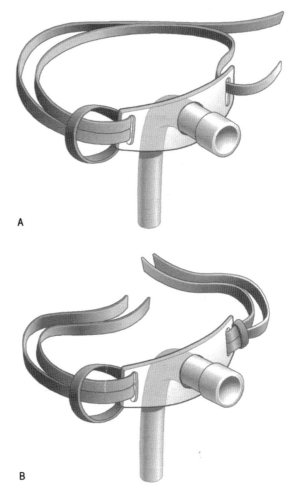

Figure 12.5 Examples of securing tracheostomy tubes.

- a tube which is a size smaller than the one in situ (in case the spare cannot be inserted)
- scissors
- suction equipment.

Humidification is normally required and is often delivered via a mask that fits over the tracheostomy.

Observation of the stoma site for signs of infection or bleeding should prevent these potential complications. Medical staff should be informed if bleeding is profuse or continuous.

The tracheostomy tube should be changed on a regular basis (often weekly), and the surgeon may ask to perform the first change.

Communication is a key nursing concern. If the tracheostomy is elective, time should be spent before surgery in establishing ways to communicate with the child in the postoperative period. Some children can be helped to vocalise by covering the tube opening, depending on the child's condition and the type of tube used.

If the tracheostomy is only temporary, the child will normally be weaned away from the need for the opening by using smaller tubes, and then blocking off the tube for 24 hours.

## LONGER TERM CARE

For those families where the tracheostomy will be left in for some time, education on the care of the child, and training in technical skills in the care of the tracheostomy are essential components of care.

Safety issues are also important: children with a tracheostomy should not go swimming or have a shower, and extreme care must be taken in the bath, with the child's head being tilted back for hairwashing. Use of talcum powder, aerosol sprays or perfumes should be avoided. Animals that shed fine hair pose a danger to these children. Parents of younger children need to be particularly vigilant to prevent foreign bodies being introduced into the tube, e.g. toys, balloons, sand, soil or dust. Clothing should not cover the opening and fluffy or furry clothing should not be worn. Young children may need to wear a bib whilst feeding to prevent liquid or food entering their airway, but plastic bibs should not be used. Very cold, dusty or smoky environments should be avoided, as should contact with people who have colds or other contagious illnesses. The value of routine immunisations and flu vaccines have been advocated for these children.

Children with tracheostomies should not participate in contact sports, and care needs to be taken

when the child is playing with others that the tube is not obscured and does not become dislodged.

There is a need for specialist equipment and constant supervision by people trained in suctioning, changing of tracheostomy tube and resuscitation, which will impact on the family's day to day life. Discharge planning should involve the family, GP and community nursing staff, nursery or school teachers (as appropriate) and the local pharmacist (for supplies). Some centres have established community liaison nursing posts to ease the transition from hospital to home. These nurses ensure that families are supported and appropriately educated to care for their child at home.

If oxygen therapy is also required, this will normally be prescribed by the GP and/or specialist nurse and supplied by the local pharmacy. Alterations to the home will be necessary to install oxygen points and concentrators. There may be a limit on the number of points which are installed (often only two) and this limits mobility within the home. Mobility outside the home will also be restricted if portable oxygen is required, in order to ensure that this does not run out. These restrictions will affect family life, and siblings often find them frustrating. The fire department should be informed if there is oxygen in the home, and it is also necessary for parents to inform their home and car insurance companies.

## ACKNOWLEDGEMENTS

Christine English and Ann Macfadyen would like to acknowledge the contribution made to this chapter by the nursing staff of the Children's ENT surgical ward, Freeman Hospital, Newcastle Upon Tyne Hospitals NHS Trust. Thanks also to Paul McDonald for the illustrations.

## References

Action for Sick Children 1996 Health services for children and young people: a guide for commissioners and providers. Action for Sick Children, London

Audit Commission 1993 Children first: a study of hospital services. HMSO, London

Caring for Children in the Health Services 1987 Where are the children? CCHS, London

Caring for Children in the Health Services 1991 Just for the day. CCHS, London

Department of Health 1990 General anaesthesia, sedation and resuscitation in dentistry – report of an expert

working party prepared for the standing Dental Advisory Committee (The Poswillo Report). The Stationery Office, London

Department of Health 1991 Welfare of children and young people in hospital. The Stationery Office, London

Department of Health 1997 Government response to the reports of the Health Committee on Health Services for Children and Young People, Session 1996–1997. The Stationery Office, London

Department of Health 2000 Modernising NHS dentistry: implementing the NHS plan. The Stationery Office, London

Department of Health 2001 The report of the public enquiry into children's heart surgery at the Bristol Royal Infirmary 1984–1995: learning from Bristol. The Stationery Office, London

Department of Health 2001 Report by the Government Operational Research Service – Risk assessment for transmission of vCJD via surgical instruments: a modelling approach and numerical scenarios. The Stationery Office, London

Chief Medical Officer Department of Health 2001. Letter Tonsil and adenoid surgery. CEM/CMO/2001/19

Department of Health 2003a Getting the right start: national service framework for children. Standard for hospital services. The Stationery Office, London

Department of Health 2003b Transmissible spongiform encephalopathy agents: safe working and the prevention of infection. Guidance from the Advisory Committee on Dangerous Pathogens and the Spongiform Tricephalopathy Advisory Committee. Online. Available: http://www.advisorybodies.doh.gov.uk/acdp/tseguidance/ [10th April, 2006]

Department of Health 2004 The national service framework for children, young people and maternity services. The Stationery Office, London

National Statistics 2003 Executive summary of preliminary findings. Children's Dental Survey. Online. Available: http://www.statistics.gov.uk/downloads/theme_health/Executive_Summary-CDH.pdf [15th September, 2006]

## Further reading

Bhaskar K 1998 Diet following tonsillectomy. Paediatric Nursing 10(9):25–27

Bisset AF 1997 Glue ear surgery in Scottish children 1990–1994: still plenty of ENT and public health challenges! Clinical Otolaryngology 22:233–238

Browning GG 1998 Is there an evidence base for the practice of ENT surgery? Clinical Otolaryngology 23:1–2

Issa A, Bellman M, Wright A 1999 Short-term benefits of grommet insertion in children. Clinical Otolaryngology 24:19–23

Scottish Intercollegiate Guidelines Network (SIGN) 2000 Clinical guideline no.47. Preventing dental caries in children at high caries risk. SIGN, Edinburgh

# Chapter 13

# Gastrointestinal surgery

Karen Evans, Elizabeth Thomas and Shelley Thomas

## CHAPTER CONTENTS

## INTRODUCTION

This chapter will consider the nursing care required by children undergoing gastrointestinal surgery. A child undergoing any gastrointestinal surgery requires skilled input from the multidisciplinary team, which may include nursing and medical staff, play specialists, physiotherapists, dietitians, stoma care nurses, the pain management team and hospital school teachers. The chapter will include an illustration of (Fig. 13.1) the normal anatomy and physiology of the gastrointestinal tract and a variety of acute and chronic conditions requiring both emergency and planned surgery. The focus will be upon complex congenital and acquired conditions such as Hirschsprung's disease and gastro-oesophageal reflux, but minor conditions such as tortion of testes will also be discussed. Some consideration will be given to the psychological effects of body altering surgery, for example the raising of stomas.

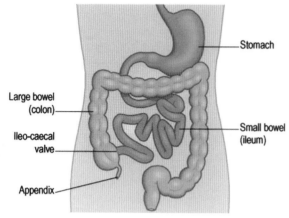

**Figure 13.1** Anatomy and physiology of the gastrointestinal tract.

## ANATOMY AND PHYSIOLOGY

### UNIVERSAL PRE- AND POSTOPERATIVE CARE

In order to ensure a safe environment (Roper et al 1996) for all children undergoing surgery, there are universal guidelines that must be incorporated into the child's plan of care (see Ch. 1). (Some further checks, such as marking of the sites of stoma settings and incisions, are patient specific.) This standardised checking procedure is necessary in order to maintain high standards of child safety and is an essential part of nursing care; its importance should not be underestimated.

Similarly, there are certain areas of standardised postoperative nursing care:

- Observations of vital signs to ensure rapid identification and treatment of hypoxia, pain, haemorrhage, hypovolaemic shock and infection.
- Regular wound checks for significant oozing. Wound closure materials are usually dissolvable to ensure neat scarring and avoid the further trauma of suture removal. However, certain wound drains are secured with nylon sutures and therefore require removing.
- Observation and recording of urinary output to ensure that urine is passed within 12 postoperative hours in order to avoid anaesthetic retention.
- The management of pain (see Ch. 6).

## FUNDOPLICATIONS

Fundoplication is the generic term for a variety of antireflux operations in which the fundus is wrapped around the lower oesophagus. The most common and well known is the Nissen's fundoplication, first described in the 1950s (Parrish & Berube 1995). More recently, there have been a number of modifications made to the operation in order to reduce the complications.

Gastro-oesophageal reflux results from a relaxed cardiac or oesophageal sphincter, which causes the reflux of gastric contents into the oesophagus. The child may suffer pain and damage to the oesophageal mucosa due to the acidity of the gastric contents. Certain groups of children are more at risk of developing reflux; these include premature infants and neurologically impaired children (75% have cerebral palsy), due to immature gastrointestinal tracts.

Symptoms of gastro-oesophageal reflux include:

- Vomiting
- Faltering growth
- Aspiration pneumonia
- Cough
- Irritability post feeding.

Gastro-oesophageal reflux is diagnosed through a combination of barium swallow X-rays and pH monitoring of the oesophagus. This will show significant time with a pH value lower than the normal level of 4. Occasionally, endoscopy is used to demonstrate oesophagitis.

Conservative treatment is the first line of management, with positioning, thickened feeds, drug therapy and early introduction of solid foods. If medical management is unsuccessful after 1 year, a surgical option is considered.

### SURGERY

The main function of an antireflux operation is to restore the competence of the lower oesophageal sphincter. By wrapping gastric smooth muscle around the oesophagus an artificial sphincter is formed. There are a variety of antireflux operations that involve either partial or complete fundal wrap in the authors' experience, two are most commonly used. First, the Nissen fundoplication (see Fig. 13.2a), which involves wrapping the fundus 360° around the lower oesophagus, restoring competence to the oesophageal sphincter. Gastro-oesophageal reflux is controlled in approximately 95% of these patients who undergo fundoplication; however, a variety of complications occur, mostly associated with tightness or slippage of the wrap. These complications may manifest themselves as dysphagia, inability to vomit or

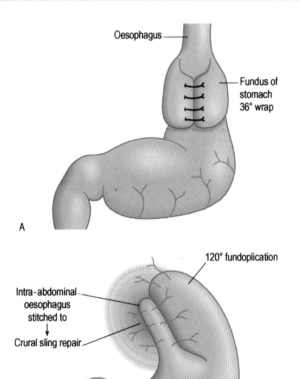

Figure 13.2 Common antireflux operations: A. the Nissen fundoplication. B. the Watson fundoplication

## RE-ESTABLISHING FEEDING AFTER SURGERY

Feeding following a fundoplication may recommence once gastric aspirate has reduced. Some children may require bolus feeds via the tube due to initial postoperative dysphagia. The stomach size may be decreased, necessitating smaller, more frequent boluses or even a continuous pump feed. If the child feeds orally, the tube should be clamped prior to feeding but may be released afterwards to vent gas. The hospital based dietitian would be involved in planning postoperative feeding and would liaise with the community nutritional support team.

## INSERTION OF GASTROSTOMY TUBES

A Foley or Malecot catheter (see Figs 13.3a and 13.3b) is used for up to 6 weeks postoperatively. If the child requires long term continuous or bolus feeds, this will then be replaced with a longer term tube such as a PEG or button tube (see Figs 13.3c and 13.3d) when a permanent tract is formed. Choice of long term tube is at the surgeon's discretion, taking into account the specific needs of the child.

A gastrostomy tube may be inserted without first performing an antireflux operation for a variety of reasons. Coldicutt (1994) lists these reasons as congenital abnormalities of the upper gastric systems, such as oesophageal atresia or tracheo-oesophageal fistula, or secondary to disorders resulting in absence or incompetence of the swallowing reflex, such as cerebral palsy. They could also be necessary in patients requiring additional nutritional support, such as in long term faltering growth or cystic fibrosis, or alternatively to ensure that enteral feeding can continue in a child who has suffered caustic burns to the oesophagus, for example following an ingestion of household cleaning solution. Finally, gastrostomy tubes are occasionally inserted in patients with diagnosed reflux in an attempt to avoid performing an antireflux operation, particularly where the patient is considered to be an anaesthetic risk.

Whatever the reason for insertion, when an antireflux operation has not been performed feeding is reintroduced after 24 hours of free drainage of gastric aspirate, providing recovery has been uneventful.

### Care of gastrostomy tubes

The importance of a taut secure tube is paramount since migration of the tube into the gastrointestinal

belch, or, more seriously, gas bloat syndrome (which has the potential to compromise respiratory effort) as noted in Parrish & Berube 1995. This can be avoided by the insertion of a gastrostomy tube (usually temporary). As well as being useful to release excess gas, gastrostomy tubes can be used for feeding purposes.

However, in response to the variety of complications experienced with complete 360° wraps, alternative solutions have been sought. One such alternative, and the second most common antireflux operation in our experience, is the Watson fundoplication (see Fig. 13.2b). Watson et al (1991) describe this as the fixing of the oesophageal sphincter below the diaphragm, thereby subjecting it to the intra-abdominal pressure, then wrapping the fundus only 120° around the sphincter with the result being improved competence without excessive pressure and consequently less complications are associated with this.

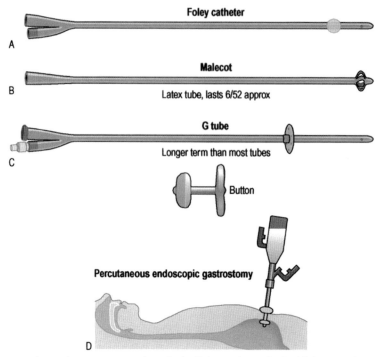

**Figure 13.3** Some commonly used gastrostomy tubes: A. the Foley catheter B. the Malecot catheter C. the G-tube and peg button D. percutaneous endoscopic gastrostomy.

system can cause vomiting, distension and ultimately abdominal obstruction or perforation.

Daily cleaning around the site with soap and water is essential as is ensuring the tube is secured adequately at all times; if pulled out, the tract will close in a matter of hours, therefore swift replacement is advisable. Skin breakdown is common due to acidic secretions that may leak around the tube site. Overgranulation of tissue often occurs, but is not inevitable and can be treated with silver nitrate.

Avoiding tube blockage is an important part of daily care and regular flushing with boiled water should be encouraged. If a blockage does occur, flushing with cola or pineapple juice can be attempted, and if this fails Clog Zapper® containing pancreatic enzymes, may dissolve it. However, this can only be used under medical supervision.

## HIRSCHSPRUNG'S DISEASE

Hirschsprung's disease is a congenital condition characterised by the absence of ganglionic cells in the distal bowel (see also Ch. 9). Harold Hirschsprung first described it in 1887, although a number of isolated reports had been published previously (Philippart 1980). The aganglionic section of the bowel has no peristalsis and therefore results in a lack of normal motility. The incidence is approximately 1 in 5000 births, with four times as many boys affected as girls. There are few associated anomalies, but congenital heart disease and Down syndrome each occur in 4–5% of cases. The disease falls into two categories, 80% involving the rectosigmoid colon (short segment Hirschsprung's) and 20% involving the total colon and small bowel involvement (long segment Hirschsprung's).

## CLINICAL PRESENTATION

The length of bowel involved and the age of the child at the time of diagnosis determine the severity of symptoms. A classic presentation in the neonatal period is failure to produce meconium stool within 24 hours of birth in the full term infant. In a preterm infant the passing of meconium may be delayed, but a delay of over 48 hours should be investigated. Constipation, bilious emesis, abdominal distension together with a reluctance to feed in the neonate are classic signs of the disease; however, often these symptoms are not constantly present and therefore a diagnosis is occasionally overlooked.

In later presentations the infant may present with a catalogue of problems, including faltering growth, alternate constipation/diarrhoea and abdominal distension. The diagnosis is often made when solids have been introduced and defecation is markedly reduced. If diagnosis is missed until childhood, the child will present with ongoing constipation and thin ribbon-like stools. Most of these cases will have ultra short segment involvement.

## DIAGNOSTIC TESTS

A rectal examination will sometimes produce an explosive stool on removal of the examiner's finger, but often there are no feces present. The anal canal feels narrow with increased tone. An abdominal X-ray will show gaseous distension. A barium enema will show a narrowing in one part of the affected colon. Barium will remain present up to 48 hours after the procedure if Hirschsprung's disease is present. If all these procedures rule out other reasons for obstruction (e.g. anorectal anomaly or colonic atresia), Hirschsprung's disease will be confirmed by the most accurate test: rectal biopsy. Suction biopsies may be taken from neonate or infant without anaesthesia; alternatively, a full thickness surgical biopsy may be taken from an older child under general anaesthesia. When looked at under the microscope these biopsies will provide a definitive answer to whether or not ganglionic cells are present.

## TREATMENT

Surgery to remove the aganglionic bowel is usually performed in two stages. Stage one is the removal of the obstruction by the formation of either an ileostomy or colostomy, so that the dilated bowel reduces in size. The formation of the stoma allows easier home care and improvement in nutritional intake. At stage two the segment of aganglionic bowel is resected and the stoma reversed. The same incision site will be used for the second stage as for the first. This second stage is carried out when the child is about 9 months old, assuming that the Hirschsprung's disease was diagnosed in the neonate or in early infancy.

The Duhamel procedure (Fig. 13.4) is the operation of choice in our experience. This describes the

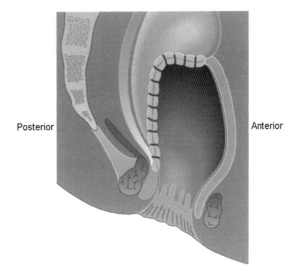

**Figure 13.4** The Duhamel procedure.

posterior pull through, with side-to-side anastamosis to the aganglionic rectum (see Fig. 13.4).

## POSTOPERATIVE COMPLICATIONS

A rare complication of the bowel resection is a leak at the anastomosis site. The child will become acutely ill with sepsis, distended abdomen, tachycardia and low blood pressure, and will show signs of hypovolaemic shock. An emergency laparotomy is required. To prevent infection, broad spectrum antibiotics would be routinely given on induction of anaesthesia, and then 8-hourly postoperatively for 24–48 hours. Obstruction may occur when there has been an incomplete resection of the aganglionic bowel or a stricture has occurred at the anastomosis site. Enterocolitis is a common problem. Incontinence may be a problem if late diagnosis has been made, as the child will have a megacolon due to years of constipation and poor bowel habit. It may take time for the bowel to develop tone. Bowel training and appropriate diet should improve this.

## STOMAS (see also Ch. 9)

A stoma is an artificial opening created in order to divert the flow of feces or urine. The stoma may either be permanent or temporary, depending on the predisposing disease/cause that necessitated the surgery. In childhood, most stomas are generally temporary (Hubbard & Trigg 2000).

Some of the conditions that may require a stoma formation are:

- Hirschsprung's disease
- Imperforate anus
- Neonatal necrotising enterocolitis
- Crohn's disease
- Ulcerative colitis
- Familial polyposis coli
- Fecal incontinence
- Trauma
- Spina bifida
- Carcinomas.

It is important to understand the reasons for stoma formation and to be able to identify the type of stoma to ensure effective management of care.

## TYPES OF STOMA

1. *Ileostomy*. A small section of the ileum is brought through the abdominal wall to form the stoma; the colon is either removed completely or is rested. Crohn's disease, ulcerative colitis and familial polyposis coli are the main reasons for ileostomy formation. The ileostomy is sited in the right iliac fossa and its output is soft and unformed.

2. *Colostomy*. This is a surgical opening into the colon. It is usually classified by the position in the bowel, i.e. transverse, descending or sigmoid colon, and its status, i.e. permanent or temporary. A colostomy is generally sited in the left iliac fossa and its output is usually formed stool, the excep- tion is a transverse colostomy where the output is often loose.

3. *Urinary diversion*. See Chapter 13.

The positions of different types of bowel stoma are shown in Figure 13.5.

It is important to remember that although the management of a stoma is fundamental, the psychological care of the child and family is also essential. These needs will be ever changing as the child moves through the developmental cycle.

## GENERAL STOMA CARE

The stoma nurse should be involved with the child and family both pre- and postoperatively to enable a trusting relationship to build up. The stoma nurse is also an invaluable resource for appliance information and for troubleshooting problems. There are many types of appliances available for stoma care, and it would therefore be impossible to mention and discuss them all. The general principles to consider for stoma care are:

- The privacy and dignity of the child is to be maintained at all times.
- The height and weight of the child need to be considered when choosing appliances as they come in a variety of sizes and lengths.
- The age and dexterity of the child need to be considered when choosing appliances, with the aim of promoting independence.

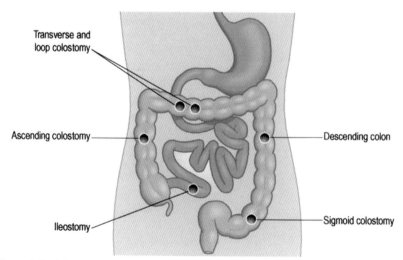

**Figure 13.5** Positions of the different types of bowel stoma.

- The size and shape of the stoma have a bearing on what is chosen for use to ensure best fit, comfort, ease of drainage and to allow the stoma to be observed.
- Skin condition must be monitored for redness/soreness and skin sensitivity to ensure the most appropriate barriers and/or lotions are used.
- As discussed earlier, the output from different types of stoma varies, therefore this has to be an important consideration in choice of appliances.

## COMMON COMPLICATIONS OF STOMAS

1. Dehydration can occur quickly, especially in those children with ileostomies. Children whose stoma output is loose or increases significantly should be encouraged to increase fluid intake.

2. Sodium depletion is a common problem in children with ileostomies, therefore regular urinary sodium levels should be taken and supplements given accordingly.

3. Prolapse is sometimes caused from excessive crying or coughing or after vigorous exercise. This is often self-resolving. If not, medical advice should be sought, and surgical intervention may be necessary.

4. Skin soreness is most commonly caused where the stoma output fluid has had contact with the skin from an ill fitting pouch. The stoma needs to be measured regularly to ensure a snug fitting flange.

Contact dermatitis can also be a problem where an obvious allergic reaction to the appliance adhesive occurs. This will follow the outlines of the adhesive shape.

5. Bleeding can occur if the stoma is knocked or scratched, and can occasionally occur during cleaning. Unless this is excessive, it will cause no further problems.

6. Stoma retraction can usually be remedied by using different shaped flanges. If this is unsuccessful, then surgical intervention is necessary.

Stoma care needs to be a partnership of care between child, family and healthcare professionals, looking not only at the physical side of care but also at the ever changing psychological and developmental needs of the child.

## MALROTATION

Malrotation (see also Ch. 9) is a congenital disorder of the intestine that is characterised by incomplete rotation of the intestines during the 10th week of fetal development. This may result in the chronic/acute, partial/complete bowel obstruction +/- volvulus. A volvulus is defined as a twisting of the bowel with obstruction and loss of blood supply.

## SIGNS AND SYMPTOMS

- Acute or chronic abdominal pain
- Faltering growth
- Diarrhoea/constipation
- Nausea – bile stained vomit, often cyclic
- Abdominal distension
- Signs of sepsis and shock.

## DIAGNOSIS

In the first instance an abdominal X-ray is performed. Findings include the 'double bubble' sign of duodenal obstruction, with distension of the stomach and generalised distension of the small intestinal loops; but malrotation +/- volvulus is easily missed on an abdominal X-ray. If symptoms persist and abdominal X-ray is inconclusive, a contrast study with follow-through is crucial. This will demonstrate abnormal placement of the duodenal C-loop, the duoden-jejunal junction lying to the right of the vertebral column and a small bowel loop on the right side of the abdomen. If volvulus is present, an abrupt cut-off of the dilated duodenum is seen and the duodenum has a 'corkscrew' appearance.

## TREATMENT

If a volvulus is determined to be present, emergency surgery is performed. Prior to surgery the child will have rapid intravenous fluid resuscitation, correction of electrolyte imbalance, decompression with nasogastric tube and administration of broad spectrum antibiotics. Surgery must be carried out as soon as possible as prolonging time will expose the bowel to an increased risk of ischaemia and bowel necrosis. If malrotation alone is diagnosed, elective surgical repair is most common due to the high risk of volvulus.

## SURGERY

Surgery is performed via a laparotomy, the volvulus is 'untwisted', and necrotic areas are resected. Then the large bowel is mobilised to the left of the abdomen and the small bowel remains on the right, as this allows better attachment, decreasing the incidence of further volvulus or malrotation. All patients also have a routine appendectomy as the caecum is placed in the upper left quadrant of the abdomen, making appendicitis extremely difficult to diagnose in the future.

## POSTOPERATIVE CARE

The child needs to have nil by mouth for 48–72 hours until bowel sounds/signs of intestinal function are determined. During this time the child should be supported with intravenous fluids, a nasogastric tube that is allowed to drain freely, plus hourly aspirations, and all losses replaced mL/mL via the intravenous route. Potassium chloride should be present in replacement fluids to ensure electrolyte balance is maintained. Analgesia is given by continuous infusion which is titrated to the child's individual level of pain. Routine observations are carried out as per infusion regime. Intravenous antibiotics are given for 7–10 days postoperatively and chest physiotherapy is given daily to prevent chest infection.

## COMPLICATIONS

If further necrotic bowel is to occur, it usually happens within 36 hours of initial surgery and will require further resection. As with all bowel surgery, there is a risk of adhesions and these will require surgery if they interfere with 'normal' bowel function. In extreme cases, where a large amount of gut is removed, the child may be left with short gut syndrome. This is a condition whereby the child may have too little gut to enable effective absorption of essential elements such as sodium, potassium and bicarbonate and may therefore require supplementation. The condition may also leave the child at risk of severe reactions to normal childhood illnesses such as gastroenteritis, thereby necessitating hospital admissions for fluid and drug administration. Those children more severely affected by short gut syndrome may require parenteral or extra enteral nutrition to supplement their oral intake to ensure that all essential salts are available to the body.

## ADHESIONS

Adhesions are usually formed after surgery when scar tissue becomes adhered to other tissue in the abdominal cavity. There are two types:

- Denovo adhesions occur as a result of a surgical procedure.
- Reformed adhesions occur where previous adhesions have been resected.

Adhesions will only become apparent if they cause intestinal obstruction. A history of vomiting and abdominal distension may be suggestive of adhesions if the child has had previous abdominal surgery.

## TREATMENT

Treatment may be conservative: the bowel is rested and a nasogastric tube is inserted to deflate the stomach and remove gastric contents. The child will be kept nil by mouth until the obstruction has resolved. Antibiotics are administered intravenously. Diet is only introduced when peristalsis is resumed. If conservative treatment is unsuccessful, a laparotomy is performed and the adhesions are divided away from the affected bowel.

## APPENDICITIS

This is the most common disease requiring surgical intervention in children. The highest incidence is between the ages of 9 and 11 years old. Incidence in children under 2 is not common. The appendix is found at the base of the ascending colon. The cause of appendicitis is generally thought to be obstruction of the appendix by feces (fecolith) or a foreign body, which allows bacteria to invade the wall of the appendix and may cause eventual gangrene or perforation.

## CLINICAL PRESENTATION

The child will complain of central abdominal pain, which localises in the right iliac fossa known as McBurney's point. This is the position on the abdomen directly overlying the appendix. When examined, this is the point that results in most tenderness in acute appendicitis (McFerran 1998). Nausea, vomiting, loss of appetite and low-grade pyrexia are also classic signs.

## DIAGNOSIS

A physical examination is carried out. Difficulty in walking is often a sign of appendicitis. The child will often complain of pain when asked to lift the right leg off the bed when lying flat. This is because the right leg is situated directly below the appendix and therefore, when bent, will put pressure on the area. Blood tests may show a raised white cell count but not always. Ultrasound scans are a useful diagnostic test to rule out ovarian cyst in pubescent girls, and a visualised appendix on ultrasound scan may indicate appendicitis. Diagnosing appendicitis is difficult as the incidence of non-specific abdominal pain is high in school age children. Also, mesenteric adenitis often presents with similar abdominal pain, although the child will usually have constantly high pyrexia and ultrasound scans may show enlarged lymph nodes. Gastroenteritis can also mimic the signs of appendicitis, with abdominal pain and vomiting.

## TREATMENT

Appendicitis is treated by surgical removal. The appendix is tied with an absorbable suture, then removed by a sharp division proximal to the clamp (see Fig. 13.6). The remaining stump is cleaned with an antiseptic solution and cauterised. The inflamed appendix is removed through an incision in the right lower quadrant of the abdomen. If the appendix has perforated, aspiration of pus and peritoneal lavage with saline will be needed. Preoperative antibiotics have been shown to minimise infection and the length of the course is dependent on the condition of the appendix at removal. Laparoscopic

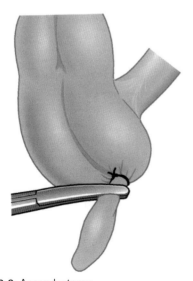

Figure 13.6 Appendectomy.

appendectomy, which enables the child to be discharged more quickly, has a decreased incidence of wound infection and increased return of intestinal function.

## COMPLICATIONS

Complications are rare but may include wound infection and adhesions. Occasionally, a collection of fluid may form in the peritoneum, which may cause a delay in recovery and is usually treated with further antibiotics.

## PYLORIC STENOSIS (see also Ch. 9)

Congenital hypertrophic pyloric stenosis is one of the most common conditions requiring surgical intervention during infancy, occurring in 1 in every 500 births, predominately in males, and is familial. It is characterised by an increase in size of the circular muscle of the pylorus, resulting in a narrow canal between the stomach and duodenum, the cause is unknown. Pyloric stenosis was first identified in 1646, and was further described by Harold Hirschsprung in 1888 (Spitz & Coran 1995), when the preferred treatment was medical due to the high mortality in surgery.

Symptoms often do not present until 2–4 weeks of age. Initial signs are non-bilious vomiting progressing to projectile vomiting, resulting in faltering growth, constipation and dehydration. The infant feeds continuously, the abdomen appears distended with visible gastric peristaltic waves, and an olive or tumour to the right of the umbilicus may be palpable during a test feed or immediately after emesis. Electrolyte imbalance is inevitable, metabolic alkalosis and potassium depletion need to be corrected, and therefore surgery is never performed as an emergency. Diagnosis is reached through a combination of physical examination, parental description of symptoms and abdominal ultrasound.

Pyloromyotomy is the treatment of choice; it was first performed in 1908 by Fredet and modified by Ramstedt in 1912 (Spitz & Coran 1995). This remains the most common approach; however, recently umbilical incisions have been used due to their improved cosmetic outcome.

Recommencement of feeds is subject to consultant preference, varying between 4 and 12 hours postoperatively. If the initial feed of dextrose solution is tolerated, the infant can progress to milk feeds on demand. Even in a successful operation, vomiting for 24–48 hours postoperatively is common due to reduced peristalsis; however, if this persists beyond 5 days it may indicate insufficient division of pyloric muscle or adhesions. Current trends advocate the application of antibiotic ointment to the umbilical wound site for 5 days to reduce the incidence of wound infection caused by staphylococcus.

## INTUSSUSCEPTION

Intussusception was first identified in 1674 by Barbette (Ashcroft & Hodder 1980), who described it as telescoping of a portion of the intestine into itself. This results in venous obstruction and oedema of the bowel wall, which if left untreated will lead to obstruction and gangrene of the proximal bowel. There have been links to gastrointestinal viruses such as adenovirus amd rotavirus, as well as Meckel's diverticulum and Henoch–Schönlein purpura.

Intussusception occurs most commonly in the first year of life, the greatest incidence being between 5 and 10 months, with a 2:1 male/female ratio. Symptoms usually occur suddenly with screaming and drawing up of the legs, secondary to abdominal pain. Vomiting is common and later a refusal to feed. One of the classic signs is a redcurrant jelly appearance of the stools, but this does not always occur. If left undiagnosed the child becomes pale, listless and quiet and may require fluid resuscitation with colloid prior to active treatment.

Diagnosis is achieved initially by abdominal examination (which reveals a sausage shaped mass), followed by ultrasound. The first line of treatment, where there is no evidence of perforation or peritonitis, involves an air enema or 'pneumatic reduction'. In the past barium was used; however, a reduced rate of infection and decreased risk of perforation has been found using air enema. Air or oxygen is delivered at 80–150 mm of mercury whilst monitoring fluoroscopically the reduction in telescoping. Currently three attempts are made to reduce by air enema (a single dose of antibiotics is given to cover this procedure), before surgery is considered.

As enemas yield such a high success rate, surgery is only considered for those children in whom radiological reduction has failed or those with the added complications of Meckel's diverticulum polyps or multiple recurrences. Surgical reduction is performed by laparotomy. The intussusception is reduced by squeezing the telescoped bowel. If the bowel is damaged or gangrenous, resection is performed.

Feeding recommences 12 hours after air enema and 24 hours after surgery, provided there are no signs of reintussusception. Intravenous antibiotics continue for 24–48 hours postoperatively following a surgical reduction. Complications that may occur are reintussusception and possible adhesions following laparotomy.

## MECKEL'S DIVERTICULUM

This was first described in 1812 by Johann Meckel (Ashcroft & Hodder 1980) as a remnant of the structure connecting the fetal yolk sac and the intestinal cavity. It is the most common congenital malformation of the intestinal tract, affecting 1–2% of the population with complications more frequently seen (3–5 times more commonly) in males (Whaley & Wong 1999). The majority of people affected remain asymptomatic; however, more than 50% of those who develop symptoms will do so within the first 2 years of life (Foglia 1980).

A symptomatic diverticulum may present with a bout of painless rectal bleeding resulting from a blood supply directly from the ileum. Bleeding usually results from the presence of gastric mucosa in the diverticulum – this is present in about 80% of patients who bleed – causing ulceration and subsequent lower gastrointestinal bleeds. The bleeding may either be ongoing and mild, resulting in dark stools and anaemia, or there may be a massive rectal bleed leading to hypovolaemic shock requiring resuscitation. An occasional misdiagnosis may occur, when the stools resemble redcurrant jelly, as this is a classic sign of intussusception. Intestinal obstruction is the second most common presentation, occurring in up to 40% of cases (Vanderbilt M. Centre 2000). It may be associated with volvulus, intussusception, hernia or torsion and it may be also mistaken for acute appendicitis.

Diagnosis may be reached through a variety of invasive tests such as rectosigmoidoscopy and barium enema to rule out alternative solutions. A technetium radionuclide (Meckel's) scan may show a Meckel's diverticulum that has gastric mucosa present; however, some may be too small to visualise. The use of cimetidine orally may inhibit the production of gastric acid, enabling improved uptake of the nuclide, thereby improving chances of a conclusive result and allowing accurate interpretation when deciding on a surgical approach.

Treatment preoperatively requires the control and replacement of blood loss and administration of intravenous antibiotics may be required to reduce postoperative infection. Surgery is subsequently indicated to perform a diverticulectomy – to resect the affected portion of bowel and also correct any associated problems.

Postoperative complications are those commonly associated with gastrointestinal surgery, such as infection, reduced circulating volume and adhesions.

## TESTICULAR TORSION

Miller (1999) described torsion as the rotation of the testicle on the spermatic cord, thereby occluding the blood supply. The cause is thought to be the absence of posterior attachments, which anchor the testicle in the scrotum.

## SIGNS AND SYMPTOMS

Torsion is characterised by acute scrotal pain and oedema, potentially radiating up to the abdomen, nausea and vomiting. Diagnosis is reached through physical examination, revealing tender scrotum with a raised testicle. Abdominal examination, urine dipstick and full blood count rule out appendicitis, urinary tract infection or sexually transmitted diseases. This surgical emergency occurs more commonly in puberty but may present in boys of any age. Doppler ultrasound suggests decreased blood flow, confirming diagnosis. The only effective treatment is surgery within 4–6 hours in order to avoid ischaemia and necrosis of the testicle. During surgery the cord is untwisted and the testicle fixed into position (orchidopexy). The area is observed for a short time to ensure sufficient blood flow has returned. The other side is checked for the presence of attachments, as the defect is often bilateral. Should the testicle be necrosed and blood supply does not return when released, then orchidectomy is performed.

Postoperatively a scrotal support may be provided to minimise oedema. A caudal block may have been administered intraoperatively for pain relief. The boy is told to observe for signs of infection and to avoid contact sports and heavy lifting for 4 weeks.

## ORCHIDOPEXY (see also Ch. 8)

During fetal development the testes develop in the abdominal cavity and only descend into the scrotum during the final trimester of pregnancy. Hutson (1995) states that in 4–5% of newborns this fails to happen on one or both sides. This incidence can rise up to 20% in preterm babies. An alternative name for undescended testicles is cryptorchidism (Whaley & Wong 1999). It is often accompanied by congenital hydrocele and hernias.

## SIGNS AND SYMPTOMS

Undescended testes are usually initially noted in neonates during the check by the paediatrician prior to discharge home. In a high number of these children the testes have descended by the age of 3 months, thereby reducing the incidence to 1–2%. If the testes have not reached the scrotum by the age of 1 year it is unlikely to occur naturally, and surgery before the age of 2 years is indicated in order to maintain optimum sperm production. Lugo-Vincente (1993) suggests that a higher incidence of malignancy, trauma and torsion are further indications for early surgical intervention. Surgery at a later age may be necessary if the spermatic cord does not grow in proportion with the child, thereby drawing the testicle out of the scrotum.

If surgical treatment under general anaesthetic is required, the child is often admitted as a day case (see Ch. 8). Two incisions are used: one in the groin to maximise the length and free the cord, and a second in the scrotum to enable the testicle to be gently pulled down. Once this has been achieved the testicle is stitched into place and the incisions closed. The child may have a caudal block for pain. Postoperatively few complications are expected; however, contact sports are discouraged for approximately 1 month to allow inflammation to reduce and sutures to dissolve slowly.

Lugo-Vincente testicular vanishing syndrome (Lugo-Vincente 1993), where the testicle does not exist or subsequently atrophies, necessitates removal as the only course of action. In this case boys are offered a prosthetic replacement in later life, purely for cosmetic reasons.

## HERNIAS AND HYDROCELES (see also Ch. 8)

A hernia is the protrusion of parts of the body through an abnormal opening in the wall of the abdominal cavity. This may become more prominent when the child cries or strains (Borkowski 1994). Hernias are one of the most common surgical conditions affecting children, and the most frequently occurring of these is the inguinal hernia followed closely by umbilical hernias. The ratio of incidence per sex is 9:1 boys to girls (Weber & Tracey 1980).

An inguinal hernia develops from the processus vaginalis (a hollow pouch of peritoneum) which is present from 12 weeks gestation (Borkowski 1994). The pouch decends through the inguinal canal to the scrotum or labia major. The opening usually closes around the time of birth; however, if this does not occur a hernia sac is left, allowing bowel, ovary or fallopian tube to descend into the scrotum or labia. If only partial closure occurs, fluid is able to accumulate forming a hydrocele. The size of the hydrocele may fluctuate and it may be single or bilateral. Hydroceles often form in association with inguinal hernias (Digital Urology Journal 2001). Figure 13.7 shows the common types of hernias and hydroceles.

All inguinal hernias will require surgical intervention to avoid potential intestinal obstruction or loss of testes/ovary. However, umbilical hernias are expected to close spontaneously by 1 year and most

surgeons would not consider surgery unless the hernia persisted beyond 2 years (Neblett & Holcomb 1980). Whilst the inguinal hernia remains intermittent, it does not necessitate emergency surgery; however, should the contents of the sac become trapped, reduction is required as a matter of urgency. Providing the hernia has not been incarcerated long enough for swelling to occur, manipulation by an experienced paediatrician may be successful. If this is not possible, surgical repair is required at the earliest possible time to avoid necrosis of the protruding component.

The surgical incision is made in the groin in a natural skin crease. The patent processus (hernia sac) is ligated and the testes manipulated into the scrotum. The hole in the abdominal wall is left to close spontaneously. Some surgeons choose to explore the second side; however, many consider that the potential risks of damage to the vas and vessels make a negative exploration unnecessary.

Postoperatively the child may have been given a caudal block with supplementary oral analgesia. An overnight stay is not often necessary; however, it may be required when there is a history of anaesthetic problems, prematurity or when the hernia was strangulated.

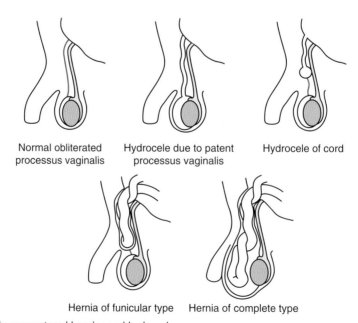

Normal obliterated processus vaginalis

Hydrocele due to patent processus vaginalis

Hydrocele of cord

Hernia of funicular type

Hernia of complete type

Figure 13.7 Commonly encountered hernias and hydroceles.

## CONCLUSION

This chapter has gone some way to providing an overview of some of the conditions, acquired and inherited, that may affect the gastrointestinal tract during childhood. Whilst the discussion of the more minor conditions such as hernias and orchidopexy can be covered fully, when dealing with complex congenital conditions such as Hirschsprung's it is impossible to be exhaustive in one chapter. We would hope that what has been provided here will be a baseline from which to progress with more in-depth reading.

## References

Ashcroft KW, Hodder TM (eds) 1980 Paediatric surgery, 2nd edn. WB Saunders, London

Borkowski S 1994 Common pediatric surgical problems. Pediatric Surgical Nursing 29(4): 551–561

Coldicutt P 1994 Children's options. Nursing Times 90(13): 54–56

Digital Urology Journal 2001 Hernia and hydrocele. Division of Urology, Children's Hospital, Boston. Online. Available: http://www.duj.com/hernia.html

Foglia RP 1980 Meckels. In: Ashcroft KW, Hodder TM (eds) Paediatric surgery, 2nd edn. WB Saunders, London

Huband S, Trigg E (eds) 2000 Practices in children's nursing. Churchill Livingstone, London

Hutson JM 1995 Orchidopexy. In: Spitz L, Coran AG (eds) Rob and Smith's operative surgery (paediatric surgery), 5th edn. Chapman & Hall Medical, London

Lugo-Vincente HL 1993 The pediatric inguinal hernia: Is contralateral exploration justified? Pediatric Surgery Update 1:1. Online. Available: http://home.coqui.net/titolugo/psuo1.htm

McFerran TA 1998 Minidictionary for nurses, 4th edn. Oxford University Press, Oxford

Miller KM 1999 Testicular torsion. American Journal of Nursing 99(6): 33–34

Neblett WW, Holcomb GW 1980 Hernias and hydroceles. In: Ashcroft KW, Hodder TM (eds) Paediatric surgery, 2nd edn. WB Saunders, London

Parrish R, Berube M 1995 Care of the infant with gastroesophageal reflux and respiratory disease: after the Nissen fundoplication. Journal of Pediatric Health Care Sep/Oct 9: 211–217

Roper N, Logan W, Tierney A 1996 The elements of nursing: a model for nursing based on a model of living. Churchill Livingstone, Edinburgh

Philippart ? 1980 Hirschsprung's. In: Ashcroft KW, Hodder TM (eds) Paediatric surgery, 2nd edn. WB Saunders, London

Spitz L, Coran AG (eds) 1995 Rob and Smith's operative surgery (paediatric surgery), 5th edn. Chapman & Hall Medical, London

Vanderbilt M/C (1998) Mekel's Diverticulum. http://www.me. vand.edu/peds/pidl/gi/meckel.htm

Watson A et al 1991 A more physiological alternative to total fundoplication for the surgical correction of resistant gastro-oesophageal reflux. British Journal of Surgery 78: 1088–1094

Weber TR, Tracey TF 1980 Hernias. In: Ashcroft KW, Hodder TM (eds) Paediatric surgery, 2nd edn. WB Saunders, London

Whaley L, Wong D 1999 Whaley and Wong's essentials of paediatric nursing. London

# Chapter 14

# The urinary system

## Karen Evans and Shelley Thomas

## INTRODUCTION

This chapter will consider childhood diseases and disorders of the urinary system. First, a brief description of urinary function and development will be given, augmented with diagrams of both the male and female systems.

The urinary system is designed to remove waste from the body (see Fig. 14.1). A complex filtration system that adapts according to the body's requirements ensures that chemical and fluid balances are maintained and excess waste removed. This filtration occurs in the kidneys, situated near the middle of the back below the rib cage. Once the appropriate level of fluid and chemicals (urea, sodium and potassium) have been removed from the bloodstream, they are passed by muscular contractions down the two ureters to the bladder (see Figs 14.2 and 14.3).

The bladder is a hollow muscular balloon which expands until full, when nerve endings inform the brain that the bladder needs to be emptied. Until that point has been reached the sphincter muscles automatically remain contracted to avoid leakage of urine. When the brain has informed the bladder that it is time to empty, the detrusor muscles contract and the sphincter muscles relax to allow the urine to be squeezed out via the urethra. This process happens automatically in babies; however, as the child's nervous system develops the messages are sent to enable control over voiding until an appropriate time.

Problems either with design or function of any of these structures may lead to problems requiring medical and surgical intervention. It is these

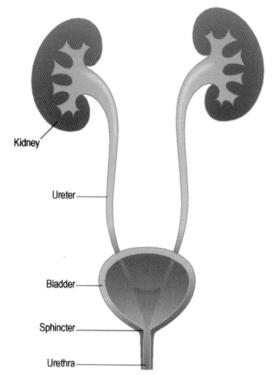

Kidney

Ureter

Bladder

Sphincter

Urethra

**Figure 14.1** Front view of urinary tract.

problems that will be considered in greater depth in this chapter.

## URINARY TRACT INFECTION

The urinary tract is one of the commonest sites for bacterial infection. Larcombe (1999) estimates that at least 8% of girls and 2% of boys will have a urinary tract infection (UTI) during childhood. Larcombe goes on to define a UTI as the presence of

a pure bacterial growth with more than 100 single species colony-forming units per mL. The name of the UTI depends on its location within the system; if it is found to be in the bladder it is known as cystitis. Alternatively, pyelonephritis refers to the potentially more serious infection higher in the system or in the kidneys. UTIs can be divided into 2 separate categories. First, a recurrent UTI is defined as a further infection by a new organism. The alternative, a relapsing UTI, involves subsequent infection with the same organism.

Most of the bacteria that result in a UTI come from the body's natural flora, usually those found in the bowel or on the skin. Heritage (1996) gave statistics comparing the underlying bacteria in UTIs of patients in hospital and those in the community. In both groups gram negative bacteria are the commonest cause, resulting in 65% of hospital cases and 84% of community instances. Of these *Escherichia coli* accounts for 3/4 of cases, whilst other gram negative infections include *Klebsiella*, *Pseudomonas aeruginosa*, and *Enterobacter*. Hospital-based patients are more at risk of contracting *Candida albicans*, due to the higher incidence of indwelling catheters.

The signs and symptoms of a UTI include:

- Urgency – an overwhelming need to micturate
- Frequency
- Dysuria – difficulty or pain on passing urine
- Cloudy or offensive urine – either due to the presence of pus (pyuria) or blood (haematuria)
- Loin pain
- Pyrexia
- Irritability
- Lethargy
- Vomiting.

**Figure 14.2** Side view of female urinary tract.

Peritoneum

Uterine tube

Ovary

Uterus

Vesicouterine pouch

Urinary bladder

Pubic bone

Labium minora

Labium majora

Vertebrae

Sigmoid colon

Rectouterine pouch (of Douglas)

Cervix

Rectum

Vagina

Urethra

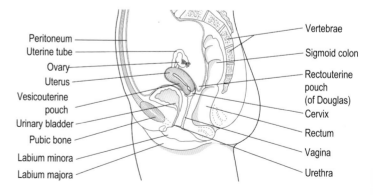

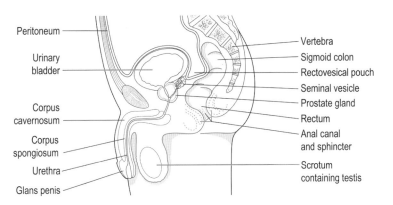

**Figure 14.3** Side view of male urinary tract.

Peritoneum

Urinary bladder

Corpus cavernosum

Corpus spongiosum

Urethra

Glans penis

Vertebra

Sigmoid colon

Rectovesical pouch

Seminal vesicle

Prostate gland

Rectum

Anal canal and sphincter

Scrotum containing testis

## DIAGNOSIS

The most common method of diagnosis is the microscopic examination of a midstream urine sample. Passing a small amount of urine prior to collection allows the removal of any bacteria from the distal end of the urethra. The method of collection of this sample is very important as if it is incorrectly done abnormal results may be found. In children not toilet trained, a sample may be obtained by placing an adhesive bag over the perineum or a collection pad may be placed in the nappy. Both of these methods are susceptible to contamination and therefore not favoured by medical staff. Urethral catheters and suprapubic aspiration are more reliable methods, producing a cleaner sample. In the older child, a sterile pot is provided for a midstream sample. The urine is then subject to microscopic examination, culture and sensitivity testing (MC&S); this reveals the presence of leukocytes (white blood cells), red blood cells, bacteria and `casts' (deposits formed in a diseased kidney and shed in urine). If evidence of an infection is found, an antibiotic sensitivity test is performed on the sample. Urine taken from a long term indwelling catheter is likely to contain bacteria and therefore the patient should only be treated if symptomatic.

## TREATMENT

This involves a course of antibiotics. Initially, broad spectrum drugs are used and then subsequently changed to bacteria-specific antibiotics once sensitivities are available. Larcombe (1999) points out that delaying treatment until sensitivities are available may be related to increased renal scarring. Generally, oral syrup or tablets will be given; however, patients who are unable to tolerate anything orally may be given intravenous antibiotics for several days. Following an isolated UTI, no further investigations or treatment will be required; however, in the case of repeated infection, further diagnostic tests may be carried out to identify any functional abnormalities.

Whilst statistics indicate a higher incidence of UTIs in females than males, both Heritage (1996) and Larcombe (1999) state that under 3 months of age boys are more susceptible due to the higher number of anatomical abnormalities of the urinary tract in infant boys. Thereafter, the incidence reverts to that usually stated, whereby the relatively short urethra in females compared to males enables easier migration of bacteria up to the bladder and beyond. Ross (1999) recommends urine culture for all male patients under 6 months and females under 2 years presenting with a pyrexia of 39°C or above.

MC & S is also considered a useful test in a patient presenting with abdominal pain in order to rule out UTI before a diagnosis of appendicitis is reached.

## DIAGNOSTIC TESTS

Following the detection and treatment of a UTI it may be considered necessary to carry out further tests beyond the scope of simple urinalysis to determine the origin of the infection. These include the following:

- 24-hour urine collections can reveal whether the kidneys are functioning efficiently at removing waste from the body.
- Blood tests may also reveal decreasing kidney function by examining the level of creatinine and urea nitrogen in the blood.

• A plain X-ray of the kidneys, ureters and bladder is helpful.

• Ultrasound uses sound waves to the detect size and shape of the kidneys, the degree of ureteric dilation and the thickness of the bladder wall.

• Intravenous pyelograms are a commonly performed test used to identify abnormalities to the urinary tract, such as any obstruction due to stones, hydronephrosis, bladder filling dysfunctions and residual urine post voiding.

• Nuclear scans, such as DMSA (Dimercaptosuccinate) and Mag 3 (Tc-labelled mercaptoacetyl triglycerine) provide a measure of the function, shape and emptying of each kidney.

• Computer tomography (CT) and magnetic resonance imaging (MRI) scans are used if a tumour is suspected, to detect the size, site and extent of tumour involvement. CT scans are also useful to look for non-opaque stones causing a filling defect that is seen on intravenous pyelogram (IVP).

• Micturating cystourethrogram (MCUG) is used to detect abnormalities of the inside of the bladder and the flow of urine as excreted.

• Urodynamic studies evaluate the storage of urine in the bladder, the flow of urine from the bladder through the urethra, and the contraction of the bladder muscles as it fills and empties. These tests are used to diagnose problems with the nerve supply and muscles of the lower urinary system.

• Cystoscopy is an evaluation under anaesthetic of the position and shape of the ureters. Although it is not widely used, some surgeons use this test to determine the likelihood of ureteric reflux spontaneously resolving, thereby negating the need for more radical surgery.

This list of investigations is by no means exhaustive; however, it does include the most commonly used tests in diagnosing urinary tract disorders in childhood.

## HYPOSPADIAS

Hypospadias is caused by abnormal development of the urethra in the embryotic stage. Hypospadias is a fairly common birth defect that affects approximately 1 in 350 male births. There is a familial trait with 8% of fathers having hypospadias and 14% of males siblings are also affected. Kallen et al (1986) reported some factors that affect the risk of hypospadias. These include:

• Maternal age. There is an increased incidence in older mothers, which significantly increases if this is their first child.

• Twin births also resulted in an increased risk, especially when both twins were male.

Hypospadias is characterised by the abnormal positioning of the meatus (see Fig. 14.4). The urethra opening is found underneath the glans, its position determining the level of severity.

## TREATMENT

Hypospadias can be surgically corrected, and the optimum age for this is between 6 and 18 months. The surgery involves refashioning and lengthening of the glans urethra. Either a stent is placed into the bladder to allow draining of urine into the nappy, or alternatively a suprapubic catheter is inserted for urine drainage and a tied stent is placed in the urethra, allowing the refashioned urethra time to heal. Silicone foam dressing which is placed around the penis in liquid form then solidifies, leaving a soft mildly compressive dressing that is waterproof. Dressings should accomplish gentle pressure on the penis to help with haemostasis and to decrease oedema formation without compromising vascularity of the repair. The dressing remains in situ for one week.

The use of low dose antibiotics whilst the stent is in place has been proven to reduce the rate of infection. Unfortunately, the stent often causes bladder spasm as it can rub on the bladder mucosa and

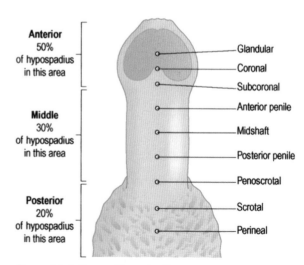

Figure 14.4 Types of hypospadias.

trigone. Most bladder spasms are minor; in those that are more severe, regular low dose oxybutynin has been found to be effective. For pain control most children will either have a caudal block or penile block whilst in theatre, which offers 4–6 hours of pain relief. This is then supplemented with oral analgesia.

Most children are discharged home after an overnight stay following surgery, returning one week post surgery to have removal of dressing. If they do not have a suprapubic catheter in situ, they can be discharged home once they have voided. If a suprapubic catheter is in situ the catheter is clamped, the stent is removed, the child then needs to void prior to the removal of the suprapubic catheter. Once this is achieved the child can be discharged home. In both cases the children will be followed up in the outpatients clinic in 3 months. Until return for the outpatients appointment, prophylactic antibiotics should be continued.

## COMPLICATIONS

Fistulas are the most commonly reported complication, reported in 1% of cases and resulting from a failure to heal at some point along the suture line. Further repair of fistulas should not be carried out for at least 6 weeks after the original surgery, to allow complete tissue healing. Another reported complication is bladder spasm. This is treated with low dose oxybutynin as mentioned above, but parents should be advised that oxybutynin can cause facial flushing.

## NEPHRECTOMY

A nephrectomy is the surgical removal of the kidney. This can be performed for a number of reasons, including cystic disease of the kidney, severe hydronephrosis due to obstruction at the pelvic ureteric junction when kidney function is severely affected, and renal tumours such as Wilms'. Heminephrectomies (partial removal) are also performed on children who have a duplicated system.

## TREATMENT

Preoperative investigations are carried out in order to establish the site, size, extent and nature of renal disease. When it has been decided that a nephrectomy is necessary, they are good indicators as to the type of nephrectomy that should be undertaken.

The surgery can be done using two basic approaches: lateral and anterior.

## POSTOPERATIVE CARE

- Fluid balance is managed by intravenous infusion but the child can eat and drink.
- Pain is managed by epidural continuous infusion.
- The wound is drained by redivac wound drain for 48 hours.
- Urethral catheter is in situ for 48 hours.
- Intravenous antibiotics are administered on induction, postoperatively for 24 hours and then continued on a prophylactic dose.

## PYELOPLASTY

This is the preferred treatment for moderate to severe hydronephrosis. In children the most common site of obstruction in the upper urinary tract is the pelvic-ureteric junction. The incidence is between 1:1000 and 1:2000 live births and it is more commonly found in boys. It has been found that in 60% of cases the left side is more commonly affected and that 5% of cases are bilateral (Spitz & Coran 1995).

## CLINICAL FEATURES

The most commonly presenting signs have been reported as recurrent urinary tract infections and non-specific back pain.

## PREOPERATIVE CARE

A nephrostomy tube is often inserted some time prior to surgery to drain the kidney and reduce hydronephrosis before surgery. Treatment doses of antibiotics are given from time of tube insertion.

## TREATMENT

Surgery is performed in order to improve the drainage of the pelvic-ureteric junction, which in turn reduces hydronephrosis and prevents further renal deterioration. During surgery, the narrowed section of the ureter as well as a small amount of the renal pelvis are excised. The remaining ureter is then divided and anastomosed to the renal pelvis (see Fig. 14.5).

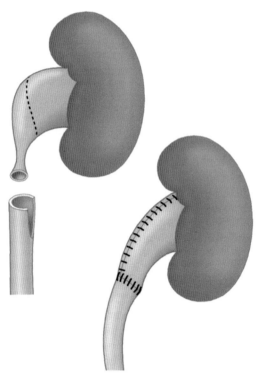

**Figure 14.5** Surgery for pyeloplasty.

## POSTOPERATIVE CARE

- Fluid balance is managed by intravenous infusion but the child can eat and drink.
- The stent is tied off at 3 days postoperatively (if pain and swelling occur then it is untied) and is usually removed after 5–7 days.
- If an internal stent (either a J tube or a Y tube) is inserted, the patient will be discharged home with the stent in situ and it will be removed after DMSA scan under a general anaesthetic after 3 months.
- The wound is drained by redivac drain for 48 hours.
- Intravenous antibiotics are administered on induction and orally until stents are removed.

## VESICO-URETERIC REFLUX

Vesico-ureteric reflux (VUR) can be defined as a permanent or intermittent backflow of urine from the bladder into the upper urinary tract, due to a dysfunction of the ureterovesical junction. This can be secondary to posterior urethral valves, neuropathic bladder or bladder outflow obstruction.

## CLINICAL SIGNS

Recurrent UTIs are often associated with VUR, with an average incidence of 21%, with a higher ratio occurring in females than males. Outcomes of VUR are extremely variable, ranging from spontaneous resolution to hypertension and renal failure. Younger children are thought to have a better chance of spontaneous resolution; this is often related to the level of growth occurring within the bladder.

## DIAGNOSIS

VUR can often be detected via ultrasound scan whilst the baby is still in utero. Diagnosis after birth occurs via investigations following recurrent UTIs. Once a diagnosis has been reached a DMSA scan is performed to determine renal function and subsequent treatment. Figure 14.6 shows the different types of vesico-ureteric reflux.

## TREATMENT

Non-operative management involves preventing/minimising infection by giving prophylactic doses of oral antibiotics and regular review of urinary culture and renal function scans. It should be stressed that alongside the above management adequate hydration, good perineal hygiene and bowel management are crucial aspects of care. If medical treatment does not improve the symptoms of reflux or reflux is severe, then surgical treatment is required. The type of surgery generally depends on diagnosis but usually involves either a pyeloplasty or reimplantation of ureters.

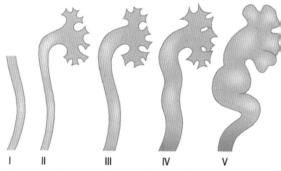

I    II    III    IV    V

**Figure 14.6** International reflux classification.

# REIMPLANTATION OF URETERS

There are various different surgical procedures to reimplant the ureters into the bladder. The basis of all procedures is to move the ureters into a higher position in the bladder, preventing reflux of urine back to the kidneys as the bladder fills.

## POSTOPERATIVE CARE

Ureteric stents and a suprapubic catheter are left in position to allow healing of the suture sites and decrease pressure on the bladder. Initially, urine drains from the stents due to swelling of the ureters, but as swelling decreases urine drains around the outside of the stents into the bladder and out through the suprapubic catheter. The child is discharged home once intravenous or epidural analgesia is no longer required. Parents are taught basic catheter care prior to discharge and told to observe for signs of infection or dehydration that may require readmission.

The child is readmitted for removal of stents and clamping of the suprapubic catheter 7–10 days post surgery. Once it has been established that the child is able to void normally, the catheter is removed and the child discharged. Prophylactic antibiotics continue until review in the outpatients department, usually 3 months post surgery.

## COMPLICATIONS

There are a number of complications of surgery:

- Bladder spasm – due to the presence of catheters. It is treated by antispasmodic drugs to prevent or minimise the spasm.
- Infection – also due to the presence of catheters. Treatment doses of oral antibiotics continue until the drains are removed. Symptoms are pyrexia, reduced or cloudy urine output and abdominal pain. If these occur then a urine sample should be taken and appropriate antibiotics and fluids given.
- Blockage of catheter – usually detected by a reduction of urinary output. The catheter is flushed with 0.9% saline to remove the blockage.

# SELF-CATHETERISATION AND URINARY DIVERSION

Intermittent self-catheterisation (ISC) is carried out to prevent incontinence and promote emptying of the bladder, thus preventing risks associated with reflux. The term is used to describe the draining of the bladder at regular intervals in a 24-hour period. There are a variety of conditions that may necessitate the introduction of intermittent catheterisation either through the urethra or an alternative route:

- Bladder exstrophy: a condition where the bladder protrudes through the abdominal wall (Retik 2001). Cosmetic surgery is performed to create an acceptable appearance to the abdominal wall and external genitalia. Bladder capacity is often reduced and surgery may be required to amend this. Some children may have a normal urinary tract and subsequently no problems with continence. Others require ISC in order to empty their bladder adequately.
- Cloacal anomaly: characterised by an open bladder, communication of bowel and bladder, imperforate anus, abdominal wall anomalies and varying degrees of spinal defects. Surgery is performed to repair any abdominal problems, create a stoma to bypass the imperforate anus and close the bladder whilst potentially forming a vesicostomy. Further surgery may be undertaken to create a rectum and enable normal bowel motions and create a continence diversion for ISC (Teliha & Pena 1996).
- Neuropathic bladder: due to either bladder exstrophy, trauma, spina bifida or sacral agenesis. The nerves are either not present at birth or damaged in some way, therefore normal voiding in response to nerve signals does not occur. Often the child will dribble urine whilst still having a residual volume in the bladder, thereby presenting the risk of infection and reflux. Therefore ISC is introduced to reduce these risks.

Lauthian (1998) highlights the problems associated with bladder drainage by catheter: trauma, UTI, blockage, strictures, perforation and encrustation. As a general rule, intermittent catheterisation is not subject to all of these; however, trauma and UTI from regular catheter insertion are the most common complications. Patients undertaking ISC generally take prophylactic antibiotics to avoid infection and continued practice will reduce the risks of trauma. Prior to introducing a patient and the family to ISC, it is important to involve the community continence advisor in order that a rapport is developed to enable effective support once at home, and to avoid learning poor habits at the outset. Once parents and child have been introduced to the procedure, they remain in the hospital until they feel confident to continue without supervision. The child will be followed up at home by the continence advisor, who will deal with continued supplies of equipment. This should reduce the need for hospital admissions to when further surgery is required, thereby allowing the family to lead a normal life.

In the event that urethral catheterisation is inappropriate, perhaps due to constant wetting, anatomical anomalies or non-compliance with catheterisation, a urinary diversion conduit may be considered as an alternative. A catheterisable port is created by channelling the appendix (or, in its absence, a short segment of bowel) from the external abdominal wall, through the umbilicus to the bladder wall, which in turn creates a valve thereby avoiding leakage through the stoma (Gibbons 1995). Ashcroft & Hodder (1980) note that experimental surgery involving the caecum and appendix was undertaken as far back as 1908. Interest waned until 1978 when a pouch was constructed out of ileum to provide a continence and antireflux mechanism. The original surgical procedure advocated the closure of the bladder neck to reduce leakage; however, often now it is left open to act as a release valve in the event of stoma blockage or catheterisation not taking place. The past decade saw the development by a French surgeon of the Mitrofanoff procedure (see Fig. 14.7), which has become by far the most popular choice of diversion in the UK (Busuttil-Leaver 1994). The Mitrofanoff procedure, combined with reimplantation of ureters, provides protection to the upper renal tract. Whilst a large capacity, low pressure reservoir is created through bladder augmentation, this is surgery to increase bladder capacity by joining a section of large bowel to the bladder.

In the initial postoperative period a suprapubic catheter is inserted to allow urine drainage and the Mitrofanoff is stented to enable healing. A vacuumed wound drain collects any oozing or blood or urine and prevents the formation of a haematoma. Inadequate fluid volumes may result in debris and clot formation, therefore fluids are often given at greater than maintenance rate to provide a flushing effect. The child will have nil by mouth for a period of days postoperatively, due to the handling of and trauma to the bowel. The suprapubic catheter is flushed regularly (frequency is determined by the size of the child) to ensure it remains free flowing at all times and to clear any debris; if the bladder neck has not been closed, occasionally urethral leakage may suggest a partially blocked catheter (Gibbons 1995).

Once eating and drinking, the child will be discharged home with the catheter in situ to be readmitted some weeks later to introduce catheterisation of the stoma. The child is given a general anaesthetic to enable the removal of the stent and parents are invited into theatre and together with the surgeon catheterise the stoma whilst the child is completely still, so that they can feel the easiest route to the bladder. The subsequent length of hospital stay depends on the ease and confidence with which the stoma is catheterised. The suprapubic catheter is removed once it has been established that the catheterising is adequately emptying the bladder.

## COMPLICATIONS

• There may be leakage of urine through the urethra if the bladder neck has not been closed. The ISC may have to take place more frequently initially, in order to avoid this problem. Occasionally, the

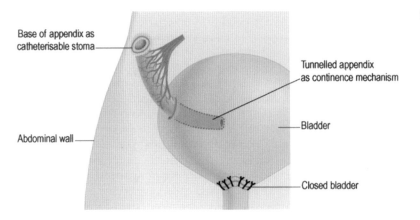

**Figure 14.7** Mitrofanoff technique.

Base of appendix as catheterisable stoma

Tunnelled appendix as continence mechanism

Abdominal wall

Bladder

Closed bladder

surgeon may be persuaded to close the bladder neck. However, most are reluctant to do this as without this release valve, if the bladder is not emptied, it may break down at the suture line, which is a surgical emergency.

- Metabolic complications may occur due to the use of bowel in diversionary surgery as the tissue continues in its secretory and absorptive functions. In order to prevent metabolic acidosis, the child is given an alkalising oral supplement such as sodium bicarbonate (Mundy 1999).
- Normal bowel bacterial flora continue to develop in the anastomosed section of bowel, thereby presenting the potential for infection. This necessitates continued prophylactic antibiotics, bladder washouts and excellent ISC technique for life (Gibbons 1995).
- Formation of bladder stones secondary to the production of mucus may be a problem. The child is advised to drink cranberry juice, which has been found to contain properties that break down mucus.

## BLADDER AUGMENTATION

A child with a neuropathic bladder poses a difficult task for surgeons, but major advances in surgical techniques have been made. A bladder augmentation involves attaching a section of bowel to the bladder to increase capacity. Urodynamics are always performed preoperatively to establish contractility and nerve supply. Currently there is no one type of augmentation suitable for all children, therefore there are certain factors that need to be taken into consideration:

- assessment of renal function
- degree of reflux
- level of outlet resistance

- history of bowel dysfunction
- need for a continent catheterisable stoma
- physical and mental capacity of child or carer to perform ISC.

The ileum is the most commonly used bowel segment for bladder augmentation; its advantages are:

- large quantity available
- ease of handling
- predictable and abundant blood supply
- lesser mucus production compared with colon
- less metabolic complications than colon.

Disadvantages may still be:

- development of loose stools due to removal of bowel
- vitamin $B_{12}$ deficiency
- metabolic acidosis
- stone formation
- mucus production
- infection.

Obviously these factors have to be weighed up before this major surgery can be considered.

## CONCLUSION

This chapter has considered the diseases and disorders that may affect the various structures of the urinary system during childhood. Whilst consideration has been given to the methods used to diagnose the disorders, preferred methods of treatment in our experience, and ongoing issues for the child in later life, this has been by no means exhaustive. There is a great deal more that could have been written and we would encourage more in-depth research if this is an area of particular interest to the reader.

## References

Ashcroft KW, Hodder TM (eds) 1980 Paediatric surgery, 2nd edn. WB Saunders, London

Busuttil-Leaver R 1994 The Mitrofanoff pouch: a continent urinary diverison. Professional Nurse Aug: 748–753

Gibbons M 1995 Urinary problems after formation of a Mitrofanoff stoma. Professional Nurse Jan: 221–224

Heritage J 1996 Urinary Tract Infections. University of Leeds, Leeds

Larcombe J 1999 Urinary tract infections in children. British Medical Journal 319(7218): 1173–1175

Lauthian P 1998 The dangers of long term catheter drainage. British Journal of Nursing 17(7): 336–379

Mundy AR 1999 Metabolic complications of urinary diversion. Lancet 353(9167): 1813

Retik AB 2001 Exstrophy of the bladder – advances in management. The Inside Edition. Digital Urology Journal. Online. Available: http://www.duj.com

Ross J 1999 Pediatric UTI and reflux. American Family Physician (Mar 15). 59(6)

Ross E 2001 Cranberry juice helps urinary tract. Medline Plus

Spitz L Coran AG (eds) 1995 Rob and Smith's operative surgery (paediatric surgery), 5th edn. Chapman & Hall Medical, London

Teliha L, Pena A 1996 Cloacal exstrophy. Pull-Thru Network News (Winter). Online. Available: http://www.pullthrough.org/ptnn.html

# Chapter 15

# Caring for children undergoing orthopaedic surgery

## Maggie Doman

## INTRODUCTION

This chapter will consider the care required by children undergoing orthopaedic surgery. This is potentially a vast topic area as paediatric orthopaedics has become a speciality in its own right. The main focus will therefore be the care of children undergoing surgery performed to correct the commoner congenital or acquired problems, such as developmental dysplasia of the hip (DDH), talipes equinovarus, Perthes' disease, slipped capital (or upper) femoral epiphysis, scoliosis and musculoskeletal problems resulting from cerebral palsy. Other treatments used in conjunction with surgery, notably traction and plaster, will also be discussed. The care of children requiring surgery for problems caused by trauma, malignant disease, metabolic disorders or more generalised genetic disorders will not be considered here, though many of the principles of care for the conditions included will apply. Previous knowledge or experience, or preparatory reading may assist understanding of this chapter, as some familiarity with orthopaedic terminology and normal anatomy, physiology and development of the musculoskeletal system has been assumed.

## BACKGROUND

The numbers of children with orthopaedic problems nursed in hospital in Great Britain have fallen dramatically in recent years, partly due to changing patterns of disease, but improved public health and social conditions have also had a major effect. In the

18th and 19th centuries, many children were affected by disease and disability caused by poverty, malnutrition and poor standards of public health and welfare, particularly in the cities. Tuberculosis, poliomyelitis, osteomyelitis and rickets were common problems, and the children who survived these conditions often grew up to become crippled and deformed adults who were unable to work and earn a living; thus many resorted to begging in the absence of welfare or treatment. In the latter part of the 19th century, the plight of the handicapped and disabled was increasingly recognised. This was also a time of philanthropy, when many hospitals were being built and the care and treatment of sick children were improving. Orthopaedic hospitals were founded in many parts of Great Britain and these usually provided inpatient treatment for children, unlike other 'general' hospitals which were often reluctant to admit children due to the perceived infection risks. Children's orthopaedic wards provided rest, treatment and nursing care combined with a better diet and environment, as the orthopaedic hospitals tended to be surrounded by pleasant grounds where patients could benefit from the fresh air and opportunities for exercise. Gradually, the facilities for children in hospital improved, with play facilities and schooling being provided. Children spent long periods of time in these hospitals which became their second homes, as they were often many miles away from their families and visiting was restricted. The eventual return home was, therefore, often traumatic for the whole family.

The last 50 years or so have seen many changes to the care of children with orthopaedic problems and the average length of stay in hospital has decreased dramatically. Whereas, for example, children with Perthes' disease could be nursed on traction in hospital for 9 months or more, many now do not even require admission to hospital. This is also true of a number of other conditions, where it is increasingly recognised that many children can receive treatment as outpatients or day cases, due to improved surgical procedures and equipment, and new investigative techniques. In addition, the improvements in public health and the availability of appropriate antibiotics have reduced the incidence of tuberculosis and osteomyelitis; immunisation programmes have helped to prevent tuberculosis and, in particular, polio; and advances in preconceptual and neonatal care and antenatal screening have contributed to a reduction in the numbers of children with myelomeningocele and

hydrocephalus, many of whom also spent long periods of time in children's orthopaedic wards. Acceptance of the recommendations of the Platt Report (Ministry of Health 1959) which highlighted the potential adverse emotional and psychological effects of separation due to hospitalisation has also led to shorter hospital stays for children with orthopaedic problems. The development and increased availability of community children's nursing teams who can provide care and support for these children and their families at home have assisted this further. Separate children's orthopaedic wards have therefore become less common, and have amalgamated with 'general' children's surgical wards in many District General Hospitals.

## CURRENT PROVISION OF CARE

Children with orthopaedic problems require skilled care and treatment from the multidisciplinary team, which may include nursing and medical staff, physiotherapist, play specialist, orthopaedic technicians and orthotists, teacher, occupational therapist, dietitian, pharmacist and social worker. It must be remembered that these children are seldom 'sick', with the acute care provided in hospital, such as that following surgery, only being required for relatively short periods of time. Instead, their needs tend to be long term, and are mainly due to restricted mobility, which in turn can affect their normal activities of living as well as impacting on all aspects of development. In addition, not all orthopaedic consultants are willing or able to manage the care of children effectively, particularly if they have rare or complicated problems. Consequently, although most of the care is provided at home, it may also be necessary for some families to travel considerable distances to access the specialist advice and treatment that their child requires.

There are, therefore, a number of psychosocial aspects that must also be taken into account in the management of care. These include effects on the individual child, such as delayed social and physical development resulting from restricted mobility, interruptions to schooling and home life, and, especially for older children, the psychological impact of wearing plasters or a brace and having an altered body image, particularly in relation to surgery. Additionally, being separated from family and/or friends and, for adolescents, being different from their peers, can be particularly challenging to cope with. These difficulties can lead to boredom, depression, non-compliance or other behavioural implications which may exacerbate the problems already experienced (Payne et al 1997). The family can also be affected. Problems such as talipes are apparent at birth, and this can be extremely distressing for parents, who may experience feelings such as shock, disbelief, anger or guilt. Although some conditions can be identified antenatally, thus providing opportunities for counselling and preparation before the child's birth, families still have the worry of coping with a child who has extra needs as well as having to handle comments from 'well-meaning' family members, friends and even strangers. Other effects on the family can include financial implications, such as travel costs or the need for alterations to the house; social restrictions, such as difficulty in finding babysitters willing to accept responsibility for their child; and the potential for altered family dynamics. In particular, there may be an impact on 'well' siblings, such as resentment of the extra attention paid to their brother or sister, anger or even guilt about possible causation. It is therefore imperative that the management of care for children with orthopaedic problems is family-centred, with children and their families being involved in all aspects of care and decision making.

It is also important to be aware that surgery may only be one part of the treatment process, with many children undergoing procedures and continuing care as outpatients both before and after surgical intervention. With the decline in separate wards or facilities for children with orthopaedic problems, and the need for staff on general children's wards to develop a broad repertoire of knowledge and skills (Doman 1998), there is the possibility that specialist skills may be diluted or lost. It is therefore essential to recognise that, as with any speciality, there is the potential for harm or complications to arise due to lack of knowledge or experience. As a result, all staff caring for children undergoing orthopaedic surgery must ensure they have the appropriate knowledge and skills (e.g. of relevant anatomy or specific nursing interventions) to provide safe, effective care whilst the child is in hospital and to support and prepare the family adequately for discharge and care at home.

The overall aims of care and treatment for orthopaedic problems are threefold:

1. to relieve pain
2. to prevent or correct deformities and

3. to achieve maximum function or mobility for the child.

Treatment may be conservative, using splints, plaster, strapping, traction, etc; surgical, including manipulation, tendon release or osteotomy; or a combination of the two. The actual treatment regimes and surgery performed may vary considerably, therefore, according to the individual needs of each child as well as surgeons' preferences. As a result, it will not be possible to describe definitive care programmes, but an explanation and overview of some of the more familiar conditions and their treatment, and the rationale for some of the commoner surgical interventions will be presented. Specific pre- and postoperative care for the different types of surgery and conditions, such as the investigations required prior to spinal surgery, and neurovascular observations and plaster care postoperatively, will then be addressed. Finally, some of the developments in the provision of care for children with orthopaedic problems, which it is hoped will benefit these children, their families and the staff involved in their overall management, will be considered.

## DEVELOPMENTAL DYSPLASIA OF THE HIP

Developmental dysplasia of the hip (DDH) was formerly known as congenital dislocation of the hip (CDH) but has been renamed as this is not always evident at birth and the hip may not be fully dislocated. DDH is an abnormal development of the head of the femur, acetabulum or both, leading to instability, subluxation or complete dislocation of the hip joint. This occurs in approximately 1:1000 live births, is commoner in girls than boys by a ratio of at least 4:1 and the left hip is more commonly affected than the right. It may be unilateral or bilateral and may be associated with another congenital abnormality such as talipes or myelomeningocele.

The exact cause of DDH is unknown, but is acknowledged to be multifactorial. There appears to be a genetic/familial component, as the condition often occurs in areas where intermarriage is common. In addition, there is thought to be a dominant inheritance of joint laxity, which is often diagnosed early, and a polygenic inheritance of acetabular dysplasia, often diagnosed late. Environmental factors may also be involved in causation. A ligament-relaxing hormone secreted by the mother shortly before birth may cross the placenta, causing lax joints in the baby for a short time. Breech delivery with the legs extended can lead to dislocation and oligohydramnios can limit fetal movement, also resulting in hip problems. Cultural practices may influence the development of the hip, for example if the legs are swaddled, dysplasia tends to be commoner than in babies whose legs are kept abducted (McCullough et al 1994).

The underlying pathology is variable, as DDH refers to a group of disorders. For the hip joint to develop normally, it is believed that the head of the femur needs to be in close contact with the acetabulum (Duckworth 1995). Babies' hips are checked routinely after birth, and if 'clicky hips' are found, or there is a family history of DDH, ultrasound may be used at 2–6 weeks of age to confirm the diagnosis. (X-rays are not of use in babies under about 3 months of age.) If problems are detected at this stage, it is often possible to reduce the hip and maintain a normal position using double nappies or a Pavlik harness. The family are taught how to care for the child in the harness, including aspects such as how to wash and dress the child without disturbing the position of the hips. The baby's progress is checked regularly and if treatment is successful, the baby is gradually 'weaned off' the harness and reviewed as an outpatient until about 8 years of age.

If treatment is unsuccessful, or diagnosis is made later, then surgical intervention is required to overcome secondary changes that may occur (see Fig. 15.1).

These changes include:

- The acetabular roof becomes defective and slopes steeply, so it is not able to hold the head of the femur securely (Fig. 15.1a).
- The ossific nucleus of the femoral head may develop late so is often smaller than the unaffected side and the femoral neck tends to be shorter (Fig. 15.1b).
- The joint capsule remains intact, but may stretch, forming an 'hourglass' shape; or the acetabular labrum may become enlarged and fold into the acetabulum, forming a 'limbus'. In addition, the ligamentum teres or stretched psoas muscle may cause an obstruction, thus preventing reduction of the head of the femur.
- In time, if not detected, the muscles from the pelvis also become shortened and tight and the femur anteverted.

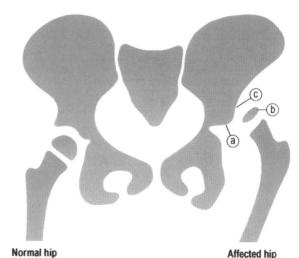

**Normal hip**　　　　　　　　　　　　**Affected hip**

Figure 15.1 Deformities associated with developmental dysplasia of the hip: a. steep roof of acetabulum, which cannot hold the femoral head; b. small ossific nucleus on affected side; c. gradual formation of false acetabulum above the true articular surface.

- After weight-bearing begins, a false acetabulum may start to form above the original fossa (Fig. 15.1c) and the child may develop a painless limp when walking.
- Bilateral problems are more difficult to recognise as there is no asymmetry or obvious limp, but there may be a widened perineum and a waddling gait when walking.

If surgical intervention is required, the child will need to be admitted to hospital. A period of traction, sometimes including gradual abduction, is often used for a week or more to help reduce the hip and stretch the muscles and ligaments prior to surgery. The type of traction will depend on the age and size of the child: babies/toddlers may be on Gallows (Bryant's) traction, while older children may be on straight leg (Pugh's) traction. The child will then be taken to theatre for an arthrogram, which involves the insertion of radio paque dye into the hip joint and examination of the hip under X-ray control. An outline of the structures of the joint can then be viewed, which will help to determine whether the head of the femur and/or acetabulum are forming properly and the presence of any obstructions which may prevent full reduction of the hip. An adductor tenotomy is frequently performed to release the tight tendon in the groin and aid manipulation of the hip. A closed reduction is preferable, and if there are no obstructions and the head of the femur can be located securely in the acetabulum, then the position is held by applying a hip spica with the hips flexed and abducted. The 'frog' position (90° flexion, 90° abduction), which was used previously has now been superseded by the 'human' position due to the potential risks of avascular necrosis of the femoral head (Benson & MacNicol 1994, Adams & Hamblen 1995). This plaster is maintained for about 6 weeks, then the child is readmitted and the cast is changed under anaesthetic, which also provides an opportunity for the position of the hip to be checked. This spica is applied for a further 6 weeks, then if the hip is stable, this is removed and the child may be placed in broomstick plasters or a brace for a further period of time to prevent adduction of the hips whilst allowing some movement and an opportunity to mobilise gently. Hydrotherapy and physiotherapy to aid the child to regain normal mobility follow removal of the plaster.

Occasionally, a closed reduction is unsuccessful, or there are structures such as the labrum, capsule or tendons causing an obstruction to the femoral head. An open reduction will then be performed to excise or move the obstructions or for reefing of the capsule to allow the head of the femur to be located in its 'normal' position (Taylor & Clarke 1998). Rarely, a femoral derotation osteotomy may also be required if the hip can only be reduced in a rotated position. This ensures that the hip joint is stabilised but the leg is straightened (Apley & Solomon 1994). A hip spica will again be applied following surgery, as for closed reduction, but the metalwork (such as plate and screws) used to fix the femur internally may need to be removed at some time in the future.

If treatment is still unsuccessful, or if the child is older, a pelvic osteotomy may be necessary as the acetabulum will not be properly formed so the position of the head of the femur cannot be maintained. Surgery may include a Salter (wedge) osteotomy or Chiari (shelf) osteotomy to provide a 'roof' over the femoral head and to deepen the socket. The position is again held by application of a hip spica, but as these children are usually older, they are often very heavy and care must be taken when helping them to move, as discussed later in this chapter.

## CONGENITAL TALIPES EQUINOVARUS

This is commonly known as talipes or 'club foot', although other similar abnormalities may also be referred to in the same terms. Talipes can occur alone or may be associated with myelomeningocele, polio or cerebral palsy. The problem occurs in about 1:1000 births, is commoner in boys than girls by about 2:1, and is bilateral in about one third of cases. Although the cause is uncertain, there appears to be a genetic link as there is a 1:35 chance of a second child being affected. Teratogenic factors have also been implicated, such as maternal infection interrupting development or intrauterine moulding due to oligohydramnios.

Talipes equinovarus is the commonest deformity, and involves an abnormal foot in an abnormal position, the 'true' form being rigid with tight tendons and ligaments and bone deformities, especially of the talus, and may include subluxation of the talonavicular joint (Kyzer & Stark 1995). There are three main components to the deformity: supination (or adduction) of the forefoot and perhaps midfoot; equinus (pointing downwards) of the foot and ankle; and varus (turning inward) of the hindfoot (see Fig. 15.2). The tibia and calf muscles may also be implicated if the deformity is severe, and the affected foot and leg will always be smaller than the other.

The overall aim of treatment is to correct the deformity within the first year in order to enable the child to walk normally. The management will depend upon the flexibility of the feet and the severity of the deformity, which should be assessed as soon as possible. Initially, treatment will involve conservative management, which includes physiotherapy (manipulation) and stretching exercises which are taught

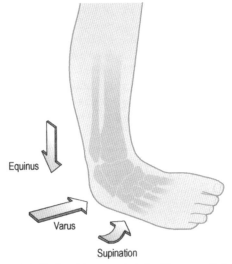

Figure 15.2 Deformities associated with congenital talipes equinovarus.

to the parents so they can continue treatment at home. If there is potential for correction, strapping is also used and this may be combined with the application of below-knee plaster boots or night splints. Progress is reviewed regularly, but if the deformity persists, at the age of approximately 6–8 months surgery will be required (though the timing may vary according to individual surgeons' preference).

Soft tissue surgery is performed initially, which involves the release or elongation of tight tendons or ligaments. Firstly, a plantar-medial release of the foot is performed, followed by postero-lateral release where the Achilles tendon is 'lengthened', in an attempt to straighten the foot and correct the plantarflexion. These operations may be carried out sequentially under the same anaesthetic, or in two stages, with about 2 weeks between them. It may also be necessary to perform other tendon releases or transfers, such as of the tibialis anterior. Following each surgical intervention, the corrected position is held by applying long leg plaster(s) which are changed under anaesthetic as required and are retained for about 3 months in total (Kyzer & Stark 1995). Once the plasters are removed, the child may have to wear specially fitted night splints or boots (e.g. Piedro boots) to maintain the correction until the age of about 2 or 3 years, and progress will continue to be reviewed in clinic to the age of 7 or 8 years.

If previous treatments are unsuccessful, once the child is over the age of at least 2 years further surgery is usually required, which may involve repeating or extending the soft tissue releases and, in older children, skeletal surgery. In more severe cases this may include osteotomies (e.g. of the calcaneum); bone resections (e.g. lateral wedge tarsectomy); or arthrodesis (e.g. of the calcaneo-cuboid joint), the position again being maintained by the application of plaster (Adams & Hamblen 1995). Additionally, procedures involving Ilizarov instrumentation, a form of external fixator, may also be necessary. This requires the child and family to be taught how to carry out the gradual distraction of the bone(s) by adjusting the appropriate nuts, as well as pin site care to prevent skin discomfort and infection. For children whose problems persist beyond about 3 years of age, follow up will continue until skeletal maturity.

## CEREBRAL PALSY

Cerebral palsy results from brain damage at or shortly after birth so the actual impairment of motor function may vary considerably. The neurological damage is usually non-progressive but orthopaedic problems arising from spasticity may worsen. As the child grows, the muscles and tendons may not grow at the same pace as the bones, leading to the development of contractures. If untreated, these can cause secondary joint problems and will impair function further. The overall aim of treatment is therefore to improve function and/or posture, but the actual surgery performed will depend on the child's individual problems (Robb 1994, Taylor & Clarke 1998).

Soft tissue surgery is commonly carried out and may involve the release of individual tendons, or there may be a multiple level approach. Interventions include tenotomy to release excessive flexion, e.g. of the wrist, or contractures, especially in the hip; tendon 'lengthening' such as release of the Achilles tendon to prevent 'tiptoeing' and allow the child to walk more easily; and tendon transfers to rebalance antagonistic muscles. Occasionally, osteotomies may also be performed. Following soft tissue or bony surgery, the child will then have a plaster cast applied to allow healing in the corrected position. For example, in the leg this may be a below-knee or long leg plaster or, for the release of hip contractures, a hip spica or broomstick plasters (Robb 1994). Physiotherapy is vital after this treatment to help the child to exercise the affected part and gain maximum benefit from the surgery, and the child and family will be taught how to continue this care at home.

## PERTHES' DISEASE

Perthes' disease, also known as Legg–Calvé–Perthes' disease, is a form of osteochondritis that affects the femoral head. It occurs more commonly in boys than girls, usually between the ages of about 4 and 8 years. For reasons not fully understood, the blood supply to the femoral epiphysis is temporarily disrupted, leading to necrosis and softening of the bone, which may become deformed (see Fig. 15.3). On X-ray the femoral head may appear more dense and there is apparent widening of the joint space, though cartilaginous growth continues. Revascularisation will occur, followed by repair and remodelling over a period of 2 to 3 years, but if a large area of the femoral capital epiphysis is damaged and flattened, this may be permanently deformed and a secondary acetabular dysplasia may develop, which in

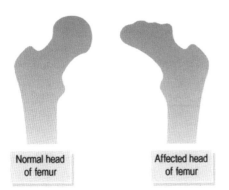

Figure 15.3 Flattened head of femur in Perthes' disease.

turn may result in osteoarthritis in adulthood. The eventual outcome will vary according to factors such as the child's age, the stage of disease at diagnosis and the degree of involvement of the femoral head (Apley & Solomon 1994, Catterall 1994).

Treatment will depend on the child's symptoms and the extent of disruption to the femoral head and/or hip joint. In the early stages, the hip is often 'irritable' and the child may limp. Assessment at this time is difficult, as muscle spasms cause movements to be restricted and painful, and X-rays may be inconclusive, though a bone or magnetic resonance imaging (MRI) scan may indicate changes. Bedrest and/or traction in conjunction with analgesia can help to relieve the symptoms in the irritable stage, then the child is allowed to mobilise before being discharged home. The child's progress is reviewed and X-rays are performed at regular intervals in the outpatient department to ensure that the femoral head is preserved and is contained within the acetabulum – a process referred to as 'supervised neglect' (Apley & Solomon 1994, Taylor & Clarke 1998). As long as the head of the femur heals well and the normal position in the acetabulum is maintained, no further treatment may be necessary. Restricted weightbearing or movement may be needed to ensure 'containment' for some children, however, and may be achieved by applying a brace or broomstick plasters to keep the hips in abduction and internal rotation whilst allowing mobility. This is often continued for a year or more, which can be very frustrating for a school age child whose activities and social life are necessarily curtailed.

Alternatively, if there are problems with compliance, or conservative treatment is unsuccessful, or if there are concerns about the integrity of the femoral head or hip joint, then surgery may be performed to ensure containment. Catterall has summarised the relative advantages and disadvantages of both methods of containment (Catterall 1994, p. 455). Femoral or pelvic (innominate) osteotomy may be performed, and the position maintained by the application of a hip spica that is retained for up to 3 months. After removal, hydrotherapy and physiotherapy are needed to help the child regain strength and mobility. As with older children requiring surgery for DDH, moving and handling a child in a hip spica can be very difficult due to the weight of the plaster and the child's restricted mobility, and must be carried out with care.

## SLIPPED CAPITAL (UPPER) FEMORAL EPIPHYSIS

As with Perthes' disease, this affects the proximal femoral epiphysis, but, as the name suggests, is a displacement from its normal position on the femoral neck at the growth plate, with the femoral head slipping backwards and downwards (see Fig. 15.4). The cause of slipped capital femoral epiphysis (SCFE) is unknown, but may be associated with hormonal changes, as this commonly affects adolescent boys (though girls may be affected) who are tall and thin or rather obese, and occurs around the time of puberty. The slip may be described as acute, chronic, or 'acute-on-chronic' as there may be a history of trauma immediately preceding the slip, or of recurrent intermittent pain in the hip or knee combined with a limp. There may be pain and muscle spasm, external rotation and some shortening, with limited internal rotation and abduction on examination. The slip is apparent on X-ray, particularly in the lateral view. The displacement may be categorised as mild, moderate or severe, but the main aim of treatment is to prevent further slippage, avascular necrosis and damage to the growth plate (Apley & Solomon 1994, Taylor & Clarke 1998).

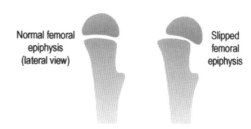

Figure 15.4 Lateral view of femoral head showing normal and slipped femoral epiphysis.

The chosen method of treatment will vary according to the degree of displacement and the surgeon's preference. Manipulation is rarely attempted, as there is a high risk of avascular necrosis, and the use of plaster (hip spica) to immobilise the hip has not been found to be effective. Surgical intervention is usually required to fix the epiphysis in situ, possibly preceded by a period of bedrest and/or skin traction. Two or three threaded screws or pins, such as Newman's pins, are inserted across the physis under X-ray control to ensure these are positioned accurately. As there is also a high risk (30% or more) of slipped epiphysis of the other hip, some surgeons may pin both hips at the same time, whereas others will observe the child closely, at regular intervals, in the outpatient department. With severe slips, it may also be necessary to perform a femoral osteotomy to correct any remaining deformity (MacNicol & Benson 1994, Taylor & Clarke 1998). After the epiphysis has been pinned, and secure fixation has been confirmed by X-ray, the child will be taught by the physiotherapist how to mobilise, non-weightbearing, using crutches. Once children are mobilising safely and their families are happy to care for them at home, they will be discharged from hospital and followed up in the outpatient department. After about 2 weeks, partial weightbearing may be permitted and full weightbearing by 6–8 weeks postoperatively.

## GENU VARUM (BOW LEGS), GENU VALGUM (KNOCK KNEES) AND INEQUALITY OF LEG LENGTH

Genu varum in infants and toddlers, and genu valgum in children between the ages of about 3 and 6 years are very common conditions, and almost part of normal development. Unless there is an underlying problem such as rickets, which should be checked for and treated, these apparent deformities will correct spontaneously in the majority of children by the age of 8 or 9 years, so the parents of younger children can usually be reassured that no treatment is required. Occasionally, genu valgum may persist beyond 10 years of age, so correction may be necessary. This is usually achieved by stapling the distal medial femoral epiphysis to slow growth and allowing the lateral side to 'catch up' (Apley & Solomon 1994). Postoperatively, children can mobilise with full weightbearing, but will usually require good assessment and management of

their pain to enable them to do so comfortably. Their progress will be reviewed in the outpatient department, and the staples removed under anaesthetic when it is deemed that the deformity has been sufficiently corrected. This is not an exact science, however, and in some cases an osteotomy may be required to correct the deformity.

Inequality of leg length may be associated with another condition such as myelomeningocele or polio, but can also be idiopathic. If the inequality is greater than 2.5 cm, then treatment is required. For minor differences, a shoe raise may be sufficient, but surgery can correct by as much as 10 cm. Two main methods are used:

1. lengthening the shorter leg by callotasis using an external fixator (usually for shorter lengthenings (Saleh & Norman 1993)), or with an Ilizarov frame (Eckhouse-Ekeberg 1994) on the femur or tibia; or
2. shortening the longer leg by arresting growth with staples around the epiphyseal plate.

If the former method is used, the child and family need to be taught how to care for the device at home. Saleh & Norman (1993) and Eckhouse-Ekeberg (1994) describe programmes of care developed for children undergoing this treatment that can last for 2 years or more.

## SCOLIOSIS

Scoliosis is a lateral curvature of the spine, normally painless, which is further classified according to the type of problem experienced. Non-structural ('mobile') scoliosis is usually a postural deformity and may occur due to muscle imbalance, inequality in leg length or pain, causing the young person to compensate for this problem. It is usually treated by correction of the underlying problem, but may become structural if allowed to progress. In structural ('fixed') scoliosis the vertebrae rotate, which in turn distorts the rib cage, resulting in a hump. There are various causes: it may be due to congenital skeletal abnormalities; it may be secondary to underlying neuromuscular problems such as cerebral palsy, myelomeningocele or polio; or scoliosis may be idiopathic. This is the largest group, accounting for approximately 80% of cases, and is further divided, according to the child's age at the time of onset, into infantile (under 3 years), juvenile (3–10 years) and adolescent idiopathic scoliosis (over 10 years), the latter category comprising the majority (Taylor & Clarke 1998).

Scoliosis is often detected by the school nurse during routine screening, or others may notice that clothes tend to 'hang' differently on the young person's body due to the rib hump or because the shoulders, waist and hips are not in alignment. This can be difficult to identify, especially if loose fitting, baggy clothes are worn. The diagnosis is confirmed by examination and X-rays.

The curve develops as the muscles and ligaments around the vertebral bodies become shortened on the concave side, leading to progressive deformity as the vertebrae and spinous processes rotate. In turn this causes compression on the ribs which crowd together on the concave side, the thoracic cage becomes narrowed and the vertebral body may become wedge-shaped and distorted towards the convex side (see Figs 15.5A and 15.5B). A secondary curve usually develops to counterbalance the primary curve. The deformity of the rib cage can lead to diminished lung volume and vital capacity, thus compromising pulmonary function. The curve can increase throughout the growth period but especially during periods of rapid skeletal growth, such as that occurring in adolescence.

Treatment for structural deformities will vary according to the severity and site of the curve and the age of the child. All children with scoliosis will be reviewed regularly as outpatients where they will be examined carefully and the curvature measured by Cobb's angle. For congenital and secondary problems, treatment will depend on the underlying cause, which may need to be managed first. If the scoliosis is severe, surgery, i.e. spinal fusion, will be required. Infantile idiopathic scoliosis often resolves spontaneously but if the curvature persists, serial plaster jackets and later a brace, which is used as an external control of the curve in an attempt to prevent further progression, may be fitted. If this treatment is not successful and the curve continues to progress, surgery may be required in adolescence to minimise the loss of height that can occur as a result of spinal fusion. Juvenile scoliosis is more difficult to treat, and surgery including spinal fusion is often necessary. A recent development is the use of 'growing rods', which are telescopic rods that can be gradually adjusted through a small incision as the child grows, thus helping to overcome the problem of height loss. Young people (more commonly girls) who present with adolescent idiopathic scoliosis will be reviewed regularly and may be taught exercises to increase the mobility of their spine. If the

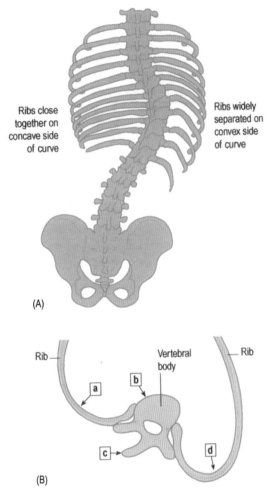

Figure 15.5A Curvature of the spine in scoliosis. B Rotated and deformed vertebra and ribs in scoliosis: a. rib on concave side of curve pushed anteriorly and laterally; b. vertebral body distorted towards convex side; c. spinous process deviated towards concave side; d. rib on convex side of curve pushed posteriorly with narrowing of rib cage.

curvature increases to between 25° and 35°, they may be fitted with a Boston brace, which they are expected to wear for up to 23 hours a day (McCullough et al 1994). Although this can be hidden under clothes, it can be very restrictive both physically and socially, especially for an adolescent who wants to be accepted by peers. Negotiation may be necessary to allow for the brace to be removed for sports and other activities, thus increasing the likelihood of compliance. Regular review continues at least until skeletal maturity, and possibly into adulthood, though progression is rare by this stage. If the angle of curvature becomes greater than 40° or is progressing rapidly, then surgery is usually required. Operations carried out include:

1.   Anterior release, whereby some of the vertebral discs are removed to improve the flexibility of the spine. This requires a thoracotomy, which can cause further problems for those with diminished pulmonary function, though the use of thoracoscopic surgery, which can reduce some of these complications, has been reported (Nymberg & Crawford 1996).

2.   Costaplasty. In this procedure, sections of rib are removed to help to flatten the rib prominence and improve the cosmetic appearance.

3.   Anterior or posterior fusion to prevent further curvature and improve function. Various devices and techniques have been developed for this purpose, e.g. Harrington or Isola rods, Dwyer (cable) instrumentation or Luque (wire) segmental instrumentation, which are all forms of internal fixation, and vertebrae are fused, possibly using bone grafts. The actual device will be selected according to the type and severity of the curve, associated problems and surgeon's preference.

Surgery may be carried out in one, two or more stages, possibly combined with a period of traction, such as halo-femoral or halo-pelvic, preoperatively or between stages. Immediately following surgery, these young people usually need to be nursed in an intensive care or high dependency unit so they can be closely monitored. They will also need help to move, to prevent twisting or bending of the spine, often accomplished by 'log rolling', though occasionally they may be nursed on a Stryker frame and turned regularly. If this is used, thorough psychological preparation is required preoperatively to overcome the fear and discomfort often associated with this equipment. When they are ready to mobilise, a brace (or occasionally a plaster jacket) is usually fitted to provide further support and prevent twisting of the spine. This is retained for 3–6 months after surgery. The physiotherapist will assist them to regain their balance and mobility, and when safe and fully recovered they will be discharged home. Depending on the procedures performed, this will normally occur after about 7–10 days, and regular review as an outpatient will continue.

## SPECIFIC PREOPERATIVE CARE

As previously stated, surgery may be only one stage in the programme of treatment for children with orthopaedic problems, with conservative management and regular review being carried out before and after surgical intervention. As a result, the vast majority of surgery will be elective, allowing time for these children and their families to be prepared physically and psychologically for admission to hospital and for all associated procedures such as traction, the operation itself and postoperative care which may include adapting to a plaster cast. In addition, the family may already be familiar with members of staff and, if several operations are required, with the ward and facilities available. Preparation can therefore be planned and provided according to the individual needs of the child, taking into account each child's age, stage of development and communication abilities. The constructive and therapeutic use of play (see Ch. 1) can be particularly effective in this process. Information provided should include details about the surgery itself, the probable length of stay and postoperative care, and negotiation regarding discharge arrangements and care at home. These issues are discussed in more detail in Chapter 1.

Safe preparation for the administration of anaesthetic and surgery will be required as for any child undergoing surgery, but there are additional aspects to preoperative care for children undergoing orthopaedic surgery. These will include ensuring that recent X-rays and, in the case of children with talipes or scoliosis in particular, photographs are available so comparisons can be made postoperatively. As haemorrhage can be a problem with soft tissue and bony surgery, blood tests are usually required to check full blood count, clotting times and blood group for cross-matching in case transfusion is needed postoperatively.

A full nursing assessment to establish normal routines and abilities, and an examination by medical staff, are also essential. These will include assessment of mobility and of the skin, as restricted mobility can predispose to the development of pressure ulcers in children. A reliable method of scoring to assess the potential for pressure damage should be used if possible, though there are difficulties associated with some scales which are not adapted for use with children. For those at greatest risk of developing problems associated with pressure, e.g. following spinal surgery, arrangements should be made for the use of a pressure-relieving mattress or other specialised equipment.

Preoperative care will also include consideration of pain assessment and management. Children and/or their families should be asked about previous experiences of pain and how this is recognised and expressed, and the use of pain assessment tools should be discussed and, as appropriate, taught to children to facilitate their involvement in the management of their pain postoperatively (see Ch. 6). If methods such as epidural or patient controlled analgesia are to be used, the child should also be prepared for these interventions. Alternatively, for infants, parents should be informed about the routes and types of administration of analgesia, such as the use of morphine by infusion or Y-can, and combinations of oral and/or rectal preparations.

Consent will need to be obtained prior to surgery, as for any operation, but for young people undergoing orthopaedic surgery there may be particular considerations. The legal age for consent to surgery is 16 years, with parents or legal guardians undertaking this role for those who are younger; but young people whom the doctor deems 'competent' may be able to decide for themselves. This entails estimating the child's ability to understand the procedure and its implications, including the potential consequences of refusing surgery, i.e. ensuring consent is 'informed' (see Ch. 3). Many young people requiring orthopaedic surgery will have a very good understanding of these issues in relation to their own problems, and even young children can be involved in decisions about their care and treatment, looking on their parents to support their wishes rather than assuming sole responsibility for consent. For an excellent consideration of a range of consent issues, including the views of children, see Alderson (1993).

If plaster is to be applied postoperatively, it is essential that children are given explanations at a level they can understand about what this entails and the length of time that may be involved, and reassurance that their arm or leg will still be there, even if they cannot see it! Again, preparation through play can be particularly effective, demonstrating the use of plaster on a doll or teddy.

Prior to spinal surgery, the above issues all need to be considered, but there are additional aspects to preoperative care and preparation. These include:

• Recording of height as well as weight so comparison can be made postoperatively.
• Evoked potentials to check spinal nerve function.
• Chest X-ray, pulmonary function tests, including peak expiratory flow recordings and monitoring of oxygen saturations, and assessment by the anaesthetist.

• Electrocardiography.
• Assessment by the physiotherapist of current mobility and preparation for postoperative exercises, such as teaching about log-rolling and turning, especially for hygiene and elimination purposes and for eating and drinking, as well as deep breathing and limb exercises.
• Assessment by the occupational therapist and dietitian may also be required.

Psychological care is also essential prior to spinal surgery, which can be lengthy and very frightening, particularly in view of the potential complications such as paralysis. Thorough explanations of all aspects of treatment and care must be given, including preparation for traction (if used), the insertion of a urinary catheter and for admission to an intensive care or high dependency unit postoperatively. If this is planned, arrangements should be made for the young person and family to visit the unit beforehand to meet staff and familiarise themselves with the environment and equipment. Privacy should also be assured, as these young people often feel very vulnerable with strangers and conscious of their deformity, as well as having to cope with the indignity of requiring assistance with hygiene and elimination postoperatively.

## PRINCIPLES OF CARE FOR A CHILD IN TRACTION

If a child requires traction preoperatively, such as prior to surgery for DDH or scoliosis, nurses caring for these children need to ensure that they are fully aware of the purpose of the traction, the type chosen (e.g. skin or skeletal traction, Gallows or Pugh's), and the maintenance and care required. It should be remembered that the focus of care should be the child and family, although the correct maintenance of the traction equipment will enhance this care.

For Gallows (see Fig. 15.6) and Pugh's traction, the colour, sensation, movement, temperature and peripheral pulse of the extremities should be checked at least 2-hourly to ensure there is no neurovascular deficit. If problems are detected, the bandages should be removed and the legs checked for restoration of circulation and movement before reapplication using less tension.

All areas prone to pressure should be checked regularly for any signs of redness. This includes heels, buttocks, sacrum, shoulders, elbows, back of

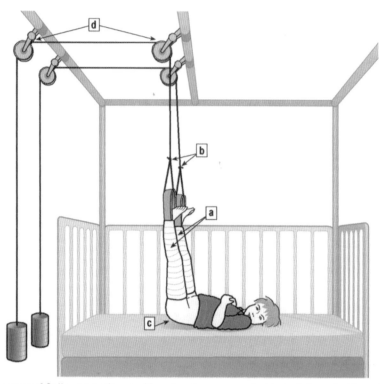

**Figure 15.6** Diagram of Gallows traction: a. skin extensions are applied to both legs; b. skin extension cords are attached to weights and pulleys on beams above the cot; c. counter traction is provided by the child's body weight and gravity, balance being achieved if the buttocks are just off the bed (it should be possible to place a flat hand under the buttocks); d. abduction is achieved by gradually moving the pulleys outwards along the beam.

head, etc. Older children should also be encouraged to change their position regularly. For infants in Gallows traction, their position (i.e. lying on their backs) can cause urine to seep into the back of their nappy, possibly leading to soreness or even skin breakdown. Nappies should be changed regularly and extra padding may be required. For toddlers on traction, elimination can be a particular problem, especially if toilet training is being established. It may be possible for the traction to be partially removed to allow the child to sit on a potty but children may not always realise that they need to use this, or may be reluctant to ask. Some staff or parents may advocate a temporary return to the use of nappies, but if the traction is only to be maintained for a week or so such a disruption to the child's normal routine may not be advisable and could have long term effects (Folcik et al 1994). Ensuring privacy and dignity for personal hygiene and elimination purposes is essential for all children on traction.

Children should be encouraged to eat a healthy, balanced diet, taking account of their likes and dislikes, to include plenty of fluids, fruit and vegetables, and protein-rich foods as far as possible. This is to help prevent problems associated with restricted mobility and prolonged bedrest, such as constipation and urinary stasis, as well as ensuring they are fit for surgery. Again, this can be difficult for children on Gallows traction, particularly if they are developing independence in eating, but offering finger foods including fresh fruit and vegetables can provide some opportunities for this process to continue.

Traction may need to be maintained for over a week, thus, usually, necessitating that children stay in hospital, yet they are likely to be feeling well and active. A child of any age on traction can become bored very quickly and can also become frustrated due to restricted mobility. These children will therefore need plenty of activities to keep them occupied, and to ensure that some degree of 'normal' life can continue. Appropriate play facilities (and education for older children) are essential, and should be provided according to the child's individual needs and abilities. Families should be encouraged to spend time with their children and to stay if possible, and they can be involved in various aspects of their child's care as appropriate. For older children and adolescents in particular, their friends should also be encouraged to visit, especially after school time and at weekends.

Maintenance of the traction equipment includes checking all parts of this at least once daily. For skin traction, skin extensions should be intact, and bandages should be reapplied regularly – firmly but not tightly – ensuring that they are free of wrinkles. The malleoli should be padded with foam, and bandages should start above these points to prevent rubbing or excess pressure (Folcik et al 1994). Skin on the limbs should be observed for reddening, irritation etc. and, if appropriate, cream may be applied to exposed dry or sore areas. If adhesive skin extensions are used, unless the traction slips or there is skin breakdown, it should not be necessary for these to be removed until the course of treatment by traction is completed. For those on skeletal traction, the pin sites should be cleaned daily, ensuring they are dry and free from infection.

Other daily checks include:

- Ensuring all connections on beams etc. are tight and secure
- Checking that all pulleys are free-running
- Checking that weights are hanging freely, are not resting on the bed or floor or suspended over the child, and that all connections are tight
- Checking all cords to ensure knots are not slipping (securing by use of knots such as a clove hitch or two half hitches should ensure this), and that no areas are rubbing or frayed.

## SPECIFIC POSTOPERATIVE CARE

As with any type of surgery, the child needs to be observed closely postoperatively to ensure that recovery is uneventful, and to recognise the onset of, and minimise or prevent, complications. Observations of vital signs including pulse rate, respirations and temperature should be recorded regularly as determined by their condition. Neurovascular observations should be carried out and recorded regularly, for example 1/2–1-hourly for the first 12 hours, 2-hourly for the next 12 hours and 4-hourly thereafter. Observations should include checking the colour, sensation and movement of extremities, and the peripheral pulse if available. Extremities should be pink and warm, with brisk capillary refill indicating good circulation, and children should be able to move their fingers or toes. Sensation can be difficult to ascertain in infants and young children due to their immaturity, but should be checked where possible. If appropriate, the affected limb should be elevated to allow the swelling to subside. Blue or cold extremities may result from swelling, so the limb may need to be elevated further. If this does not relieve the problem or it is not possible to demonstrate movement of the extremities, the nurse and/or doctor in charge of the child's care should be informed, as it may be necessary to split the plaster to relieve constriction.

Although attempts are made to minimise blood loss during surgery, this can be considerable following many orthopaedic operations, especially osteotomies and spinal surgery. A wound drain such as a redivac may be inserted to prevent blood accumulating at the operation site or a haematoma from forming, and this should be checked regularly to ensure it is draining and the vacuum is maintained. If the wound is visible, it should be inspected regularly and further padding applied as necessary. If bleeding is excessive, medical staff should be informed. A blood transfusion may also be required and the child should be monitored carefully throughout. If a plaster has been applied, the wound cannot be inspected so the plaster should be checked for any oozing of blood through it. If present, the outer edge should be marked, the time recorded and regular observation continued. Again, if bleeding is excessive or oozing persists, medical staff should be informed and, if present, the wound drain should be checked to ensure that it is functioning normally. The blood count may be checked again to ascertain whether further treatment is required. Dissolvable sutures are normally used under a plaster, but staples or sutures requiring removal may be used for closure of other wounds. The details should be recorded to ensure sutures are removed at the appropriate time, either in hospital or following discharge.

If a thoracotomy is performed for anterior spinal release or fusion, or a costaplasty, chest drains will also be inserted postoperatively. These should be checked regularly to ensure they are functioning correctly and will remain in place until the lungs have reinflated. Deep breathing exercises should be encouraged and care taken when turning to prevent further problems.

Good pain management is also essential postoperatively. A variety of routes and methods are available and should be selected according to the needs of the child (see Ch. 6). The use of peripheral local anaesthetic blocks during surgery has increased and these are particularly effective for hip and foot surgery. Epidural pain relief is also effective, and is becoming more popular, especially following spinal (Kester 1997) and lower limb surgery. These methods can affect sensation, however, so this should be taken into account when recording neurovascular observations. For older children and especially following spinal surgery, a continuous intravenous opioid (usually morphine) infusion, perhaps combined with patient-controlled analgesia, can be very successful. Respiratory rate and depth must be monitored carefully with all these methods, however, as respiratory depression can occur. The use of intermittent intramuscular opioids is seldom effective at providing consistent relief, as well as being painful and unpopular with children, their families and nursing staff, though morphine may be administered via a Y-can prior to the withdrawal of epidural or continuous infusion. Oral analgesia should also be prescribed, the drugs of choice being paracetamol, ibuprofen and/or diclofenac and a muscle relaxant such as diazepam may be prescribed to help prevent muscle spasm. Check X-rays will be taken postoperatively to ensure the desired position has been achieved and is being maintained. Appropriate positioning and careful turning postoperatively are also important. Restricted mobility is inevitable, so there is considerable potential for pressure sores. Preventative measures such as regular turns, including log rolling after spinal surgery, and the use of pressure-relieving devices or mattresses should be taken. The child's position, especially if a plaster has been applied, may also affect sleeping patterns and this can be exacerbated by a loss of normal routines such as bedtime rituals or the ability to curl up or change position unaided. Effective pain relief, the use of muscle relaxants and ensuring, where possible, that bedtime routines are continued may assist this.

Intravenous fluids may be given until the child is able to drink a sufficient amount orally, and diet will also be reintroduced as the child's appetite returns. Although a nutritionally balanced diet should be encouraged to aid healing and recovery, the child's likes and dislikes (ascertained during preoperative nursing assessment) need to be taken into account for this to be successful. Following spinal surgery, paralytic ileus may occur so oral intake should be delayed until bowel sounds are present, and mouth care should be provided until the child is able to drink again. Food can be difficult to manage as initially the child is unable to bend or sit up and will have to eat lying flat on his back or side. Gradually, children will be assisted to sit and stand, but will still not be able to bend.

Similarly, elimination can be a problem postoperatively. Problems with eating and drinking combined with restricted mobility can lead to urinary stasis or constipation. A urinary catheter is usually inserted for a few days following spinal surgery so this will also require care to prevent infection. For these young people, however, having to request assistance, and fears about the preservation of privacy and dignity, can cause embarrassment and possibly exacerbate their problems. Once they are able to use a 'slipper' bedpan or sit out of bed on a commode, the catheter can be removed, though assistance will still be needed to prevent bending or twisting.

There are many aspects to psychosocial care postoperatively. Ensuring privacy, especially for hygiene and elimination purposes, is imperative for children of all ages. The effects of separation from family and/or peers, and boredom once they have recovered from the initial effects of surgery, can have behavioural implications for children, and again play, education and spending time with family and friends are essential activities to help them to deal with their frustrations. Re-establishing a normal routine and choosing fashionable clothes that can fit over a plaster, fixator or brace can assist in helping them regain some degree of normality in their lives.

## PRINCIPLES OF CARE FOR A CHILD IN PLASTER

Many children will have a plaster applied following surgery or manipulation, to maintain the required position. Plaster of Paris, which is composed of gypsum-impregnated bandages, is still used, as it is much easier to mould this to the required position. This may only be used in a single layer, or to create a backslab, however, and the cast may be completed using a synthetic material such as Dynacast. In addition to the lighter weight and durability of these materials, they are also produced in a range of colours, including red, blue, green, pink, and red or green and white stripes. This can allow children some choice, so they can select a colour that matches their outfit, their favourite colour, or to advertise their support of a particular sports team!

It is essential that children receive adequate pain relief both prior to the application of a plaster and afterwards to help to ensure they remain comfortable. Pain may arise due to the surgery, due to swelling and consequent constriction, or as a result of dents, sharp edges or infection of a wound, so any complaints of pain should be investigated as well as being treated appropriately. Muscle spasm is also a common problem, so a muscle relaxant such as diazepam should be prescribed and administered alongside analgesia, particularly in the early postoperative stages and at night.

The plaster should be allowed to dry naturally, without the use of hairdryers or heaters as this may lead to cracking or softening of the plaster. Preferably, the plaster should be placed on a pillow and towel, and the position changed regularly, turning from side to side (e.g. for long leg plaster) or front to back (for hip spica or plaster jacket) to allow air to circulate all around the plaster.

The plaster should be handled carefully with flat hands to prevent moulding with fingers whilst damp, and checked for any dents, as these can cause localised pressure to the underlying skin, possibly resulting in blisters or pressure sores. The edges should be checked for constriction or sharp areas as these can also rub. Talcum powder should not be used around plasters as this can cause irritation and lead to skin reactions.

The plaster should not be allowed to get wet with anything. This includes not writing or drawing on the plaster until this is completely dry as it may cause damage. The plaster should be supported well to prevent cracking or softening, especially at joints, for example, a long leg plaster can be supported, particularly under the knee, with pillows when resting. It is also important to watch for signs of wear or crumbling, again around joints such as the hip or knee. If this occurs the plaster may need reinforcing or replacement.

Nothing should be put down inside the plaster (e.g. small toys or knitting needles), especially to try to scratch, as this may cause skin damage or wound infection. The child should be observed for signs of soreness, e.g. rubbing, itching, smells and oozing, and a child's complaints of pain anywhere should be taken seriously. These signs may indicate the presence of a wound infection or even a plaster sore, especially over prominences. If this occurs the child will need to return to the clinic or ward for

examination, and either a 'window' may be removed from the plaster over the affected area, or the whole plaster may need to be changed under anaesthetic.

Hip spicas are often applied immediately following hip surgery, e.g. for DDH or Perthes' disease, to immobilise the joint and maintain the reduced position. For infants and young children the plaster extends from the waist down both legs to the ankles (see Fig. 15.7). In older children, the whole of the affected leg will be encased in plaster but it may stop above the knee on the unaffected side to allow some degree of mobility.

Children in these plasters need careful handling as they may be very heavy and need lifting and turning regularly to prevent pressure sores and for toileting purposes. The bar (if present) is placed to help maintain the correct position of the hips and therefore should not be used for lifting, as this may weaken the plaster. Once dry, the edges of the plaster around the groin should be covered with a waterproof dressing to help keep the plaster dry and relatively unsoiled. A foam pad may also be placed at the back to prevent rubbing. Small nappies can be tucked into the sides of the plaster to try to keep the edges dry and should be changed frequently. For older children using bedpans, the use of a pad or toilet paper to help aim the flow of urine can help to protect the plaster.

Broomstick plasters may be used in the treatment of DDH or Perthes' disease following or as an alternative to surgery. The plasters may be in the form of a cylinder applied to both legs from thigh to ankle, or just below the knee and again the position is

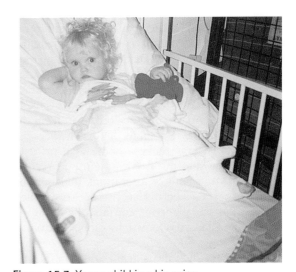

Figure 15.7 Young child in a hip spica.

maintained using a bar. The aim is to keep the hips abducted, again to protect the position of the femoral head, but this also allows the child some degree of mobility.

Plaster jackets, if applied, also need special care. A 'porthole' may be made in the plaster to enable the child to breathe and eat normally, without causing problems. It is important to ensure that the plaster is not restricting the child, and to observe for signs of excessive vomiting, which may be due to overstimulation of the vagal nerve.

## PREPARATION FOR DISCHARGE

The family needs to be fully informed, and verbal and written advice about ongoing care, and who to contact in case of problems, should be provided for them prior to their child's discharge. Robinson & Miller (1996) highlight the importance of ensuring this is written in a format suitable for 'lay' people, i.e. parents and children, by avoiding jargon or ambiguities, using the example of the care of children in a hip spica. Outpatient appointments and medicines to take home should also be arranged prior to discharge and explained carefully to the family.

For children in plaster in particular, parents need to be taught how to help their child mobilise, or how to lift and move them safely. This process can be aided by the use of a mobile hoist for older or bigger children, which can often be borrowed from the hospital occupational therapy department. Young children can be seated comfortably in a bean bag chair which supports them well, and can also be transported in a wide buggy or pushchair. It can be difficult to secure them in car seats, however, although special seats can be obtained, and a seat belt exemption certificate may also be required.

For older children, it may be advisable for their beds to be moved downstairs. A wheelchair is likely to be required and can often be obtained from the local Red Cross medical loans depot. The occupational therapist may make a home visit prior to discharge to assess the environment and recommend any equipment or alterations that may be needed. As it may be difficult to access a toilet, urine bottles and bedpans can also be obtained through the Red Cross for use by older children at home.

The primary healthcare team and community children's nurses should be informed of the child's discharge so they are able to provide support and care, such as removal of sutures or regular plaster checks at home. For school age children, their school should also be informed, though it may be necessary for home tuition to be arranged through the Local Education Authority. The hospital school should be able to assist in this process prior to the child's discharge.

Regardless of the surgical intervention, children should not be discharged home until their family feels able to cope with their care. Occasionally, especially for some older children whose needs are complex or who are heavy to lift, it may be necessary for them to stay in hospital for longer periods of time, but the aim is for all children to go home, perhaps with extra professional support, as well as the support of their family.

## FURTHER DEVELOPMENTS IN THE PROVISION OF CARE

Teamwork is vital in the care of children undergoing orthopaedic surgery, and each member of the multidisciplinary team has an important role in this. Nursing staff, as well as providing care, are often responsible for liaison with and coordination of the team, and the development and increasing use of integrated care pathways may facilitate and enhance this aspect of their role. These are being developed in many areas, and there is considerable potential for their use in coordinating the care of children with orthopaedic problems, as this can ensure consistency in approach and of information provided for families.

There is also an increase in the numbers of clinical nurse specialists, or of advanced nurse practitioner roles. Courses are now available to prepare nurses for history-taking and preoperative assessment and clerking of children, which suggests that the considerable potential of such roles has been recognised, and a further expansion in numbers is likely. The Chief Nursing Officer's 10 key roles for nurses in the NHS Plan (Department of Health 2000, p 83–84) include requesting X-rays, taking bloods/cannulation, prescribing, history-taking, nurse-led clinics, and receiving and making referrals. Some nurses are already taking on such roles, including in the field of children's orthopaedics, which is an ideal speciality for extending the scope of nursing. If managed successfully, they can improve the continuity and consistency of care, improve liaison between hospital and community services and the provision of a seamless service, cut down on waiting times, especially in clinics and pre-admission, and avoid repetition. This does not entail taking over junior doctors' roles but rather extending the nursing role to improve services for children and their families. Currently there is little research available evaluating the effectiveness of such roles, but the potential is considerable (see Dearmun & Gordon 1999, Rushforth et al 2000).

## CONCLUSION

This chapter has considered the care of children undergoing orthopaedic surgery. Various conditions and treatment options have been outlined, as well as the nursing care required. These are often long term problems, and surgery may only form a part of their treatment, so family-centred care and effective teamwork are essential. New developments are evolving all the time, with the potential for exciting new nursing roles and improvements in services for these children and their families.

## ACKNOWLEDGEMENTS

I wish to thank Julia Judd and Liz Wright, Paediatric Orthopaedic Nurse Practitioners, Sister Nikki Critchley and the staff of Ward G3, Southampton General Hospital, for their assistance in the preparation of this chapter.

## References

Adams JC, Hamblen DL 1995 Outline of orthopaedics, 12th edn. Churchill Livingstone, Edinburgh

Alderson P 1993 Children's consent to surgery. Open University Press, Buckingham

Apley AG, Solomon L 1994 Concise system of orthopaedics and fractures, 2nd edn. Butterworth Heinemann, Oxford

Benson MKD, MacNicol MF 1994 Congenital dislocation of the hip. In: Benson MKD, Fixsen JA, MacNicol MF (eds) Children's Orthopaedics and Fractures. Churchill Livingstone, Edinburgh, p 415–442

Catterall A 1994 Legg–Calvé–Perthes' Disease. In: Benson MKD, Fixsen JA, MacNicol MF (eds) Children's orthopaedics and fractures. Churchill Livingstone, Edinburgh, p 443–457

Dearmun AK, Gordon K 1999 The nurse practitioner in children's ambulatory care. Paediatric Nursing 11(1): 18–21

Department of Health 2000 The NHS plan: a plan for investment. A plan for reform. Department of Health, London

Doman M 1998 Nursing children in a range of hospital settings. Paediatric Nursing 10(1): 10–11

Duckworth T 1995 Lecture notes on orthopaedics and fractures, 3rd edn. Blackwell Science, Oxford

Eckhouse-Ekeberg DR 1994 Promoting a positive attitude in pediatric patients undergoing limb lengthening. Orthopaedic Nursing 13(1): 41–49

Folcik MA, Carini-Garcia G, Birmingham JJ 1994 Traction: assessment and management. Mosby, St Louis

Kester K 1997 Epidural pain management for the pediatric spinal fusion patient. Orthopaedic Nursing 16(6): 55–62

Kyzer SP, Stark SL 1995 Congenital idiopathic clubfoot deformities. Association of Perioperative Registered Nurses Journal 61(3): 491–512

McCullough FL, Andrews MM, Mooney KH 1994 Alterations of musculoskeletal function in children. In: McCance KL, Huether SE (eds) Pathophysiology: the biologic basis for disease in adults and children, 2nd edn. Mosby, St Louis, p 1482–1509

MacNicol MF, Benson MKD 1994 Slipped capital femoral epiphysis. In: Benson MKD, Fixsen JA, MacNicol MF (eds) Children's orthopaedics and fractures. Churchill Livingstone, Edinburgh, p 459–470

Ministry of Health 1959 The welfare of children in hospital. (The Platt report.) HMSO, London

Nymberg SM, Crawford AH 1996 Video-assisted thoracoscopic releases of scoliotic anterior spines. Association of Perioperative Registered Nurses Journal 63(3): 561–575

Payne WK, Ogilvie JW, Resnick MD, Kane RL, Transfeldt EF, Blum RW 1997 Does scoliosis have a psychological impact and does gender make a difference? Spine 22(12): 1380–1384

Robb JE 1994 Orthopaedic management of cerebral palsy. In: Benson MKD, Fixsen JA, MacNicol MF (eds) Children's orthopaedics and fractures. Churchill Livingstone, Edinburgh, p 255–274

Robinson A, Miller M 1996 Making information accessible: developing plain English discharge instructions. Journal of Advanced Nursing 24(3): 528–535

Rushforth H, Bliss A, Burge D, Glasper EA 2000 Nurse-led pre-operative assessment: a study of appropriateness. Paediatric Nursing 12(5): 15–20

Saleh M, Norman A 1993 Hope for legs: limb lengthening for deformities. Professional Care of Mother and Child 3(4): 101–104

Taylor GR, Clarke NMP 1998 Orthopaedic Surgery. In: Atwell JD (ed) Paediatric surgery. Arnold, London, p 800–824

# Chapter 16

# Burns and plastics

## Alyson Methven, Orla Duncan and Margaret Chambers

## BURN INJURIES IN CHILDREN

### INTRODUCTION

This chapter has been written as a resource for those wishing to gain a current and comprehensive basic knowledge of nursing practice within the field of burn injury in children. A burn injury arises when thermal energy is applied to the skin at a rate greater than that at which the energy can be dissipated.

Burn injuries are a unique form of trauma, in that they are capable of inflicting massive body insult, effecting a cascade of multisystem events in the affected individual. It is this sequence of events that creates the greatest challenges in caring for a burn injured patient. Major burns can affect all body systems, therefore an understanding of the systemic response is vital to ensure the optimal management of the burn injured child. The systemic effects of a major burn injury are often more life threatening than the local effects.

Best care of the burn injured child requires a multidisciplinary team approach. Members of the team will include the burns surgeon, nursing staff, physiotherapist, dietitian, occupational therapist, psychologist and pharmacist. This 'burn team' configurement is the vital key in providing the holistic care required to assure optimal recovery. The nature of the injury and the child as an individual will determine the volume of input required from any given member of the team.

In recent years advances in burn care have led to decreased mortality and morbidity (Settle 1996), thus nurturing a shift in the ethos of care to one of a good quality survival. To facilitate this we, as care providers, must understand the multiple dynamics often involved in managing a child with a burn injury. To ensure best possible recovery, an understanding of both the local and systemic effects of a burn injury, combined with a good understanding of the principles of effective wound management is required. These are the key elements in promoting quickest possible healing and recovery times, ensuring good form and function and thereby facilitating the best possible overall rehabilitation of the child. For a nurse the ability to promote and influence the outcome of rehabilitation cannot be underestimated; the nurse is pivotal to the child's care, providing wound care and contemporary communication with all team members, therefore providing continuity and coordination of all aspects of care from admission to discharge.

## EPIDEMIOLOGY

It is estimated that 1.4 million people worldwide are burned each year, with medical attention being required because of the injuries sustained. 50% of these burn injuries occur during the formative and productive years, in children ranging from 1–5 years and in men from the ages of 17–30 (Wilson 2000).

In the UK it is estimated that 175 000 individuals per year attend an Accident and Emergency Department with a burn related injury. About 13 000, that is one in every thirteen burn injured patients, require

hospital admission. Of these, 1000 are 'major' burn patients requiring intravenous fluid resuscitation and it is estimated that half of these are children (National Burn Care Review Committee 2001).

70% of burns in the child population occur in children under 5 years, most commonly between the ages of 1 and 2 years, with a boy to girl ratio of 3:2 (Bosworth 1997). In the Glasgow Burns Unit, around 130 children are admitted with thermal injuries every year. Around 90% of these injuries are caused by scalding agents. A review of the literature proposes that the majority of thermal injuries in the child population are caused by scalding, i.e. injuries caused by hot liquids. A Birmingham study suggested that children are 36 times more likely to sustain a scald than an adult is, with the majority of these injuries occurring in the home (Lawrence 1996).

The high incidence of burn injury in the child population can be attributed in part to an underdeveloped ability to sense, and therefore avoid, danger. A link with poor socioeconomic circumstances has also been found (Child Accident Prevention Trust 1991). In acknowledging these factors we can begin to appreciate the significance of the health professional's role as educator with regard to child safety and accident prevention. Recognition of the importance of data collection for audit purposes is vital in identifying emerging patterns of child safety issues, if we are to successfully shape a burn service that will adequately meet the requirements of burn care in the years ahead. Issues regarding this can be viewed in the report of the National Burn Care Review Committee (2001).

## TYPES OF BURN INJURY – CAUSATIVE AGENTS

Injuries that may be encountered in the clinical setting may be due to:

- Explosion and flame
- Scalding water/oil
- Contact
- Electrical sources
- Chemicals
- Friction
- Radiation.

First, to understand the effects of burn injury on the skin it is important to be aware of the structure and function of normal skin. A brief review follows.

## ANATOMY AND PHYSIOLOGY OF NORMAL SKIN

The skin is the largest organ of the body and its role is diverse. It is crucial to the maintenance of homeostasis. It offers protection from the external environment: for example, it acts as a barrier to invading pathogenic microorganisms. It is essential in heat regulation, excretion of water and salts, and the synthesis of important chemicals and hormones. It also protects many underlying structures, as well as being host to many sensory receptors that allow us to be aware of important external factors, such as temperature, touch, pressure and pain.

The skin's structure is thin and relatively flat. It is composed of two layers: the *epidermis*, which is the outer thinner layer comprising several types of epithelial cell, and the *dermis*, the inner thicker layer consisting of connective tissue (see Fig. 16.1).

The epidermis consists of stratified (layered) squamous (flat) epithelium. It measures less than 0.17 mm thick in most areas. Exceptions to this are the hands and feet where it is notably thicker, measuring 1–1.3 mm (Thibodeau & Patton 1993). It is avascular, and comprises several types of epithelial cell. Keratinocytes are the most significant and plentiful. These form the main structural element of the outer skin. Epidermal cells can be found in up to five distinct layers. The epidermis undergoes continuous regeneration – complete epidermal renewal occurs around every 2 months (Wysocki 2000).

The dermis is the thicker layer of the skin, averaging 2 mm thick. It comprises two layers: a thin **papillary** layer and a thicker **reticular** layer. As a general rule dermis is thicker on the posterior surface of the body. In comparison with the multicellular epidermis it is sparsely populated, primarily by fibroblastic cells. These cells synthesise and secrete proteins. Other cells present are macrophages and lymphocytes.

The dermis forms a supportive matrix for the epidermis. The point at which the epidermis and dermis join is known as the **basement membrane zone or dermal–epidermal junction.** This is the area that is affected in blister formation. The dermis has a rich supply of blood vessels, sensory nerves, muscle fibres and proteins. The main proteins are collagen and elastin. The skin's mechanical and tensile strength arise from the dermis. Also in the dermis are the hair follicles, sweat and sebaceous glands; these are epidermal structures, sometimes referred to as the adnexal appendages. These penetrate deep into the dermis. They are significant in that, as they are lined with epidermal cells, they are capable of regenerating the epidermal layer if they remain intact following burn injury.

Unlike the epidermis, the dermis does not go through a continuous cycle of regeneration, replacing like for like. Only in the event of trauma does the dermis replace itself by the body's main healing mechanism, one of repair, not regeneration. New blood vessels are produced and fibroblasts reproduce forming an atypical dense mass of new connective tissue fibres. Wound repair is complicated in deep dermal or full thickness injuries. There is disruption in the wound healing mechanism resulting in the formation of extensive scar tissue. This tissue does not possess the same functions or strength as normal skin (Waldrop & Doughty 2000)

## DEPTH OF BURN INJURY

Depth of injury is dependent upon the duration of time the causative agent is in contact with the skin and the intensity or concentration of the burning agent (Bosworth 1997).

Many factors affect the skin's ability to absorb and dissipate thermal energy. These include its thickness, blood supply and water content, and also the time over which the energy is delivered. These variables will determine the level of skin damage. A child's skin is thinner than that of an adult

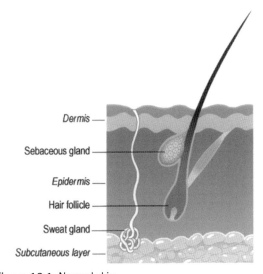

Dermis —

Sebaceous gland —

Epidermis —

Hair follicle —

Sweat gland —

Subcutaneous layer —

**Figure 16.1** Normal skin.

(Arturson 2000) and therefore has less resistance to tissue damage. This couples significantly with a delay in, or failure to respond to the painful stimulus, as may be demonstrated in a young child whose instinct is underdeveloped.

It is not always easy to determine the depth of a burn injury in the immediate post-burn period unless it is particularly deep or superficial. Heat damage causes an increased permeability within the burn wound, making it oedematous and difficult to assess. This capillary permeability returns to normal after a period of around 36 hours (Muir et al 1987). Burn wounds do not necessarily present with a uniformity of depth but more usually with a mix of depth. Ascertaining wound depth is essential in planning appropriate management. Terms used to describe the depth of a burn injury may vary from country to country and classifying a burn injury by degrees can be confusing (Marsden 1996). Commonplace terms are:

- Superficial injury
- Partial thickness injury, which is further divided into two sub groups: superficial partial thickness or deep partial thickness
- Full thickness injury. (see Fig. 16.2)

## EVALUATION OF THE BURN INJURY

Jackson's burn wound model (see Fig. 16.3) demonstrates three distinct zones, which are also three dimensional (Jackson 1983). These are a zone of

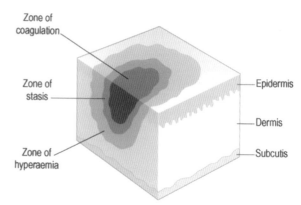

Figure 16.3 Jackson model of a burn wound.

coagulation, a zone of stasis and a zone of hyperaemia. Each zone represents a different degree of cell damage.

The *zone of coagulation* is the region where greatest destruction has taken place. It is the area that has been closest to the heat source and is usually found in the centre of the wound. It is the area where heat could not be conducted away quickly enough and so the cells are heat coagulated, resulting in cell death. This is the deepest part of the burn wound. It may or may not heal by itself. This is dependent upon the depth to which cell damage extends. The fewer epidermal appendages left intact post burn, the higher the requirement for burn tissue excision and grafting.

The *zone of stasis* surrounds the zone of coagulation and the heat damage here is less severe. The tissue remains viable but has decreased perfusion due to effects of the injury on the local vasculature. The risk of further cell death from ischaemia is a distinct possibility. However, with the correct management this area should remain viable. Adequate fluid management, with avoidance of wound bed dessication and contamination are important factors in maintaining viability of this area. The zone of stasis should stabilise within 36 hours and there will be no further cell death. Inadequate management may result in continuing cell death, creating an extension of the zone of coagulation.

The *zone of hyperaemia* is the zone of least damage. It surrounds the zone of stasis, and is essentially normal skin with a temporary increase in blood flow. Cells usually recover within 7–10 days. This area of skin damage is red, bloated, hot and painful (Wilson 2000).

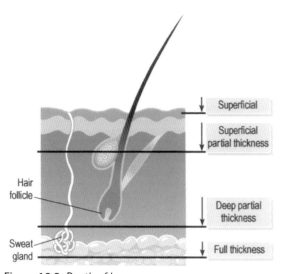

Figure 16.2 Depth of burn.

## BASIC OVERVIEW OF WOUND HEALING

Normal wound healing (see also Ch. 4) is an integrated chain of processes that occur in a timely sequence in response to skin injury. The process can be separated into four active stages. These stages are:

- the vascular response
- the inflammatory response
- the proliferation phase
- the maturation phase. (Flanagan 1999)

Similarly with other wounds, a burn injury progresses through these defined stages of wound healing.

In a major burn injury, however, there may be disruption in the normal healing process, caused by the inability of the cells required for healing to interact efficiently (Kearney 1997). Tissue damage immediately results in a localised increase in blood supply and cellular activity. Injury of the skin, extending to the dermis or beyond, triggers a coagulation cascade controlling blood loss and providing a preliminary fibrin matrix which helps to trap bacteria at the wound's surface.

In response to both tissue damage and the vascular response, the inflammatory response is initiated, resulting in the release of inflammatory mediators, for example histamine. This causes vasodilation and increased permeability in the capillaries, allowing a leak of fluid from the capillaries into the surrounding tissues resulting in oedema and swelling. Vasodilation facilitates the migration of leukocytes into the area of injury. The first to arrive are neutrophils. Their role is to engulf and digest, or phagocytose, bacteria in the initial injury period. More importantly, macrophages arrive at the wound bed by the third day. These are large mobile cells that are able to destroy bacteria and devitalised tissue. In essence, they provide a clean wound bed. They also release important growth factors essential to the attraction of fibroblasts, the cells from which connective tissue develops to allow repair of tissue defects. Macrophages are also initiators of the process of angiogenesis by which new blood vessels are formed (Bosworth 1997). Essentially, the macrophage regulates the entire wound repair process. They are present throughout all stages of the healing process and without them wound healing stops (Westaby 1985).

The breakdown of necrotic tissue stimulates the proliferative period, occurring between the third and twenty-fourth days post injury (Bosworth 1997). Vascular integrity is restored by the process of angiogenesis and fibroblast cells begin to synthesise strands of collagen, filling the defect with new connective tissue. The processes that occur during this phase are interdependent, each relying on the supportive mechanisms of the other (Waldrop & Doughty 2000). In this phase the wound decreases in size by a combination of the production of granulation tissue, collagen synthesis/wound matrix deposition, wound contraction and re-epithelialisation. Wound contraction is caused by the contractile forces of fibroblasts pulling wound edges together and is seen more predominantly in the healing of larger open wounds. Re-epithelialisation across the wound surface is seen during the final stage of proliferation (Flanagan 1999).

Finally, the maturation or remodelling stage usually occurs at around day 20 post injury. This period may last for many months or may even take years (Flanagan 1999). This phase concerns the simultaneous processes of wound matrix destruction and wound matrix synthesis. The cells that control these processes are the fibroblasts. The structure of scar tissue is remodelled, increasing its tensile strength. The red, raised and itchy scar tissue that often complicates deep burn wounds (known as hypertrophic scarring) is believed to be caused by an imbalance of matrix production and matrix destruction. Following initial overproduction of matrix, blood supply decreases as scar tissue matures leaving it paler, flatter and smoother. Maturity of scar tissue may take around 2 years.

Deep dermal or full thickness burn wounds will progress through all of these stages of wound healing. Each stage is superseded by the next at variable rates, depending on the nature and the management of the injury. Wound healing is a complex activity. In view of this, our aim should be to promote optimal conditions to facilitate it.

## PATHOPHYSIOLOGY

Having identified that there are different depths of burn injury, we can now look at the local effects of each depth of burn injury.

In a superficial burn (e.g. sunburn), only the surface layers of the epidermis are involved. It is characterised by redness, pain, heat and swelling. The release of vasodilating prostaglandins in response to the burn injury causes the capillaries in the dermis to become dilated. Fluid then leaks out of the capillaries into the surrounding tissues, causing a rise in interstitial pressure, i.e. the pressure in the spaces between the cells. This stimulates the nerve endings, causing pain.

There is no blister formation and normal skin function remains intact. After a few days a superficial burn will heal without scar formation. There will usually be an episode of skin peel as the outer layer of damaged cells shed themselves, revealing a new layer of healthy cells. Healing occurs quickly by regeneration from the basement layers of the epidermis.

A partial thickness burn involves the epidermis and a variable depth of the dermis. If the thermal damage is limited to the papilary dermis there is presence of a blister. The skin forming the cover of the blister is dead. When the burn blister is removed it is important to prevent the introduction of infection, and any drying of the wound bed. Both of these factors are damaging to the dynamics of wound healing, particularly in the early stages of burn injury. Inappropriate care may lead to further loss of viable tissue, which would otherwise revert back to a healthy state. Pain is also a significant feature in this depth of injury as the sensory nerves are exposed. For this reason also, it is important to protect the wound from unnecessary exposure to the air and extremes of temperature which will cause further discomfort.

Healing by epidermal regeneration is usually rapid in superficial partial thickness injury. The adnexal structures in the dermis facilitate this type of healing as epithelial cells are able to reproduce and can provide epidermal resurfacing by means of migration upwards through the dermis. A moist wound environment speeds the process; this will normally take place within a 10–14 day period. Scarring should be minimal or absent.

A deep partial thickness injury will result in delayed healing due to the loss of a significant depth of dermis, with consequential damage and destruction of the adnexal epithelial structures. A deep injury is likely to result in significant scarring as the characteristics of normal skin are lost, resulting in a wound repair lacking in elasticity and of poor tensile strength. Hypertrophic scarring will often occur some weeks later. Partial thickness wounds are therefore capable of healing by self-regeneration, but in deeper partial thickness wounds where there is significant loss of dermis and some of its inherent structures, it is often prefer-

able to skin graft. Failure to graft can result in very prolonged healing times, resulting in a wound repair of unacceptable quality both functionally and cosmetically.

A full thickness burn involves the epidermis, the dermis and all of its structures. The injury may also extend into the subcutaneous layer, penetrating underlying muscle, bone and tendon. The blood vessels of the dermis are coagulated by the heat source so that the tissue is devoid of vasculature. Nerve endings are also destroyed in this depth of burn injury, which is insensate to needle prick testing. It is important to remember that no burn wound is completely painless. Full thickness injuries will heal only at their margins as they have lost all or much of their deep rooted epithelial structures, removing the ability to regenerate acceptable quantities and quality of epithelium. Skin grafting is therefore required to prevent unacceptable wound healing times and the complications of this, such as contractures resulting in loss of function.

Wound depth, characteristics and healing potential are summarised in Table 16.1.

## ADMISSION CRITERIA

The criteria for admission of a child to a specialist burns unit for assessment and care have been defined by many experts in the burn field. Box 16.1 encompasses those criteria.

## ADMISSION – AN OVERVIEW

The admission of a child to hospital is a traumatic and stressful event at any time, and especially so if the injury might have been avoided. Not only are the needs of the child high, but those of the parent or carer are also likely to be elevated (Kemble & Lamb 1987). Admission to a paediatric unit is an important step in being able to provide the holistic care required (Reid 1997). Prior to admission onto the ward, the child should have a full assessment of airway, breathing and circulation in the Accident and Emergency Department.

Obtaining a full history, and undertaking a head to toe examination will help to rule out any other injuries. Estimation of burn size should be undertaken as this will dictate the decision to give intravenous fluids. If fluid resuscitation is required the child ideally should have insertion of at least one

**Table 16.1** Classification of burn depth

| Burn depth | | Structures affected | Characteristics | Healing |
|---|---|---|---|---|
| Superficial | | Epidermis | Skin intact, red, blanching, swollen, may blister | Painful. Heals within 7 days |
| Partial thickness: | superficial dermal | Epidermis and superficial dermis | Blistering present, red to pink wound bed. Capillary return brisk. Wound bed moist to wet appearance | Painful. Heals in around 14 days |
| Partial thickness: | deep dermal | Epidermis, deeper dermis sparing hair follicles and sebaceous glands | Blistering present, wound bed has a red, wet or waxy appearance. Capillary return absent | Mostly painless. Healing may take months. Skin grafting indicated for early wound closure |
| Full thickness | | Epidermis and dermis destroyed, may extend into the subcutaneous fat layer, fascia and bone. Epidermal appendages are destroyed, all skin function is lost | Blistering absent. Charred, leathery white, brown, or cherry red appearance. Absence of capillary return. Presence of thrombosed vessels | Painless. Requires skin grafting due to the destruction of the skin appendages capable of regeneration |

---

**Box 16.1  Admission criteria (Marsden 1996, Pape, Judkins & Settle 2000)**

- Thermal injuries which are superficial but affecting 10% or more of the child's body surface area, or deeper dermal and full thickness injuries affecting > 5% of a child's body surface area.
- Thermal injury to the eyes. Opthalmology opinion should be sought as quickly as possible prior to onset of swelling which makes assessment difficult.
- Facial burns, all of which have the potential to swell and may compromise the child's airway.
- Burns to the outer ear where there is no fat protection, and the ear is at risk of necrosis.
- Injuries affecting hands, feet or flexure surfaces, particularly of the neck and axilla.
- Thermal injuries to the perineal or buttock area, which are often difficult to keep clean and dressed, particularly in a young child.
- Injuries that are circumferential which have the potential for circulatory embarrassment, compromising the neurovascular state of limbs and extremities.
- Electrical burns which require special management including 24 hour ECG monitoring and care of both exit and entry wounds. There may be deep tissue injury which the visible wound may not necessarily indicate.
- Suspected non accidental injuries.
- Chemical or radiation injuries.
- Other criteria include children under the age of five, the presence of pre-existing illnesses, and other associated injuries.

---

large bore intravenous cannula, preferably into an area of unburned skin. Failure to cannulate promptly delays fluid resuscitation. The resulting shut down of the child's peripheral circulation, caused by hypovolaemia, increases the difficulty of cannulation.

Blood samples ideally should be taken at the time of cannulation, both to minimise patient distress and to provide a timely baseline on which to manage the child's fluid replacement most effectively. Analgesia requirements should be assessed. Intravenous (IV) opiates are the drug of choice in a child with a major injury as they can be titrated against the child's pain.

On admission to any unit/ward, a designated, experienced nurse should meet the child immediately and carry out a 'glancing assessment' (British Burn

Association 1996), paying particular attention to the child's airway, breathing, circulation and neurological status. The initial assessment in the Accident and Emergency Department may underestimate the severity of burn injury, and signs of inhalational injury may be missed (Driscoll 1993). After this initial assessment, it is important to ensure any IV infusions in progress are running appropriately, and that cannulae are secure. Affected burn areas can be covered with cling film to reduce both heat loss and pain (Lawrence 1977). Vital signs including blood pressure should be recorded. The child's weight should be obtained if possible, to permit accurate calculation of IV fluid resuscitation and drug therapy requirements.

The initial admission details and history should include the time and cause of the injury and a note of any first aid given, together with details of any pre existing conditions, allergies, current medications and immunisation status, for example tetanus.

Total body surface area (TBSA) affected by the injury is estimated using the formula designated. The child's pain is assessed and managed appropriately, ensuring any drugs already given are noted. As much reassurance and information as possible are given to both the child and family. Suitable dressings are applied. All necessary documentation is completed.

## NON-ACCIDENTAL INJURY (NAI)

Staff working with children who have sustained burn injuries should be alerted to the possibility of NAI by any child whose injuries are clearly demarcated or inconsistent with the history given by the carer, or if there has been a delay in presentation of the child. An established diagnosis of NAI is important if the child is to be protected from further risk, but it is also important to avoid misdiagnosis as this can lead to a catalogue of difficulties (Reid 1996). Clearly defined procedures should be available for all staff caring for a child with a suspected NAI.

## AIRWAY AND BREATHING

Any thermal injury affecting the airway either directly, or one that has the potential to affect the airway, should be assessed by an anaesthetist. If the airway is compromised, intubation and mechanical ventilation should be considered. Airway damage should be suspected in any child who has suffered smoke inhalation or who has a thermal injury directly to the face or neck. Useful indicators of airway damage are abnormal respiratory rates and sounds and decreased oxygen saturation levels. Other measures in managing a child with inhalation injury include tracheobronchial lavage, physiotherapy, antibiotics, bronchodilators and on occasion steroids (Judkins 1996).

For a child with a major thermal injury, first aid should include 100% oxygen therapy, which will improve hypoxia secondary to hypovolaemic shock and assist in optimal tissue perfusion. Oxygen also alleviates the poisonous effects of carbon monoxide.

## CIRCULATION

Loss of fluid occurs both at the burn surface as blister fluid and exudate, and into the surrounding tissues in the form of oedema. The main constituent of this fluid is plasma, and loss continues until the capillaries start to recover at around 36 hours post injury (Bosworth 1997).

When the size of the burn injury exceeds 20–30% TBSA, the process of fluid leakage becomes more generalised, leading to the formation of diffuse body oedema. Hypovolaemic shock quickly follows. Time is of the essence in obtaining IV access in a child with a compromised circulation, and cannulation should not be delayed.

Thermal injuries involving near or fully circumferential insult to the chest, neck or limbs require frequent observation to allow detection of any circulatory compromise. Any reduction in colour, sensation and temperature of the area affected requires immediate assessment and intervention by the burns surgeon. Circumferential chest wounds mandate close monitoring of breathing pattern. These injuries may require escharotomy to relieve pressure and circulatory compromise.

## ASSESSMENT OF BURN SIZE

Various methods of assessing the extent of a burn injury are in use. One commonly applied tool to determine burn size is the rule of nines, which essentially divides the body surface into parts that represent 9% or multiples of 9%, with the exception of the perineum which is estimated at 1%. This, however, may lead to miscalculation of the burn size in children as their body surface proportions differ to those of an adult. The 'rule' is adapted as in Figure 16.4 to allow for changing proportions with age.

The Lund and Browder method relies on accurate hand drawn replications of the burn wound onto a chart depicting the different ratios of head to body and limbs. The sections are then added together to give the total body surface area affected, as shown in Figure 16.5.

A useful method to estimate smaller 'dotted' areas of burn injury is to use the palmar aspect of the patient's hand, which is deemed to be approximately 1% of the child's body surface area (British Burn Association 1996).

Getting the calculation right is vital for correct IV fluid resuscitation and all of these methods are subject to error.

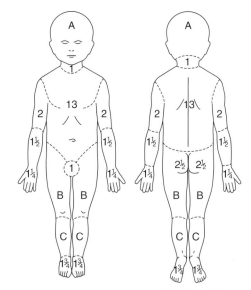

Figure 16.4  Paediatric rule of nines (age 1 year).

Figure 16.5  Lund and Browder chart.

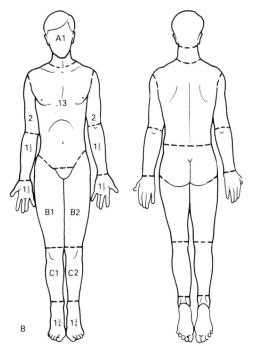

Percentage of body surface at various ages

Percent of areas affected by growth

|  | 0 | 1 | 5 | 10 | 15 | Adult age |
|---|---|---|---|---|---|---|
| A = ½ head | 9½ | 8½ | 6½ | 5½ | 4½ | 3½ |
| B = ½ one thigh | 2¾ | 3¼ | 4 | 4¼ | 4½ | 4¾ |
| C = ½ one leg | 2½ | 2½ | 2¾ | 3 | 3¼ | 3½ |

To estimate the total of the body surface area burned, the percentages assigned to the burned sections are added. The total is then an estimate of the burn size.

## FLUID RESUSCITATION

The threshhold at which fluid resuscitation is required in children is lower than that for an adult. This is because children have a greater surface area to mass ratio in comparison with adults, and more limited physiological reserves.

There is debate about which fluid resuscitation regime should be used. The two best known are the Muir and Barclay formula and the Parkland formula. The latter is the internationally recognised choice for the initiation of fluid resuscitation (British Burn Association 1996).

In the UK, the Muir and Barclay formula (which gives human albumin solution 4.5% [HAS] for replacement) is still used. To utilise the formula the patient's weight and the TBSA of injury are required.

The volume of HAS to be transfused is given by the formula: total percentage of burned body surface area multiplied by patient weight in kg/2 = R.

The volume arrived at (R) is then transfused over six allocated time periods (4 h, 4 h, 4 h, 6 h, 6 h and 12 h) together with normal maintenance fluids (i.e. 4 % glucose in 1/4 normal saline). For example, if 10% of the child's body surface area is affected by the burn injury and the patient weighs 10 kg, then 50 mL of HAS should be given over each of the six time periods of the formula. It is important to start the regime from the time of injury. By 4 hours post injury the child should have had 50 mL of HAS transfused intravenously. Therefore, if the child presents 2 hours post injury the rate of HAS infusion will be adjusted to ensure that the delay between burn injury and initiation of fluid resuscitation is compensated for.

After each of the allocated time periods of the fluid resuscitation, the patient's condition should be reassessed. If it is satisfactory, then the formula can be followed as presented. If the child's condition is unsatisfactory, then adjustments to the fluid resuscitation will be required.

The Parkland formula utilises Hartmann's or Ringer's lactate solution. For a child 4 mL of this solution per kg multiplied by the size of the burn injury is transfused over a 24 hour period. One half of the calculated amount is given over the first 8 hours post injury and the other half is given over the subsequent 16 hours. This resuscitation fluid is given in conjunction with 4% glucose in 1/4 normal saline maintenance fluid, as in the Muir and Barclay formula. In the second 24 hours post burn injury, albumin may be required to help restore circulating volume. It is important to remember that these formulae are guidelines and may require some tailoring to meet the individual child's fluid resuscitation needs.

Monitoring the condition of the child is met by observation of the child's general appearance, capillary return, skin colour and by measuring core and periphery temperature difference, urinary output, blood pressure, pulse, blood gases, urea, creatinine and electrolytes.

The insertion of a urinary catheter is advocated by the British Burn Association in those children presenting with a major thermal injury that is greater than 10–15% TBSA. This facilitates accurate monitoring of urine output which should ideally be 1 mL/kg/h; the acceptable range is between 0.5 and 2 mL/kg/h (Pape et al 2000). If urine output is maintained at these levels then satisfactory organ perfusion is maintained. A low urine output indicates inadequate tissue perfusion and increases the risk of further cellular injury. Conversely, a large urine output indicates excessive fluid resuscitation with the risk of increasing oedema formation.

## PAIN MANAGEMENT

A thermal injury is a painful experience as even if sensation is lost at the site of the injury, the surrounding area is often painful. The initial analgesic drug of choice in a patient with a major injury is usually IV morphine sulphate. Small increments of morphine are given until the pain experienced is controlled (Judkins 1996). In children over the age of 3 months, a loading dose of 100 µg per kg can be slowly administered over a 3–5 minute period, an interval of 10 minutes before reassessment should be allowed before administering a further bolus. An infant of 1–3 months should receive half this amount. No more than three boluses within a 2 hour period are recommended. In infants under 1 month a dose of 5 µg per kg is recommended, with diligent assessment before administering any further boluses, and total dose should not exceed 25 µg per kg (Lawson 1998).

Subcutaneous or intramuscular routes of administration are best avoided during the first 36 hours post injury. At this time there may be poor peripheral blood supply resulting in poor tissue absorption. Initial inadequacy of pain control is later followed by a risk of respiratory depression when peripheral blood supply is restored. Respiratory depression may occur even with therapeutic doses of morphine and therefore consciousness level and Sa O$_2$ level should be monitored closely for several hours post administration.

Pain management should be considered in the initial injury period, during and between dressing changes and following surgical intervention such as skin grafting. Nonsteroidal anti-inflammatory drugs, for example diclofenac sodium, are also useful analgesics, these can also be used in conjunction with oral opiates to give very effective analgesia. Paracetamol is only used if pain is minimal (Orr 1997).

The control of pain presents its own challenges and to facilitate the optimal recovery it is important to manage pain both safely and effectively. Pain assessment in children is often more challenging than in adults. Children's parents or carers should, if possible, be involved in the process of pain assessment. Their judgement as to whether pain is being effectively managed is helpful. However, it is important to recognise that the carer is in an unfamiliar place and situation and may not be able to make accurate judgements.

Skills in assessing both pain and the child's response to any given pain relief are essential for the health professional. A withdrawn child may be interpreted quite differently by medical or nursing staff who are not familiar with the child's normal behaviour. Burr in 1993 reported some common, ill founded assumptions that, for example, pain always results in a crying child, or that a quiet child is a pain free child. She argues that children do not always tell the truth about their pain for fear of being given an injection.

Pain is subjective and personal, no two people will experience it in the same way. Before assessing a child's pain it is important to think about the variables that may affect pain response or perception. They may include past experiences of pain, how well prepared in advance the patient is for any necessary procedures and, of course, cognitive level. Taking a holistic view of a child should afford health professionals greater ability as pain assessors (see Ch. 6).

## DRESSINGS

When considering dressings for any burn wound, several factors are considered:

- Creation of the optimal wound environment to facilitate healing
- management of burn exudate
- prevention of wound contamination
- patient comfort and safety.

The suitability of dressings for any burn wound is dependent upon the nature, size and depth of injury, the volume and type of exudate and the location of injury. Appropriate selection depends on an understanding of wound physiology.

Available dressings include:

- contact layer dressings
- foam dressings
- hydropolymer dressings
- vapour permeable adhesive film dressings
- hydrocolloids and hydrogels
- alginates and hydrofibres
- medicated dressings.

A contact layer dressing is commonly advocated for initial burn injury. It permits the passage of wound exudate through the mesh formation, and is particularly useful for large burn injuries. It is used in conjunction with an absorbent secondary dressing that can be easily removed and replaced without having to touch the contact layer dressing itself. If there is leakage of exudate through the dressing it must be repadded or replaced as this creates an access route for invading microorganisms, and causes wound contamination.

Another benefit of contact layer dressings is that they do not distort the appearance of the wound bed and therefore, in the early stages of burn injury, wound inspection and assessment can take place without difficulty. Various brands are available, at varying prices. A disadvantage of this type of dressing is that it may adhere to the wound bed, and therefore on removal may cause further trauma.

After the initial exudative period (approximately 48 hours post injury), the wound should be reassessed and the type of dressing may need changing. No single dressing is suitable for all wounds; the depth, size, location, tissue type, volume of wound exudate and presence of infection are all determining factors in the wound product selection process. Hydrocolloids or hydropolymer dressings are good alternatives to contact layer type dressings if the wound bed is appropriate.

Topical creams are often avoided in the initial period as they may mask the appearance of the wound bed. Thereafter, where antibacterial cover is required, the topical, white cream, silver sulphadiazine 1%, is commonly used. It both prevents and treats infection in burn wounds.

Different wound cleansing solutions may be used, for example sterile saline, sterile water, chlorhexidene aqueous solution, or tap water. The solution should be warmed to avoid wound bed cooling which inhibits cell mitosis, potentially delaying the healing process. The removal of bacteria from the wound bed is the gold standard by which wound cleansing is judged. Wound irrigation under high pressure does this best; it also reduces infection rates (Miller & Gilchrist 1997).

Removal of blisters covering large burns reduces the risk of infection. This is because burn fluid within the blister is rich in nutrients, and is an ideal environment for bacteria to thrive (Bosworth 1997). Smaller blisters may be left intact, to act as a biological dressing (Wilson 2000).

Bandaging secures primary dressings and promotes effective circulatory return if it is applied firmly and evenly. Used in conjunction with splinting it helps to maintain functional positioning and prevents contractures and deformity.

Circumferential injuries require frequent assessment in the acute phase of the injury, and bandaging inhibits this. Dressings that permit frequent observation are indicated. Exposure of circumferential burns is not recommended unless specialised facilities are available (Pape et al 2000).

Face, ears, perineum, digits, joints and flexor surfaces require special consideration. Facial burns are difficult to dress and are better left exposed (Marsden 1996). The exudate is allowed to dry and coagulate in a warm environment. Olive oil or soft paraffin may be applied over crusted areas, to enable removal of crusting and dead skin. This coagulum should not be removed prior to its independant separation or healing will be damaged. Removal occurs at around 7–14 days.

Eyes (conjunctiva) should be protected with saline lavage and 1% chloramphenicol ointment.

Ear injuries require application of creams or ointments, for example Flamazine, to ensure cartilage is not permitted to dry out. Otherwise ear deformity and the increased risk of infection arise.

Injuries over joints, digits or flexor surfaces should be managed in conjunction with an experienced physiotherapist and occupational therapist. These areas are subject to risk of contracture, with loss of function and range of movement.

Perineal injuries are at increased risk of infection. Cleansing and redressing is needed each time the patient passes urine or feces. Bladder catheterisation may be required to prevent urethral obstruction by oedema and urinary retention. Relative constipation can be induced (if required) by slowing bowel transit using antimotility drugs (codeine phosphate or loperamide).

## NUTRITION

The aim of nutritional support in a thermally injured child is to help provide both the optimal environment for wound healing and to maintain normal growth requirements. It is well documented that a good nutritional status in the critically ill patient reduces the likelihood of problems such as poor wound healing and infection and helps to reduce length of hospitalisation (Wallace 1994).

In the past, thermal injury resulted in hugely elevated energy requirements giving rise to a hypermetabolic state. Advances in both medical and nursing management such as earlier wound coverage, improved pain and infection control, and control of ambient temperature have led to reduction of the catabolic effects of burn injury (Childs 1995, Bosworth 1997). Energy requirements in children with burns are now thought rarely to rise above the estimated normal basic requirements post burn injury (Childs 1994); normal body weight can be maintained by giving normal energy requirements (Childs 1995). Laitung 1996 is supportive of this and reports that provision of normal daily recommended allowance in children is adequate. However, there is an increased need for provision of protein (Cunningham et al 1995).

In children with less than 10% TBSA burns, early reintroduction of dietary intake should be encouraged. Where possible, milky fluids should be substituted for juices. If the child is not achieving the required dietary intake as estimated by the dietitian, the use of dietary supplements such as calorie fortified drinks and puddings should be considered. If the child cannot take sufficient oral supplementation, nasogastric feeding should be implemented.

Children with major burns, that is greater than 10% TBSA, should normally be commenced on nasogastric feeding. Enteral feeding commenced within the first 6 hours of burn injury reduces the occurrence of paralytic ileus, and gives protection to the mucosal lining of the gastrointestinal tract, which when damaged may permit the translocation of bacteria across the gut wall into the blood stream. Even a very small hourly volume can provide this protective effect. Other benefits include improvement in wound healing times, improved immune status (Childs 1995) and better restoration of haemoglobin.

Mineral and vitamin supplementation are important in wound healing processes. In a patient with a major burn, vitamin, mineral and trace elements should be monitored on a weekly basis until total healing occurs. Most burn units advocate oral administration of iron and multivitamins (Laitung 1996).

Monitoring the child's progress is important in the quest for excellence in nutritional support. The child should be weighed on admission and thereafter during dressing changes, i.e. without dressings. Stool pattern should be monitored, indicating frequency and consistency. Diarrhoea may be a consequence of enteral feeding and may necessitate reduction in volume or concentration.

Modifications in nasogastric feeding should also be made as the child's wound decreases in size and as the child's oral intake improves (see Ch. 7).

## SKIN GRAFTING

'Skin grafts are biological tissue harvested from a donor area and applied to the recipient bed. In order to survive, the graft requires a good exchange of nutrients.' (Cowell 1995) Skin grafts are performed to restore skin coverage, and to reconstruct deformity and malformations of tissue. They may be full thickness or split thickness.

Full thickness grafts are useful for small tissue defects in areas with an important function such as the face and fingers. The donor site (groin or post-auricular) is repaired by primary closure or, if necessary, by secondary split skin graft from another site.

Split skin grafts are most commonly used. Autografts (the patient's own skin) are harvested with a knife (dermatome), which is adjusted to allow for variable thickness of graft. Graft is prepared as either a sheet or a mesh. Sheet grafts are stronger and are more cosmetically pleasing whilst meshed grafts cover larger areas in circumstances where donor sites are restricted. The meshed appearance persists after healing has taken place which makes it an unsatisfactory option for areas such as the face.

The graft 'takes' by a three stage process of imbibition, inosculation and capillary ingrowth. Imbibition occurs within a few hours of 'grafting' and is bonding by fibrin adhesion. Inosculation is establishment of a primitive blood and lymphatic supply in 3 days. Finally, capillary ingrowth from the recipient into the graft occurs within 5 days (Cowell 1995).

Management of the skin graft includes the prevention of fluid accumulation or haematoma formation between the graft and the recipient site. Otherwise, disruption of the graft taking process and failure of the graft are inevitable. Prevention of infection by meticulous hand washing by health personnel is paramount. Graft trauma should be minimised by careful thought when positioning, washing and providing pressure care for the patient. Nutrition and adequate hydration are essential during the process of graft healing. Skin grafts become stable 10–14 days after grafting (Wilson 1997).

It is dependent upon the surgeon's preference whether the child's grafted site is bandaged or exposed. If the grafted area is exposed it is easier to monitor for complications and so early intervention is facilitated. The child with an exposed graft is nursed in a heat regulated environment to maintain ambient body temperature, which optimises wound bed perfusion and promotes graft take. Sedation and pain control requirements need regular reassessment.

Bandaged grafts should be inspected after five days, taking great care with dressing removal. Daily replacement until no longer required is best thereafter.

Following harvesting of the split skin graft, bleeding occurs at the donor site from the remaining dermis. It is controlled by a haemostatic dressing, for example Kaltostat, an alginate dressing that provides a matrix supportive of clotting.

A donor site is essentially a superficial partial thickness wound and may be reharvested following healing, several times if necessary. Care of the donor site involves control of haemorrhage, prevention of infection and promotion of epithelialisation by adequate hydration and nutrition. It should heal within 7–14 days. Delayed healing and presence of infection will result in scarring.

Alternative grafting techniques include:

- techniques such as the use of a dermal regeneration template (Integra), combined with the use of split skin grafts
- use of laboratory cultured sheets of epithelial cells.

## AFTERCARE AND REHABILITATION

The main aim of burn treatment is to promote early healing, reduce scarring, and promote function in the affected area, so reducing the need for future surgery. Preparation of the child and carer for the aftercare of the burn injury is important. After deep burn injury or skin grafting, scarring is inevitable. Scar tissue will never look or behave like normal skin, but with good aftercare the end results can often be very satisfactory. Burn scars require gentle washing, moisturising and massage several times per day until scar maturity at around 18–24 months.

Scar tissue is made up of many small fibres of collagen laid down in an unorganised fashion. Massaging helps to separate the fibres, and improve the appearance and texture of the scar tissue. At least 30 minutes in total per day is recommended. It is best to avoid soaps and moisturisers that are highly perfumed, as these may irritate the skin. Aqueous cream BP and E45 (Crookes) are amongst those commonly used. Moisturising the skin after bathing or swimming is important, as these activities dry out and tighten the skin.

As split skin grafts do not include all of the structures associated with normal skin, they will look and feel different. Hair follicles, sweat and sebaceous glands will be damaged or destroyed in deep dermal injuries. Loss of some or all of the sebaceous glands causes the skin to become very dry and loss of the sweat glands will make the scar tissue more sensitive to changes in temperature. Therefore, it is advisable to wear cool cottons in warm weather and adequate warm clothing in the winter.

## HYPERTROPHIC SCARRING

Normal smooth skin exerts an even pressure on the loosely connected subcutis. In a deep burn injury this is lost and the process of the production and

breakdown of collagen is disrupted. Red, raised and hardened areas of hypertrophic scar tissue result. Pressure garments, silicone therapies and massage help to control this process.

## PRESSURE GARMENTS

Pressure garments are made to measure from strong stretchy Lycra® material. They are worn continuously under normal clothing, and taken off only to allow for washing, moisturising and massage of the skin. They are indicated for any post burn healing area with significant scarring and are designed to exert an even, continuous, gentle pressure. Their use should be continued for approximately 2 years and may be combined with silicone application.

## CONTRACTURES

If contractures or bands of scarring develop, particularly in areas of the neck, axilla and hands, surgical release may be needed to restore full function. Controlled exercise under direction of a physiotherapist is recommended to minimise contracture. Splints are also helpful in the prevention of loss of function, particularly over joints. Swimming is a good form of exercise, once wounds are healed, as it promotes good range of movement.

## EXPOSURE TO SUNSHINE

In the first year or two after a burn injury it is vital to protect a child's skin from the sun's strong rays as the healed skin is highly sensitive to sunlight and will burn very easily. Care of the donor site is the same. Protect the skin with high sun protection cream (sun protection factor 20 or above) and light loose clothing. Pigmentation of skin will eventually return in scar tissue, although perhaps not completely.

## ITCHING

Itching can be a significant and distressing problem after a burn injury. Two contributing factors are dryness through decreased oil production and dilatation of the blood vessels, causing an increased blood flow through the affected area. Unfortunately, there is no single effective cure but antihistamines, for example chlorphenamine (chlorpheniramine) maleate, give symptomatic relief. Regular moisturising, cool clothing and environment, and the wearing of pressure garments all help.

## SKIN INTEGRITY POST HEALING

It is not unusual for small water blisters to appear on grafted skin, previously burned areas or donor sites. This is often caused by friction or by small knocks causing mild trauma. This should cease after a few months following healing. Blisters should be burst using a cotton bud, then antiseptic solution and a small dry dressing can be applied. Skin breakdown may be infection related and, if wound cultures are positive, antibiotics may be required.

## TOXIC SHOCK SYNDROME

This rare but potentially fatal condition that can occur in burn injured patients, even those with the smallest of injuries, is caused by the toxic shock syndrome toxin (TSST) of a strain of *Staphylococcus aureus*. Characteristic manifestations are fever, diarrhoea, vomiting, hypotension and a diffuse erythematous rash. Onset is sudden and treatment consists of prompt antibiotics and fluid resuscitation (Pape et al 2000). A less threatening manifestation is toxin mediated disease (TMD), consisting of fever and rash without hypotension and major system disturbance.

## PSYCHOLOGICAL AND SOCIAL CARE

Burn injury is a traumatic, sudden and painful experience. It may be disfiguring or life threatening. The initial period post injury can often be fraught. The care of a burned child is intensified by the needs of the child's family, who often themselves require considerable support.

To promote psychological wellbeing, health personnel need to have an empathetic non-judgemental approach, and an appreciation of the extreme feelings of guilt parents or carers may have.

Information regarding the child's care should be clear and ongoing. Support should be sought from all necessary sources. Social workers, play thera-

pists, school nurses and psychologists are essential members of the multidisciplinary team on the road to optimal recovery for both the child and family (Hollinworth 1996).

## PLASTIC SURGERY

The term plastic is derived from the Greek word 'plastos' which means to mould. Plastic surgery is used to reconstruct abnormal tissue, due to congenital conditions, disease or trauma. In order to deliver optimal care, it is vital that nursing staff are aware of the fundamentals of plastic surgery nursing.

The aim of the second part of this chapter is to give an overview of the more common forms of plastic surgery, and to outline the important points in the care of children undergoing this surgery.

The most common forms of surgery to be seen on a paediatric plastic surgery ward and which will be discussed in this chapter are:

- Otoplasty (correction of prominent ears)
- Tissue transfer
- Finger-tip injuries
- Tissue expansion
- Cleft lip and palate.

## OTOPLASTY

In our increasingly image conscious world, having prominent ears may be a source of embarrassment for many children. Prominent ears are the most common deformity of the head and neck, with an incidence of 5% in the Caucasian population (Bardach 1986). Some suffer teasing to such an extent that surgery becomes an option. The most common deformities of the ear are:

- poorly developed or absent antihelical fold
- abnormally large concha. (Stucker et al 2003)

A detailed preoperative consultation between the child (where appropriate), parent and surgeon is essential. When preschool children are reviewed in outpatient departments, it is usually the parent's opinion that the child requires surgery. The procedure may, however, be carried out after the age of 4, as the ear growth is almost complete at this stage (Ely 1881).

There are many aspects of surgery that require careful discussion and consideration before the decision to undertake surgery is taken, including possible complications which are:

- Infection
- Haematoma
- Wound dehiscence
- Scarring – possibly hypertrophic or keloid
- Recurrence of the prominence
- Ischaemia over the antihelix
- Asymmetry.

The parents and child are also informed of the need for compliance from the child, to help ensure that the postoperative pressure bandages remain undisturbed until their official removal after approximately 7 days.

Older children may opt for the procedure to be carried out under a local anaesthetic.

## SURGICAL TECHNIQUE

The otoplasty procedure was first described in 1881 and has continued to evolve ever since (Caouette-Laberge et al 2000). The original surgery involved skin excision only, which led to poor long term results.

There are varying techniques currently in use. The most common types are:

- Folding of the cartilage and the insertion of permanent sutures, to preserve the folding
- Scoring of the cartilage on the anterior surface to allow it to fold
- Cartilage excision
- A combination of the above.

Controversy exists, however, as to which technique is superior for primary ear correction. Once the surgery is complete, a non-adherent dressing is placed between the ear and the cranium, and a pressure bandage is carefully applied and securely fixed in place. This will ensure the newly moulded ears stay in an optimal position.

The surgeon takes care not to place undue pressure over the antihelix–conchal cartilage as the skin is particularly thin at this point and is susceptible to ischaemia.

The head bandage must not be disturbed during the postoperative period, unless complications are suspected.

The postoperative nursing care will include:

- Analgesia and antihistamine medication. Itch may be more of a problem if the environment is particularly warm.

- Frequent observation until the child is fully awake and recovered from the anaesthetic, to ensure the bandage remains undisturbed.
- Regular pain assessment, using an appropriate paediatric assessment tool. If the child complains of persistent moderate/severe pain, the possibility of the presence of a haematoma should be explored. The bandages are carefully removed and any obvious haematoma expressed. This may require a general anaesthetic. Severe pain may also be an indication of ischaemia over the newly formed antihelix, due to the bandage having been applied too tightly.

Postoperative nausea and vomiting are a recognised complication of any surgery. It has been reported that patients who undergo the otoplasty procedure are more prone to postoperative nausea and vomiting (Honkavaara & Pyykko 1999). This is due to the stimulation of the auricular branch of the vagus and auriculotemporal nerves, both of which have parasympathetic fibres. This stimulation may induce vomiting (Mansour 1989).

Once the bandage has been removed and the sutures removed or trimmed, depending on the type used, the child and parents are reminded that a head band or bandage must be worn at night, usually for a minimum of 4 weeks. The purpose of this is to ensure the cartilage adopts its new position and does not 'spring' back to the original position. The band is also recommended for sports during this period. Parents are instructed in scar management techniques, which will include twice daily gentle cleansing, moisturising and massaging of the area, with a mild non-perfumed moisturiser.

## TISSUE TRANSFER

The body has an amazing ability to repair itself. When there is a significant tissue loss, however, whereby the body is unable to repair the deficit alone, a method of wound closure will be chosen. One method of selecting the correct surgical procedure is the concept of a reconstructive ladder. This is a systematic approach whereby a technique is chosen, depending on local wound needs and complexity. It begins with the simplest method of direct closure and skin grafts (as discussed previously), progressing to more complex methods of local and distant flaps. A flap is the name given to tissue transferred from one area of the body to another.

The possible conditions that may require such a flap are:

- Traumatic tissue loss, where tissue is torn from the underlying structures and may be devascularised
- Reconstruction of scar tissue
- Congenital deformities e.g. giant naevi (birthmarks)
- Disease
- Tissue deficit due to surgery.

Flaps differ from skin grafts in that they retain a blood supply during the transfer, except for a free flap where the circulation is severed before reattachment to the circulation at the recipient site. Flaps are also more durable than grafts and do not contract in the same manner as split thickness grafts. They are therefore desirable for areas such as the face, where cosmetic results with minimal scars, (which tend to contract) are of particular importance.

Preoperative planning is essential to the success of any flap. The recipient site will require (where possible) tissue that is of similar colour, texture and with similar concentration of hair follicles. It is important to understand the circulation of the flap to be able to give the correct postoperative care, and to recognize potential complications quickly and act accordingly.

Flaps can be categorised into 2 types:

- Random pattern flap
- Axial pattern flap.

## RANDOM PATTERN FLAP

The random pattern flap is so named because it is not based on an anatomically recognized arteriovenous system. In theory, the circulation may be reduced by four-fifths. The random pattern flap is usually named according to the:

- Shape, e.g. bilobed, rhomboid
- Movement, e.g. rotation, advancement, transposition, or
- Both of the above, e.g. Z-plasty, commonly used to release contraction scars.

They may also be named according to their anatomical source, for example a musculocutaneous (muscle and skin) flap may be named a latissimus dorsi or pectoralis major flap. In this type of flap, the arterial supply tends to be more effective than the venous return. One would therefore expect the appearance to be pink, with the skin blanching under pressure. The capillary return is usually similar to the adjacent skin. Complications that occur usually do so with the venous return. Cyanosis becomes evident, starting at the distal margins. There may be increased congestion and an abnormally brisk capillary return may be apparent on the epidermis.

## AXIAL PATTERN FLAPS

The circulation of this type of flap is anatomically recognised. They have a large artery at the pedicle, therefore theoretically should have a more reliable blood supply. The commonly used term 'free flap' is in fact an axial pattern flap as both the artery and vein are identified, but in this case they are divided and tagged early on in the surgery, and re-attached at the recipient site, with the aid of a microscope.

Flaps may consist of varying composites of tissues:

- skin only
- muscle only
- muscle and skin.

## POSTOPERATIVE NURSING CARE

The postoperative nursing care will include observing for the factors that may affect the flap circulation:

- Haematoma. Depending on its size, a haematoma may cause sufficient distension to interrupt the blood supply. An unresolved haematoma may also become a focus for infection.
- Tension. When the vessels are stretched, the lumen of the vessel narrows, disrupting blood supply. This may become evident as a white area in the flap.
- Kinking. This will have a similar effect to tension, but the pallor may become evident more quickly if due simply to an inappropriate change in the child's position.
- Pressure. The blood supply will be interrupted if pressure is placed upon the vessels, e.g. from fixators or due to poor patient positioning.
- Venous thrombosis.

These complications may be resolved by the following measures:

- Careful repositioning of the child may relieve the tension, kinking and pressure on vessels. If the flap fails to respond, the sutures may be removed or if the circulation does not improve, the child may be returned to theatre for surgical intervention.

• The haematoma may be evacuated by gently rolling an appropriately sized piece of gauze from the haematoma site to the nearest flap margin. If this is unsuccessful, the sutures may be removed to aid the removal of the haematoma.

The environmental temperature is monitored, as peripheral blood supply is affected by variances in temperature. An IV infusion of a low molecular weight fluid, e.g. dextran, may be used to improve perfusion of the flap as it increases capillary blood flow and reduces blood viscosity, thereby reducing the risk of venous thrombosis (Lineaweaver et al 1991). Fluid balance is closely monitored to ensure adequate hydration with IV fluids being adjusted accordingly.

If there is an adequate arterial supply, but a problem with the venous drainage, leeches may be used to relieve the congestion. Leeches were first used in Egypt around 1500 BC to treat various conditions ranging from gout to nosebleeds (O'Hara 1991). They were not in favour again until the 1960s when plastic surgeons began advocating their use for the treatment of venous congestion. The most commonly used leech is the Hirudo medicinalis. The leech has suckers at both ends to facilitate attachment whilst feeding. The mouth is on the narrower end. The leech will feed for up to 60 minutes and ingest 5–15 mL of blood (Kocent & Spinner 1992). Its saliva contains 3 substances, which make the leech a suitable treatment for venous congestion:

• a natural local anaesthetic that renders the attachment painless. (Rivera & Gross 1995)
• a vasodilator, which ensures a good flow of blood from the puncture site during feeding
• hirudin, a natural chemical anticoagulant.

The leech, therefore, not only gives almost immediate relief from venous congestion through ingesting blood, but also provides continuing relief through a slow continuous ooze once the leech has detached. It is a relatively safe, effective and economical treatment for a congested flap. Antibiotics are administered to reduce infection risk (Utley et al 1998).

Leech therapy may be used several times in the course of treatment and continues until a collateral venous drainage system is established. Children and their families may, however, find the idea of leech therapy upsetting. Detailed but appropriate explanations are essential for both parents and the child, with time allowed for questions. They are assured that this therapy is a well documented form of treatment. The nursing staff need to be confident in their handling of leeches to ensure minimal emotional reaction to the treatment (Kowalczyk 2002).

The flap may be attached by means of sutures or staples, which are removed after approximately 1 week. If staples are chosen, a return to theatre is considered for their removal, as the procedure may prove too painful for analgesia alone.

Once the flap has established a blood supply, a protective dressing may be applied, depending on the site and age of the child. After discharge, the child is reviewed regularly at the consultant clinic. If the flap is deemed to be overly 'bulky', a surgical procedure such as liposuction may be required to reduce the thickness of the flap, thereby improving the cosmetic appearance. Parents are instructed in skin care and scar management as previously discussed.

## FINGERTIP INJURIES

### EPIDEMIOLOGY

As the fingertip is the most distal part of the hand, it is most susceptible to injury. Fingertip amputations are the most common type of injury seen in the upper limb (Hans et al 1998), and among the most often met cases at a plastic surgery unit (Russell & Casas 1989). The age of the child and the anatomy of the portion of finger affected will directly affect the successful outcome of treatment. The most common mechanism of fingertip injury in children is a closing door or a falling object such as a brick, resulting in a crush type injury and occasionally amputation or incomplete amputation. Guillotine-type amputations are ideally suited to replantation, but are uncommon in children (Michalko & Bentz 2002). The success rate of reimplantation is directly related to an adequate venous outflow. A clean sharp injury will have a better prognosis than the crush or avulsion type (Martin & Gonzalez del Pino 1998).

### TREATMENT

There are a broad range of options to consider in the treatment of fingertip injuries. These range from the conservative approach of secondary wound closure or a simple surgical technique of shortening the bone with wound closure, to more extensive techniques which may involve replantation of the tip. The fingertip may be reconstructed using local or regional flaps (Lister 1993). In some cases, microsurgical tissue transfer is used, in the form of a skin flap (Logan et al 1985, Tsai et al 1989). The treatment option chosen should speed the healing process and minimise the time of functional impairment (Martin & Gonzalez del Pino 1998). An acceptable cosmetic result is also a consideration.

Fingertips, which are amputated distal to the lunula of the nail, maybe suitable for suturing as a composite graft. Vascular anastomosis is not usually necessary, as there is reasonable expectation of a good result (Michalko & Bentz 2002). The ideal result from reconstruction of fingertip injuries is to preserve finger length and restore good sensation with minimal pain.

If the nail has been avulsed, it will, where possible, be replaced, but as a splint only. If the nail is not available, a piece of shaped foil may be used as a replacement. This will maintain a flat surface upon which the new nail may grow. The replaced nail (or foil) will dislodge as the new nail begins to grow, and the sutures that have held it in place are either removed or they absorb (Martin & Gonzalez del Pino 1998). The child and parents are informed that the nail may regrow with a ridge or may be misshapen. Fingernails grow at a rate of 0.1 mm per day. After an injury there is a delay in growth of 21 days. This is followed by an increase in growth for 50 days. Three to four nail growths are needed to observe the maximum improvement.

The postoperative dressing applied to the finger will require careful consideration, regardless of the treatment chosen. A non-adherent primary dressing is essential. There should be sufficient padding to protect the digit from the expected minor trauma in the everyday life of a child. In a very young child, a boxing glove dressing, where the whole hand is enclosed, is preferable. Initial dressing changes may be traumatic, as the child may have clear memories of the accident. Any dealings with the finger may provoke a negative and distressing reaction.

Once the final dressing has been removed, instructions are given in the care of the nail bed area, which includes moisturising as previously discussed.

## TISSUE EXPANSION

When skin is needed to reconstruct a damaged area of the body, the most common method is to use a skin graft or flap. This has the disadvantage of creating further scars and the new skin, in particular skin grafts, may be a poor match for the surrounding area.

Tissue expansion is a method of 'growing' extra skin, which is becoming increasingly popular in reconstructive surgery. It has evolved as a safe and reliable technique in tissue reconstruction (Menard et al 1991). The method has the advantage of providing the surgeon with large flaps of tissue, which is colour, thickness and texture matched. It is particularly suitable for the treatment of areas of alopecia, as the stretched skin will continue to grow hair.

At the time of surgery, a deflated balloon-like implant is placed beneath the skin or muscle. Saline is injected at regular intervals through an injection port, placed at an appropriate site adjacent to the expander. Care is taken at each injection time to ensure the optimal volume is inserted. Pain may indicate kinking of the expander or undue pressure on the overlying tissues, leading to ischaemia. The saline injections continue until there is sufficient tissue to cover the defect. This type of surgery does, however, carry a significant risk of complications. The most common complications following the insertion of an expander are infection, necrosis at the margins and extrusion (Elias et al 1991, Gibstein et al 1997). Prophylactic antibiotics are commonly administered, with the area carefully observed for signs of infection.

Once the surgeon considers that there is sufficient tissue available to reconstruct the deficit, the child is returned to the operating theatre and the expander removed. The abnormal tissue is excised and the newly 'grown' tissue placed over the area and sutured or stapled in place.

## CLEFT LIP AND PALATE

### EPIDEMIOLOGY

Cleft lip and/or palate is a congenital abnormality affecting 1 in 700 children (Sullivan 1996, Sandberg et al 2002). It is more common in boys than in girls (Devlin 1995). The cause is unknown, although it has been reported that heredity may play a part, with siblings of a child with cleftings having a 40% risk (Denk & Magee 1996). Other authors have cited medications, for example phenytoin sodium, and parental age, with an increased incidence where the parents are over 30 years of age (Eliason et al 1991).

Presenting in a number of combinations, cleft lip and palate is due to failure in the fusing process of the lip, palate or mouth in early fetal development (Thompson 1999). Cleft lip can occur with or without cleft palate and is due to failure in the fusion of the lip during the 5th week of embryonic life (Thompson 1999). It ranges from a notch in the lip to a complete cleft which involves the floor of the nose and can be unilateral or bilateral, complete or incomplete (Oxley 2001). Cleft palate may occur with or without cleft lip, and ranges from a bifid uvula to a complete cleft, and may also be unilateral or bilateral. It results from failure of the palatal shelves to fuse during the 7th or 8th week of fetal life (Thompson 1999, Oxley 2001). It should be noted that clefts may be submucosal and may be part of a syndrome, for example Pierre Robin anomaly (see Ch. 9) (Adcock & Marcus 1997). Feeding difficulties and impaired speech development are amongst the long term problems associated with clefting.

## MANAGEMENT

The main aims in the management of cleft lip and palate are:

- Promotion of bonding
- Normal appearance and function in order to improve the child's self image
- Normal feeding
- Normal speech
- Normal hearing

Parents of a child born with cleft lip and palate may be very distressed and feelings of guilt, inadequacy, shame and resentfulness are not uncommon. These feelings may affect the bonding process (Sandberg et al 2002). Unless the condition has been diagnosed before birth, giving the parents time to adjust and make plans, they may also experience grief for the normal baby they were expecting to be born. Therefore any preoperative care must include the ongoing support of the parents by the multidisciplinary team, which includes the surgeon, the dentist, the orthodontist, speech and feeding specialist and specialist nurses amongst others. Surgery may take place during the neonatal period (Sandberg et al 2002) or, more usually, the lip is repaired between 6 and 12 weeks of age and the palate by the age of 12–18 months (Clinical Standards Advisory Group 1998, The Cleft Lip and Palate Association 2004).

## PREOPERATIVE CARE

During the preoperative period airway and feeding issues are addressed. Where the infant has a cleft lip without cleft palate, or with a small and narrow cleft palate, breast feeding may be attempted (Thompson 1999). However, if the infant is unable to suckle prior to surgery, breast milk may be expressed and the infant fed by another method. A number of feeding devices are available for feeding formula or expressed breast milk and the parents are best referred to a feeding specialist for expert advice.

Otherwise, general preoperative care as described in Chapter 1 is required. The infant may be fed up to 4 hours prior to surgery.

## POSTOPERATIVE CARE

The principles of postoperative care in cleft lip and palate repair are:

- Maintenance of the airway
- Early detection of haemorrhage and shock
- Management of pain
- Protection of the operation site.

The lip and palate are very vascular, and the suture line should be observed and any swallowing actions which may indicate blood swallowing noted. Pressure and ice compresses to the suture line will usually reduce bleeding (Sandberg et al 2002). Pain may be managed by both pharmacological and non-pharmacological methods, such as comfort from the parents (see Ch. 6). The infant may be fed following surgery and this will help to promote the bonding process between parent and child. The suture line may be gently cleansed after feeding, using sterile saline solution.

The traditional use of splinting following surgical repair, as a method of protecting the suture line, is controversial (Oxley 2001). O'Riain (1977) suggested that the use of splints may be unnecessary and that babies were more comfortable without them. Furthermore, the question of the psychological care of the child and family needs to be considered and the use of splints or restraints may be distressing to both. In cleft lip repair, reduction of strain to the suture line is crucial and the elimination of splints and early discharge may reduce the damage caused by crying (Oxley 2001). Whilst healing takes place over several months, the child is normally discharged 2 or 3 days after surgery.

Corrective surgery of the original repair may be required for complete clefts of lip and palate as the child grows. This may include pharyngoplasty for speech improvement (Devlin 1995) and bone grafting to correct misalignment of the top jaw (CSAG 1998). Further surgery may continue into the teenage years and adulthood as required (Oxley 2001).

There are a number of agencies that inform, support and advise the parents of children with cleft lip and/or palate and searching the internet may be a bewildering experience for them. The cleft lip and palate association (CLAPA) can be found at: http://www.clapa.com/question-treatment.html

ration between the families and the multidisciplinary team is imperative to the long term success of the surgery. Preoperative preparation is essential to assess previous treatment experiences. The child may already have had many hospital admissions and may have to endure further years of surgery and procedures. Each admission is carefully planned and evaluated. The play specialist will play an important role in preparing the child through play.

The child and parents are kept well informed of the care plan and treatment at each stage. Families are given a clear forecast of the outcome of the surgery, ensuring that expectations are realistic.

## CONCLUSION

The care of children undergoing plastic surgery is both challenging and rewarding. Effective collabo-

## References

Adcock S, Marcus AF 1997 Mid-facial growth following functional cleft surgery. British Journal of Oral and Maxillofacial Surgery 35: 1–5

Arturson G 1996 Mechanism of injury. In: Settle JA (ed) Principles and practice of burns management. Churchill Livingstone, Edinburgh

Bardach J 1986 Surgery of congenital and acquired malformation of the auricle. In: Cummings CW, Fredrickson JM, Harker LA et al (eds) Otolaryngology: head and neck surgery. Mosby, St Louis, p 2861

Bosworth C 1997 Burns trauma. Baillière Tindall, London

British Burn Association 1996 Emergency management of severe Burns (EMSB) Course Manual, UK version. The Education Committee of The Australian and New Zealand Burn Association

Burr S 1993 Myths in practice. Nursing Standard 7(25): 4

Caouette-Laberge L, Guay N, Bortoluzzi P et al 2000 Sc.N. Otoplasty: anterior scoring technique and results in 500 cases. Plast Reconstr Surg 105(2): 504–515

Child Accident Prevention Trust 1991 Burns and scalds. CAPT, Milton Keynes

Childs C 1994 Studies in children provide a model to reexamine the metabolic response of burn injuries in patients treated by contemporary burn protocols. Burns 20: 291–300

Childs C 1995 Feeding the burned patient: energy requirements, timing and effects of dietary intake. British Journal of Intensive Care May: 157–161

Clinical Standards Advisory Group (CSAG) 1998 Services for children with cleft lip and palate. A summary by CSAG of its report on standards of clinical care for people with cleft lip and/or palate. CSAG Secretariat, London

Cowell L 1995 Care after burns injury. The Journal of Wound Care Nursing 7(5):

Cunningham J et al 1990 Calorie and protein provision for recovery from severe burns in infants and young children. American Journal of Clinical Nutrition 51: 553–557

Denk MJ, Magee MP 1996 Cleft palate closure in the neonate: preliminary report. The Cleft–Palate Craniofacial Journal 33: 57–61

Devlin HB (ed) 1995 The treatment of cleft lip and palate: a parents' guide. The Royal College of Surgeons of England/Cleft Lip and Palate Association, London

Driscoll P 1993 Trauma resuscitation. The team approach. MacMillan, Basingstoke

Elias DL, Baird WL, Zubowicz VN 1991 Applications and complications of tissue expansion in pediatric patients. Journal of Pediatric Surgery 26(15):

Eliason MJ, Hardin MA, Olin WH 1991 factors that influence ratings of facial appearance for children with cleft lip and palate. The Cleft-Palate Craniofacial Journal 28: 190–194

Ely ET 1881 An operation for prominence of the auricles. Arch Ophthalmol Otol 10: 97

Flanagan M 1999 The physiology of wound healing. In: Miller M, Glover D (eds) Wound management: theory and practice. Nursing Times Books, London

Gibstein LA, Abramson DL, Bartlett RA et al 1997 Tissue expansion in children: a retrospective study of complications. Annals of Plastic Surgery 38: 358

Han SK, Lee BI, KimWK 1998 The reverse digital artery island flap: clinical experience in 120 fingers. Plast Reconstr Surg 101: 1006

Hollinworth H 1996 Teamwork in burn care. Nursing Times in conjunction with Wound Care Society 8: 1

Honkavaara P, Pyykko I 1999 Effects of atropine and scopolamine on bradycardia and emetic symptoms in otoplasty. Laryngoscope 109(1): 108–112

Jackson D 1953 The diagnosis of the depth of burning. British Journal of Surgery 40: 588–596

Judkins K 1996 Burns management. In: Settle JAD (ed) Principles and practice of burns management. Churchill Livingstone, Edinburgh

Kemble JVH, Lamb BE 1987 Practical burns management. Hodder and Stoughton, London

Kocent LC, Spinner SS 1992 Leech therapy: new procedures for old treatment. Pediatric Nursing 18(5): 481

Kowalczyk T 2002 A low-tech approach to venous congestion 65(10): 26–31

Laitung G 1996 Metabolic responses and requirements. In: Settle JAD (ed) Principles and practice of burns management. Churchill Livingstone, Edinburgh

Lawrence J 1996 Burns and scalds: aetiology and prevention. In: Settle JAD (ed) Principles and practice of burns management. Churchill Livingstone, Edinburgh

Lawson RA 1998 Opioid techniques. In: Morton NS (ed) Acute paediatric pain management a practical guide. WB Saunders, London

Lineaweaver WC et al 1991 Clinical leech use in a microsurgical unit: the San Francisco experience. Blood Coagulation and Fibrinolysis 2 February: 189–192

Lister G 1993 The hand diagnosis and indications, 3rd edn. Churchill Livingston, Edinburgh, p 121–183

Logan A, Elliot D, Foucher G 1985 Free toe pulp transfer to restore traumatic digital pulp loss. British Journal of Plastic Surgery 38: 497

Mansour NY 1989 Auriculo-emetic reflex? Anaesthesia 44: 934

Marsden A 1996 Accident department. In: Settle JAD (ed) Principles and practice of burns management. Churchill Livingstone, Edinburgh

Martin C, Gonzalez del Pino JM 1998 Controversies in the treatment of fingertip amputations: conservative versus surgical reconstruction. Clin Orthop 353: 63–73

Menard RM, Moore Mark HF, David J 1999 Tissue expansion in the reconstruction of Tessier craniofacial clefts: a series of 17 patients. Plast Reconstr Sur, 103(3): 779–786

Michalko KB, Bentz ML 2002 Digital replantation in children. C0[-=Care Med, 30(11)

Miller Gilchrist 1997 Understanding wound cleaning and infection. 'Understanding' series. Professional Nurse emap Healthcare London.

Muir IFK, 1987 Burns and their treatment, 3rd edn, Butterworth, London

National Burn Care Review Committee 2001 Standards and strategy for burn care, a review of burn care in the British Isles. Committee Report.

O'Hara MM 1991 Beauty and the beast: nursing care of the patient undergoing leech therapy. Plastic Surgery Nursing 11: 101–104

O'Riain S 1977 Cleft lip surgery without post-operative restraints. British Journal of Plastic Surgery 30: 140–141

Orr J (1997) Thermal injuries in children – nursing and related care: Journal of Child Health Care 1(2): 68–72

Oxley J 2001 Are arm splints required following cleft lip/palate repair? Paediatric Nursing 13(1): 27–30

Pape SA, Judkins K, Settle JAD 2000 Burns: the first five days, 2nd edn. Smith and Nephew

Reid C 1996 Paediatric burns. In: Settle JAD (ed) Principles and practice of burns management. Churchill Livingstone, Edinburgh

Rivera ML, Gross JE 1995 Scalp replantation after traumatic injury. AORN Journal 62(2): 175

Russel RC, Casas LA 1989 Management of finger tip injuries. Clin Plast Surg 16:405

Sandberg DJ, Magee WP, Denk MJ 2002 Neonatal cleft lip and palate repair. AORN Journal 75(3): 488, 490–499, 501, 503–504, 506–508

Settle JAD (ed) 1996 Principles and practice of burns management. Churchill Livingstone, Edinburgh

Stucker FJ, Vora NM, Lian TS 2003 Otoplasty: an analysis of technique over a 33-year period. Laryngoscope 113(6): 952–956

Sullivan 1996

The Cleft Lip and Palate Association 2004 http://www.clapa.cpm/question-treatment.html

Thibodeau G, Patton K 1993 Anatomy and physiology, 2nd edn. Mosby, St Louis

Thompson J 1999 Cleft lip and palate. Community Practitioner 72(10): 334–335

Tsai TM, McCabe SJ, Maki Y 1989 A technique of the fingertip. Microsurgery 10: 1

Utley D, Koch RJ, Goodie RL 1998 The failing flap in facial plastic and reconstructive surgery: role of the medical leech. Laryngoscope 108(8)(Part 1): 1129–1135

Wallace E 1994 Feeding the wound: nutrition and wound care. British Journal of Nursing 3: 662

Waldrop J, Doughty D 2000 Wound-healing physiology. In: Bryant RA (ed) Acute and chronic wounds: nursing management, 2nd edn. Mosby, St Louis

Westaby S 1985 Wound care. Heinemann, London

Wilson R 2000 Massive tissue loss: burns. In: Bryant RA (ed) Acute and chronic wounds: nursing management, 2nd edn. Mosby, St Louis

Wysocki A 2000 Anatomy and physiology of skin and soft tissue. In: Bryant RA (ed) Acute and chronic wounds: nursing management, 2nd edn. Mosby, St Louis

# Chapter 17

# Care of the child undergoing ophthalmic surgery

## Jilly Bradshaw

## INTRODUCTION

In 1953 Dr John Bowlby published *Child Care and the Growth of Love* (Bowlby 1953). This unique book, seen as a pivotal milestone in child psychology, explained how and why children thrive and examined their emotional needs. It identified the vital importance of maternal presence and love to the growing child, especially in the first years of life. Subsequent nursing and medical research and further legislation, namely the Children Act (Department of Health 1989), *The Patients' Charter* (Department of Health 1996) and recently the NHS Service Framework (Department of Health 2003), have striven to improve the rights and care of children in hospital.

All children require all their complex needs to be met with understanding and love. This is especially important in times of stress, such as coming into hospital. The strength and wellbeing of any family unit depends on the welfare of all its members – each parent, siblings, extended family and other significant carers. Paediatric nurses therefore need to be aware of this and extend their remit of caring to all the family. Parents know their own child best, and are indispensable to that child. The nurse can complement this role, as 'an expert, not the expert' as Nethercott (1993) states. Parents' observations of their child's state of health should always be taken seriously; parents can sense very subtle shifts in their child's behaviour and appearance, which may well not be apparent to others, including health professionals. Children should be consulted about their health, treatment and care, within the limits of their understanding, in a respectful, rights-led approach (Charles-Edwards 2003). It is important that the holistic care of the child is discussed and negotiated directly with the child and family, in an open and honest way, if truly family-centred care is to be achieved.

## KEY DIFFERENCES

Paediatric ophthalmology differs from other paediatric specialities and these differences must be taken into account by the paediatric nurse:

- The child's eyes are still growing.
- The child's visual system is immature and still developing up to the age of 8 years.
- Any ocular disorder may impact on the developing eye and visual system.
- The child may have a systemic condition that involves an ocular disorder.

The nurse should also bear in mind the following important points, many of which relate to the psychological fears of children and their parents – indeed, parents can often be more concerned about the proposed surgery and treatment than their children.

- Vision is our perceived main faculty.
- Most people, if asked, would say that they 'live' in their eyes; it is therefore harder to tolerate or distance oneself from pain or discomfort in the eyes.
- Many people feel very squeamish about eyes.
- The cosmetic appearance of the eyes is particularly important to the overall look of the child; eyes convey emotion and expression and contribute much to the dynamic appearance of the face.
- Parents frequently become emotional and even tearful when discussing eye surgery, and will voice real concerns about subjecting their child to such a delicate operation.
- If the child has a squint or a cyst on the eyelid, for example, they often receive negative comments and criticism from passers-by, friends, or even members of their own families. Children whatever their age may be teased, sometimes severely, by other children – even at preschool. This may make the child unhappy, withdrawn or aggressive. Sometimes children become so self-conscious that they will literally hang their heads.

- There are fears about the surgery itself, for example, will there be a successful visual and cosmetic outcome? Many people think that the eye will need to be removed during surgery and are terrified at this prospect.
- Some parents may have irrational fears about ophthalmic surgery, perhaps relating to macabre films that they have seen in the past. It may be hard for them to rid their minds of these images when their own child is to have an operation.
- Some parents express fears about an operation on such a small structure as the eye, especially since it is so close to the brain.
- Fears may be expressed about having the operation on the wrong eye.
- There may also be anxieties regarding the interruption of the child's vision postoperatively, and how this will have a bearing on the child's mobility and safety.
- Parents of a child whose vision may not be improved or regained, or may indeed be lost, may have deep-seated fears about how they and their child will cope.
- There is often a strong family history of squints and parents and indeed grandparents may have had treatment or surgery on their eyes as children themselves and express unpleasant memories of the experience.

It is therefore vital for the nurse to care for the child patient and the whole family in a sensitive and understanding way. It is easy for clinical staff to feel that elective eye surgery is rather routine and minor, but for the families concerned the opposite is true.

## ANATOMY AND PHYSIOLOGY OF THE NORMAL EYE (see Fig. 17.1)

The human eye is a highly specialised sense organ. The structures within the eye must be clear and correctly aligned for light to travel through the eye. The eye is positioned in the bony orbit, cushioned by fat. Further protection is offered by eyebrows, eyelids and the blink reflex. Six fine extraocular muscles coordinate eye movements with the sclera forming the tough outer layer of the eyeball. The sensitive cornea is the 'window' into the eye that forms part of the anterior surface of the eye and the conjunctiva is a membrane that lines part of the eyeball and the eyelids. Behind the cornea is the anterior chamber that contains clear aqueous fluid while the posterior segment contains a vitreous jelly-like substance that helps maintain the shape of the eye. The intraocular pressure is kept within physiological limits and balanced by the constant production of aqueous fluid by the ciliary processes and an intricate drainage system. The iris is the structure that gives individuals their eye colour, and adjusts the amount of light entering the eye. The central area of the iris is a hole that appears black when viewed from the front, known as the pupil.

In a normal eye, light entering the eye is focused by the cornea and the lens onto the highly sensitive retina. This in turn transmits the two images, one from each eye, to the brain via the optic nerve, which interprets the two received images into one clear image.

## COMMON CONDITIONS IN CHILDREN REQUIRING SURGERY

### CATARACT

The normal lens of the eye is made of water and protein and is transparent. The biconvex lens trans-mits and refracts light rays on to the retina. An opacity of the lens is known as cataract (see Fig. 17.2). It stops light entering the eye and therefore diminishes vision. A cataract is usually defined by its location, size and density, and may occur in one or both eyes (Stollery 1997).

### Incidence

A study in the USA showed an incidence of 1.2–6.0 cases per 10 000 births (Lambert & Drack 1996). Both sexes are equally affected. Cataract may be a congenital or acquired condition. Infantile cataracts continue to be one of the most common causes of blindness in developing countries, but are less common in developed countries.

### Causes

- Abnormal fetal development of the eye
- A remnant of hyaloid membrane left from fetal life can be associated with a posterior pole cataract
- Malnutrition during the first trimester of pregnancy
- Intrauterine infection such as rubella syndrome

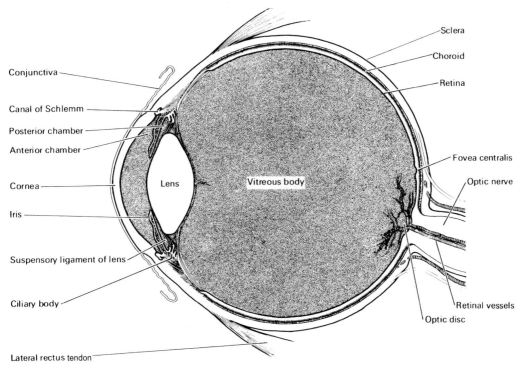

Figure 17.1 Normal anatomy of the eye.

- An inborn error of metabolism such as galactosaemia
- It is associated with Down's syndrome and other chromosomal abnormalities and syndromes.
- Following infection such as varicella, herpes simplex or cytomegalovirus
- Treatment with steroids
- Associated with retinopathy of prematurity
- Following trauma or electric shock or exposure to radiation

(Lambert & Drack 1996)

## Presentation

If the cataract is unilateral, or if bilateral cataracts are small, the baby may appear to see adequately. However, a white or cloudy pupil may be noticed by parents, friends or relatives or on a routine examination with a healthcare professional. The infant may exhibit nystagmus or photophobia or a squint may develop.

## Diagnosis

A careful and full history of the pregnancy and birth is taken and the infant undergoes a thorough examination of the eyes. The cause of a white pupil must be diagnosed as soon as possible, to differentiate it from other serious conditions. A paediatric assessment will be sought, especially if the cataract appears to be part of a systemic condition, and this will include blood tests for infection and antibody titres. A B-scan (ultrasound scan) gives a two-dimensional view of the eye and may be necessary because the fundus of the eye cannot be seen through an opaque lens. The scan is performed to identify any other ocular abnormality – for example,

a retinal detachment or retinoblastoma, a highly malignant tumour of early childhood.

## Management

It is important that cataracts, if visually significant, are removed as soon as possible to prevent amblyopia developing in the affected eye. This is a condition whereby visual acuity is reduced, due to sensory deprivation. The child's age and clinical status are fully assessed before planning surgery.

## Aim of surgery

The aim of surgery is to successfully remove the cataract. Early surgery and optical correction for infants have improved the outcome of this condition.

## Surgery

The operation consists of aspirating the lens, as it has a soft consistency in children under 15 years of age. If there are bilateral cataracts, two sequential operations are carried out to reduce the risk of bilateral infection (endophthalmitis) occurring simultaneously. An intraocular lens may be inserted at this time or during a second procedure.

## Complications

- Haemorrhage
- Astigmatism (uneven curvature of the cornea)
- Glaucoma
- Hyphaema (a bleed into the anterior chamber)
- Endophthalmitis.

Postoperative complications are more frequent in infantile cataract than in adult (glaucoma is very common following cataract surgery in neonates), and may not develop until years later.

## Follow-up

Aphakia exists following cataract removal, and is the term used to denote the absence of the lens. The eye needs a lens and this can be provided in one of two ways:

- Contact lenses. These can be used in babies and children, and give a full field of vision. However, problems include intolerance of the lenses, infection, poor compliance and loss of the lenses.
- Intraocular lenses. These are increasingly used for children, either as a primary procedure or secondary at a later date. Problems include uveitis

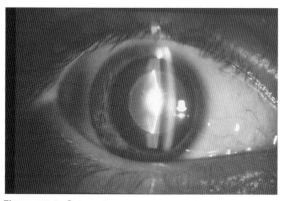

Figure 17.2  Cataract.

(inflammation of the uveal tract), glaucoma and dislocation of the lens (Stollery 1997).

Following cataract surgery children need long term ophthalmic follow-up. Visual impairment varies, depending on the size and type of cataract, the presence of other ocular abnormalities and the age optical correction began. The vision in both eyes needs to be closely monitored, and treatment given as required. Better vision may be obtained in infants with two affected eyes, than in infants with a unilateral cataract, where the visual outcome may be poor (Lambert & Drack 1996).

Nurses should teach parents about contact lens hygiene and insertion. Families whose children have any form of visual impairment need ongoing help and support from a variety of healthcare agencies. Genetic counselling may be offered to the family and the child may be registered as blind or partially sighted as appropriate. This varies from country to country.

# GLAUCOMA

During intrauterine life, the anterior chamber of the eye is filled with membranous tissue. Where there is a defect or blockage of the drainage angle by this tissue, or rarely, an absent canal of Schlemm, the intraocular pressure is increased, causing congenital glaucoma. This may adversely affect the optic disc and reduce visual fields and visual acuity.

## Incidence

This is a rare condition, occurring in approximately 1 in 10 000 births, with more boys than girls being affected (Stollery 1997). Approximately half of all cases are genetic in origin, and the condition is more common in third world countries.

## Causes

Glaucoma in childhood is usually due to anterior segment dysgenesis and although it may exist at birth, it may not present until later. It may be an isolated ocular condition or associated with rubella syndrome, aniridia, Sturge-Weber syndrome and other ocular or systemic developmental anomalies.

## Presentation

The symptoms can vary in severity. Raised intraocular pressure can occur rapidly in some cases, causing severe pain, with a restless, crying baby. Epiphoria (watery eye) and photophobia are often present. The cornea will appear hazy, with thin, bluish sclera and the baby's eyeball may look enlarged, due to stretching of the cornea and sclera, sometimes termed buphthalmos – Greek for 'ox eye'. Unilateral glaucoma usually presents earlier, as the difference in corneal size is more apparent (see Fig. 17.3).

## Diagnosis

Early detection is vital in order to limit permanent damage to the visual system. A full history of the pregnancy and birth is taken and a paediatric assessment may be sought, to eliminate systemic illness. The baby will undergo a thorough optical assessment. The normal pressure of the eye is 10–20 mmHg. This may be raised to 45 mmHg or higher. The corneal diameter is measured and the anterior chamber viewed via a gonioscope if possible.

## Management

Diagnostic tests are performed at intervals to assess progress. Initially medical treatment is used for glaucoma but patients usually require surgical intervention. If the condition is unilateral, occlusion therapy may be required to prevent amblyopia in the unaffected eye.

## Aims of surgery

Surgery aims to reduce intraocular pressure.

## Surgery

A goniotomy, an operation to open up the drainage channels in the eye, is performed under general anaesthetic. A repeat procedure may be needed in the future. A trabeculectomy, a drainage operation, may be performed if the canal of Schlemm is absent or the intraocular pressure remains high. Corneal grafting may also be needed at a later date (Phillips et al 1994).

## Complications

- Hyphaema (a bleed into the anterior chamber)
- Cataract formation
- There may be under- or overcorrection of the drainage system

## Follow-up

Prognosis depends upon the severity of the condition and at what age the child was diagnosed.

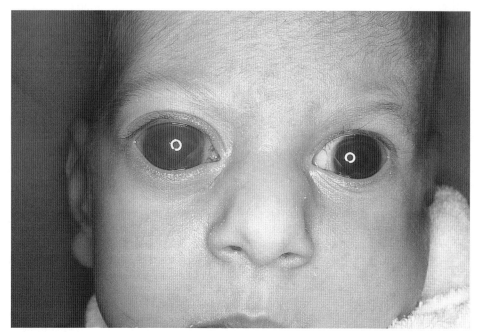

**Figure 17.3** Glaucoma/buphthalmos.

Visual impairment can be severe and the family needs long term help from social services regarding toys, books, nursery and school provision. The parents may be eligible to receive financial assistance, e.g. carer's allowance. In the UK the Royal National Institute for the Blind (RNIB) offers a wide variety of advice and practical help to families. Ongoing emotional support to the whole family is obviously necessary.

## SQUINT (STRABISMUS)

Strabismus, a common condition in early childhood, is where the eyes do not work properly together. Normal vision using both eyes correctly is termed binocular vision, and includes the ability to perceive depth of vision. Binocular vision begins to develop before the age of 1 year. If a squint is present, the brain receives two different messages, but will only recognise the stronger image and will suppress the other. Visual acuity in this eye is then reduced, a condition known as amblyopia or 'lazy eye', present in many children with strabismus.

### Incidence

The condition occurs in approximately 5% of the population (Ryder 2006). A positive family history is common and both sexes are equally affected.

### Causes

Three pairs of extraocular muscles are attached to the eyeball and enable the eye to move within the eye orbit; these are coordinated by the brain via the cranial nerves III, IV and VI (see Fig. 17.4). Strabismus is commonly due to an abnormality of nerve or muscle, a refractive error or a central neurological cause. It is also associated with Down syndrome, cerebral palsy, trauma to the eye, cataract, intracranial tumours, glaucoma and hydrocephalus.

### Presentation

A squint may be noticed by a parent or relative, or a health professional during a routine check. The

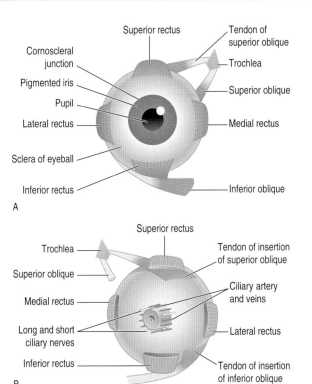

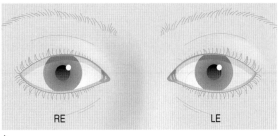

A

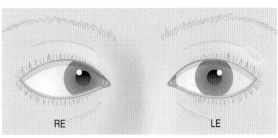

B

**Figure 17.5** Corneal Reflections (A) Symmetrical corneal reflections-no squint present. (B) Asymmetrical corneal reflections-squint present

**Figure 17.4** (A) The extraocular muscles: anterior. (B) The extraocular muscles: posterior.

squint may be continuous or intermittent, convergent or divergent, with an upward or downward deviation, manifest or latent (Fig. 17.5). The child should then be referred to an ophthalmologist for a full visual assessment.

## Diagnosis

A careful family history is taken and a full clinical assessment made of the visual system. This includes examining the eyes, noting 'visual attentiveness', ocular movements and head posture. Visual acuity is measured, although this is not always easy in the pre-school child. A cover test, in which each eye is covered in turn and any movement in the uncovered eye is noted, is carried out in conjunction with testing the corneal light reflex (asymmetrical in children with squints) to determine the presence of strabismus. A cycloplegic refraction test will be performed to disclose any refractive error, i.e. long or short sight or astigmatism.

## Management

The aim is to achieve binocular vision and prevent or reverse amblyopia, using corrective glasses if

there is a refractive error. Occlusion therapy may also be needed to improve the vision of the amblyopic eye. These measures should be underway to improve vision before surgical intervention.

## Aims of surgery

The aims of surgery are to create normal alignment of the eye, to try to achieve binocular vision (which may not recover once lost) and to improve the cosmetic appearance of the child.

## Surgery

This is the most common ophthalmic operation performed on children (Mills 1998). One or more pairs of muscles in one or both eyes are resected (shortened) and recessed (placed further back on the eye to weaken the effect of the muscle). This may be done in stages over a period of time.

## Complications

● Postoperative nausea and vomiting
● Infection

- A slipped muscle from the operation site requiring immediate surgical intervention
- Double vision (diplopia), which normally passes within 48 hours
- Over- or undercorrections of the squint
- Severe loss of vision caused by a retinal perforation or detachment (rare).

## Follow-up

The child will be seen regularly in the orthoptic clinic and by the consultant over several years as necessary. The need for further surgery is common.

## THE LACRIMAL SYSTEM: OBSTRUCTION OF THE DUCTS

Tears are produced by the lacrimal gland, which lies in the upper lateral part of the orbit. Tears are produced constantly, providing about 1 ml./24 hours, except in neonates when tears are minimal.

Tears have various actions – lubrication, provision of a smooth corneal surface, cleansing and prevention of infection by the enzyme lysozyme. Tears flow across the eye and are spread by blinking. They then flow via the two puncta to the lacrimal sac and on down the nasolacrimal duct into the nose (see Fig. 17.6).

## Incidence

It occurs in both sexes and up to 6% of infants are affected (Olitsky & Nelson 1998).

## Causes

Congenital nasolacrimal obstruction commonly presents within the first year of life, and is usually due to failure of complete canalisation of the most distal end of the lacrimal drainage system. This may be due to the presence of a membrane, or in rare cases the puncta or part of the system may be absent.

## Presentation

There is a common story of a constant, watery, sticky eye since birth with one or both eyes affected, becoming worse when the child gets a cold. Frequent apparent eye infections, which clear briefly with antibiotic eye drops but which return quickly, are due to reflux of material from the stagnant lacrimal sac. Parents and infant often feel weary with the very frequent cleaning of the eye(s) and the skin beneath the eye can quickly become red and sore.

## Diagnosis

Diagnosis is made on the history and clinical examination.

## Management

Parents are instructed to massage the lacrimal sac area and clean the eye carefully with sterile gauze and boiled, cooled water. This is accompanied by a 'wait-and-see policy' as normal growth during the first year of life may improve the condition. Surgical intervention is considered if the symptoms persist beyond the first year of life.

## Aim of surgery

Surgery aims to assess the lacrimal system and overcome any blockage, thereby alleviating symptoms.

## Surgery

A fine probe is passed via the lower or upper punctum into the nasolacrimal duct, and fluorescein or sterile water is then syringed through to assess patency. This is done under a general anaesthetic.

If the first operation is unsuccessful, further procedures may be carried out. If the obstruction cannot be overcome, an operation called a dacryocystorhinostomy may be performed to create a new channel from the sac into the nose.

## Follow-up

The child may attend as an outpatient so the condition can be monitored, as directed by the ophthalmologist.

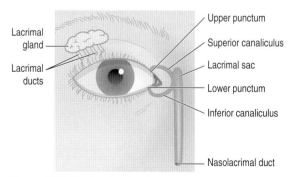

Upper punctum
Lacrimal gland
Superior canaliculus
Lacrimal ducts
Lacrimal sac
Lower punctum
Inferior canaliculus
Nasolacrimal duct

Figure 17.6 The lacrimal system.

## MEIBOMIAN CYST

A meibomian cyst (or chalazion) is a cystic swelling of one or more of the 20–30 meibomian glands that lie in the eyelid and produce the oil layer on the tear film which prevents evaporation of tears. The ducts open just behind the eyelashes and may become blocked by sebaceous secretions (see Fig. 17.7).

### Incidence

The cyst may develop at any time during childhood. Recurrent cysts may be associated with another problem, for example blepharitis, inflammation of the lid margin or a skin disorder.

### Presentation

There is an obvious pink or red swelling at any point on or inside the upper or lower lids. The cyst can fluctuate in size and disappear and reappear. The swelling may become infected, commonly with *Staphylococcus*. The cyst may be sore and irritating, which encourages the child to rub the eye making it more painful. Unfortunately, the child is commonly the victim of teasing.

### Diagnosis

Diagnosis is made on clinical examination.

### Management

The parent is shown how to clean the eye effectively using cooled, boiled water, sterile gauze and careful hand-washing techniques. The parent may be advised to apply a warm flannel to the area to reduce swelling and ease discomfort. Antibiotic cream is prescribed followed by a 'wait-and-see' policy, as some cysts will resolve on their own. Surgery is indicated if lesions are obstructing vision, discomfort is great or continual teasing is experienced.

### Aim of surgery

The aim of surgery is to remove the cyst(s).

### Surgery

A simple procedure of incision and curettage is performed under general anaesthetic. Larger lesions may require suturing.

### Complications

- Infection
- Cysts may return at any time.

### Follow-up

Clinic appointments are attend as directed by the surgeon.

## THE NURSING CARE OF CHILDREN UNDERGOING OPHTHALMIC SURGERY

### PRE-ADMISSION ASSESSMENTS

Children and their families must be prepared effectively for admission to hospital.

Children need to be cared for in a specially designated, safe area, away from adult patients, on a children's ward. The ward should be bright, colourful and as homely as possible. Toys and games should be plentiful, varied and suitable for all age groups. This is in accordance with all recent legislation for children and helps minimise the inevitable stress of coming into hospital. It has long been recognised that children should be cared for by specially trained children's nurses who promote child focused, family-centred care (Department of Health 1991, Thornes 1991).

Many children undergoing elective eye surgery do so as day cases and they should receive the same high standard of care as any paediatric inpatient (Dearmun 1994). So, whatever their age, all children and their families need a pre-admission assessment visit or a visit to a pre-admission club run by some children's units, with children's nurses, to prepare them for the admission. Effective pre-admission assessments should not merely be a swift filling in

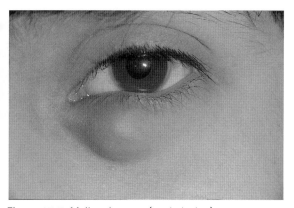

**Figure 17.7** Meibomian cyst (or chalazion).

of a nursing plan, but a real opportunity to exchange information, promote health and start building a trusting relationship with the family (Kelly & Adkins 2003).

On arrival at the unit, the child should be greeted by name, the family allowed to settle in and the child encouraged to start playing. Drinks may be offered. The atmosphere should be calm and cheerful to help the family feel at ease.

Significantly, according to Beringer (1991), parents believe that nurses provide them with the best preoperative information and, as shown by Caress (2003), it is important to discuss everything in detail, tailored to individual needs, and provide written information for families to refer to at home. An information sheet for parents, such as that in Figure 17.8, is very useful. It is important to ensure that a parent/main carer attends with the child, rather than a distant relative or friend, in order that accurate details are obtained and to achieve effective communication throughout the admission period. The nurse should advise the family that they may like to share the information provided with other significant adults who regularly care for the child so all plans go smoothly in the perioperative period. Throughout the visit, plenty of time should be allowed for questions from the child and family members. An interpreter may be needed if the family speak/understand limited English and information leaflets should be available in languages appropriate for the client group.

An appropriate medical and social history of the child should be obtained, including likes and dislikes, normal diet and daily routine. The day's events are discussed in detail, including the surgical procedure, the methods of anaesthesia and the parental role during the day, especially when the child is being anaesthetised – a very stressful time for parents. Plenty of time is needed for this and the nurse should be aware of how much information each family actually wants at each stage. Important points may need to be repeated several times and drawings can be done as necessary, for example to explain anatomy. Parents may well become emotional and need patience and reassurance from the nurse. They may also voice various concerns and bad experiences of their own or of other family members. The nurse needs to be tactful and sensitive in handling these issues. Care must be taken not to allow young children to overhear conversation that may frighten them, as most children will react negatively if they see a parent upset or crying. If the children do react in this way, a simple explanation can be given and distraction with toys will usually help to settle them again.

The following points should be discussed with parents, teenagers, and other children as appropriate:

- Preoperative fasting and how best to manage this at home. A minimal starvation period for children decreases the likelihood of postoperative dehydration and hypoglycaemia, which itself seems to make them feel nauseated (see Ch. 1). Parents can be very anxious about this, but if the child is given plenty to eat and drink the evening before admission and woken at the correct time in the morning for a last drink before being assigned 'nil by mouth', problems need not arise. However, parents should be advised to have breakfast or at least a drink themselves before travelling to hospital.

- Methods of anaesthetising the child. This is either via a gas induction using a face mask or using intravenous medication, following application of local anaesthetic cream to veins on the hands and cannulation. One parent may accompany the child into the anaesthetic room. Parents should be told how this anaesthetic process is carried out, and how they may best support their child, with the nurse's help. It is also helpful to tell them how the child is likely to respond to the procedure. For children who suck their thumb or fingers, it is beneficial to leave the appropriate hand free. The child's own 'snuggly' blanket and teddy will also be a comfort.

- The need to talk to the child at home about the forthcoming admission. Depending on the character of the child, this may be discussed a day or two prior to the operation or before then. Children's questions should be answered truthfully, whilst acknowledging their worries or concerns. Parents should be advised, again, to be careful of voicing their own concerns at home in a way that may be misinterpreted by the child, who may be frightened or confused by what is heard.

- Behaviour management throughout the operative period. The stress of a hospital admission is known to cause behavioural change in some children and parents need to be made aware of this. Parents should plan to have a few quiet days at home following surgery, to normalise life effectively and quickly (see 'Advice on care of the child at home' below).

## PAEDIATRIC CARE INFORMATION FOR PARENTS AT PRE-ASSESSMENT

| A. Things to bring in for admission | B. Reminders |
|---|---|
| Dressing gown | Bath and hairwash night before operation |
| Slippers/non slip sox | No nail varnish on finger or toe nails |
| Favourite teddy, toy, photo, etc. | No jewellery, studs or cosmetics |
| Hat with a brim (i.e. baseball cap) | Child to wear loose fitting top |
| Bottle, special beaker or cup | Cotton knickers/pants may be worn on day of surgery |
| 'Snuggly' blanket, dummy | Girls not to wear cosmetics for 1 week prior to surgery and |
| Nappies + wipes | 2 weeks afterwards. |
| Medication – checked + labelled | Hair should be tied well back with non-metallic band |
| Red book for under 5's | |
| Afternoon lists – overnight bag for child and 1 parent | |

## ARRANGEMENTS AT HOME

√ The legal form for consent to surgery must be signed by a parent. This may be done in clinic or on the day of surgery. Please ensure the parent is available on the operation day to sign it. NB. If parents are not married the mother may sign, or the father if his name is on the birth certificate after December 2003.

√ The child's parent or other adult very well known to the child should be free to look after the child for at least the first 48 hours after discharge, the child should not be left alone. Jobs outside the home may need to be rearranged.

√ It is advisable that 2 adults are in the car going home. We advise against children travelling home by bus.

√ Talk to your other children about the forthcoming admission, so they do not worry. Arrange for them to be looked after for the whole admission day.

√ Time off school/playschool. Squints – 1 week. Other surgery 1–7 days. Your nurse will advise you.

√ No swimming or ball games whilst the eyes still look red. Approximately 3–6 weeks for squint. Other activities and sports can be discussed with your nurse.

√ Please plan to have a few quiet days at home following surgery to allow him/her to settle back into routine. Young children in particular may be quite unsettled at home following even a day in hospital.

√ There must be an appropriate time for the recovery of the eye before holidays are taken, especially beach/swimming type holidays.

√ Ensure a good supply of Paracetamol syrup or tablets at home. You will be advised on the regime. Paediatric Ibuprufen is expensive but may be used if your doctor/nurse advises.

√ Remind your child about his/her admission 1–2 days beforehand. Deal honestly with any questions they ask, and in a positive way.

√ If your child becomes unwell for any reason, or develops a cough, sore throat or runny nose, please ring us for advice. The surgery may need to be postponed.

√ Be careful not to allow your child to overhear any talk about your own/family/friends negative or bad experiences whilst at home or on the telephone. Young children in particular may be confused or frightened by what they hear. Try to be straightforward and positive, and reassuring with your child. Young children are often very excited at the prospect of a hospital stay, but older children may be a little anxious.

√ You will need money to pay for the Car Park.

√ Food and drinks – Tea and coffee may be taken on the Ward, but no hot drinks are allowed in the Children's Room. Two resident parent(s)/family will be offered meals free of charge. There is also a WRVS canteen in Eye OPD, one in Main OPD and a dining room on the other side of the hospital.

√ Telephones – Mobile phones must be switched off and only used outside the building. There is a public telephone on the ward.

√ If you wish to make a comment or suggestion about the care you have received, please either talk to your nurse, put a comment in our Blue Book, or in the special red box on the ward, or write to the Chief Executive of the Hospital. We value you and your child's comments, as we are always looking to improve the service we provide.

Please ask us for any other advice you may need–we are happy to help!

Figure 17.8 Information for parents at pre-assessment.

*Pre assessments (cond.)*

- Parents are understandably concerned about their child feeling pain. The type of discomfort that is likely to be felt should be explained: e.g. sutures might feel prickly or itch; the eye may feel odd and uncomfortable. Types of analgesia that will be used should be discussed with parents and with the child too, where appropriate, and written information should be given. A pain tool must be used. (see 'General postoperative care' below).
- The comprehensive plan for discharge and care at home (see Fig. 17.9). This should be discussed so that the parents can start making appropriate arrangements, for example to re-arrange their jobs, ask friends or family to help with school 'runs' and so on. It is important that a parent is free and able to carry on the nursing of the child at home after surgery for the time required.
- It is not advisable for a child who has undergone eye surgery to go swimming until the eyes have completely healed. This makes going on a beach/camping type holiday inappropriate within the estimated time of recovery of the eye, depending on what surgery was carried out.
- The importance of involving other children in the family in the forthcoming event. Even very young siblings can become anxious, and their behaviour may reflect this if they are not given appropriate information about what is going on. Their help can be sought in caring for their sibling at home, to make them feel useful and included. Older children in the family require a straightforward explanation of what is happening and need to be given regular updates.
- Concurrent illness. Elective surgery will be postponed if the child is febrile or unwell for any reason, particularly with upper respiratory problems.

Giving clear information about what is going to happen, and instructions as to their role, actually helps children to relax and feel 'more' in control. After obtaining verbal consent from the parents and the child, the nurse can give them a simple, clear, methodical explanation of the day's events, using short sentences and language and detail appropriate to the child's age, stage, culture and life experience. It is prudent to avoid using emotive words; for example, try 'tube' instead of 'needle'. Teddies and dolls can be used to model the equipment the child will encounter, for example a theatre gown and cap, a plastic cannula ('tube'), name bands, a substitute blob of 'magic cream' (a local anaesthetic cream called Ametop), syringes, eye patches,

stethoscope, and anaesthetic equipment – tubing, face mask and the 'green balloon' (see Ch. 1). Therapeutic play, which the children usually enjoy, can then be used, under close supervision, to familiarise the child with key procedures:

- Explain that the child will need to be asleep for the doctors to 'mend their eye' (most young children do not realise this).
- Squeezing or huging the arm for the insertion of the cannula.
- Practicing keeping the arm very still.
- 'Anaesthetising' teddies or family members, using the mask, tubing and blowing up the green balloon.
- Playing with the stethoscope and syringes.
- Covering an eye to see how it feels to wear an eye patch.
- Practicing grimacing and relaxing the face.

If there is one available, the nurse could offer to show a specialist video about children and hospitals, e.g. *Judy Bear Goes to Theatre* (Donnelly 1995). This can help children understand accurately, but without stress, what will happen to them.

Young people aged 11–18 years have particular needs and when facing ophthalmic surgery will often express concerns about the appearance of their eyes afterwards. Teenagers can often seem rather preoccupied with how they look to their peers and friends and it is also important to them not to look 'different'. The nurse will need to offer information and reassurance. If resources allow, older teenagers may be offered a choice of being looked after in the adult section or children's ward; in the author's experience, most choose the paediatric area but some hospitals do have adolescent units.

Young people usually want and need to be given greater detail about the whole hospital admission, including the points above. Such knowledge helps to lessen feelings of powerlessness and loss of control, promotes trust and confidence, and aids the process of informed consent. It is also important to understand a teenager's often off-hand or abrupt manner, as this may well mask fear, pain or anxiety, which require sensitive handling. When awkward issues are raised, for example smoking, medication (the contraceptive pill, perhaps) or the use of rectal medication, discretion must be used. Teenage girls who wear eye make-up are asked to avoid this for one week prior to surgery, which is not usually a popular request!

## NHS TRUST

# PLAN FOR DISCHARGE OF CHILDREN ON EYE WARD-AND CARE AT HOME

Date.......................................    Date ...........................................

**DISCUSS AT PRE-ASSESSMENT**

- ☐ Main carer(s) present with child for first 48 hours post operatively.
- ☐ 2 adults in car on discharge.
- ☐ Transport arranged.
- ☐ Time off school/playschool.
- ☐ Domestic arrangements, job, etc.
- ☐ Advice re support of siblings.
- ☐ Advise quiet few days after surgery.
- ☐ Activities – especially swimming lessons and ball games.
- ☐ Holidays!  Suitability and timing.
- ☐ Behaviour management.
- ☐ Pain management at home.
- ☐ Paracetamol Elixir – supply at home.
- ☐ PR medication – consent obtained.
- ☐ Prescribe Ametop/Emla cream.
- ☐ Red/blue health record book – to be brought in.
- ☐ Bring in hat with a brim on op day.
- ☐ Ensure parents confident about giving eyedrops at home
- ☐ Consent – who has parental responsibility
- ☐ Give information sheet to family
- ☐ Overnight bag

**PRIOR TO DISCHARGE**

- ☐ Tolerating drinks.
- ☐ Eaten a snack.
- ☐ Passed urine.
- ☐ Up and about, playing.
- ☐ Op discussed by Dr/nurse/anaesthetist.
- ☐ Orthoptist visit- squints.
- ☐ IV Cannula removed.
- ☐ Give Star Chart (Reward scheme) Explain its use to parents.
- ☐ Advice given re care at home:
  - General childcare    ☐
  - Care of eyes    ☐
  - Give advice leaflets    ☐
- ☐ TTOs
- ☐ Complete Liaison Community Nurse form
- ☐ Give copy of the form to parent
- ☐ Arrange post op call for the following day
- ☐ Complete notes
- ☐ Time home
- ☐ Contact with HV/School Nurse/GP

**Sign** .....................................................

**Sign** ...........................................

Review Paediatric Team 4/06.

Figure 17.9 Plan for discharge and care at home.

The family should be shown around the ward and the available facilities explained. This orientation is important, as the children's eyes and perception will be affected by the operation and they may feel disorientated. Where desired by the family, they may visit the anaesthetic room; this can be very helpful in their preparation for admission. It is easy for nurses and other clinical staff to forget how frightening the 'highly technical' anaesthetic room can seem to others.

Parents should be advised that it is vital to the child's wellbeing that a parent, or close relative known to the child, stays with the child throughout the day of admission. Parental participation in the care of the child is encouraged, with help and support from the nurse.

Parents should be given a comprehensive list of items to bring in, particularly a favourite toy, cup and 'snuggly' blanket. The child should wear a loose top on the day of admission, so as not to drag clothing across the face when dressing to go home, and long hair must be tied well back. Parents are advised to bath their child and wash their child's hair the evening before admission.

For children with eye disorders, squints in particular, an orthoptic and/or consultant assessment are usually required during the month before surgery. The nurse should ensure that this is arranged. The nurse should also liaise with the anaesthetist or doctor if any significant health issues are identified with the child at the pre-admission visit, i.e. sickle cell disease or thalassaemia, significant respiratory, cardiac or systemic disease, or concerns with the child's medication. No problems should be left outstanding before the proposed admission in order to ensure smooth running of care for each family.

An appropriate risk assessment must be carried out if the child or parent has any increased health need, for example regarding mobility or manual handling. If any concerns arise at this or any other stage regarding child protection issue, the nurse should contact the senior nurse on duty and follow the hospital's child protection procedures.

Before going home the child can be given some colouring sheets to colour and bring back, or some stickers, to endorse a positive approach. Younger children are often very excited by what they have seen and heard during their visit! A visit to hospital appears to increase their 'street cred' with their friends and a nurse's theatre cap or mask is also a popular memento at 'show and tell' sessions at school.

## THE DAY OF ADMISSION

Parents require reassurance and help throughout the day in order to minimise their inevitable anxiety. When families arrive for admission they should be greeted by name, shown the allocated bed and encouraged to settle in, and the child to relax and play. Other families are introduced, whilst maintaining necessary confidentiality. Wherever possible, continuity of nursing care should be planned, so children do not see too many new faces during their admission.

Details from the pre-assessment are checked for significant changes and name bands may be placed around ankles, leaving the hands free. The family and child are then reminded of the morning's plans and are given the place and approximate time on the operating list. Every effort should be made to place children first on the list, on morning lists if at all possible, to limit their fasting period and waiting time.

The child is then prepared for theatre. This requires a calm approach. All procedures, however small, are undertaken after an explanation to the child and with a parent present to support the child. Young children, in particular, do not respond well to being rushed and it is worth developing the skill of working with time pressing, yet not rushing. The nurse should then enable the parents to participate in caring for their child as much as they feel able to during the day (Coyne 1996).

## PREPARATION FOR THEATRE

Some hospitals permit children to wear their own clothes to go to theatre but if not children should be unable to undress in private, whatever their age, and be able to put on a colourful theatre gown. These two seemingly small points often make the difference between keeping the child's cooperation and losing it. Children also need to know how they will look and feel after surgery and an explanation appropriate to their age and stage should be given.

A baseline set of vital signs is recorded. A local anaesthetic cream is then applied to veins, either on the back of the hands or the upper, outer aspect of the feet. Careful consideration should be given as to whether to apply cream with toddlers, as they may be very determined to get it off their hands or eat it. The cream is toxic to mucous membranes, so parents should be made aware of this and their vigilance sought. Applying the cream to the veins on the feet enables socks or soft slippers to cover the area and may solve the problem. A funny face may be drawn on the outer edge of the plastic covering over the cream, which the children enjoy. The nurse should discuss any concerns about the use of this cream with the anaesthetist.

Families are encouraged to play games and puzzles with their child and keep busy, or else time can pass slowly and a bored child is less likely to be happy or cooperative. Friendships may be quickly forged between children going through similar experiences and this, coupled with the general bustle of the ward, can be a welcome distraction for everyone.

A brief medical history and an examination of the child to confirm fitness for surgery will be carried out. Distraction with toys may facilitate this with young children. At this point, the affected eye is marked with an arrow on the forehead. On a busy ward with many children racing around, the child must be correctly identified. In children with squints, the doctor may not finalise the eye or eyes to be operated on until the day of surgery and the nurse needs to be very alert regarding the consent obtained and eye marked.

Informed consent is obtained from the child and the parent with parental responsibility, with information-giving and discussion, the process starting at the pre-admission visit. The anaesthetist also visits each family to discuss the anaesthetic, pain management (see Ch. 6) and any other concerns. It is common for parents to express fears about the anaesthetic and they should be given accurate information and reassurance. The pain tool will be shown to the family and its use explained. The recovery nurse should visit each family on the ward, as theirs is often the first face and voice the waking child will recognise. Teenagers may wish to be involved in these discussions about themselves and they should be treated with understanding and respect for their views and requests.

There may be preoperative eye drops to administer. These are often well tolerated by older children, but it may require much patience and ingenuity to successfully give them to younger children! Distraction with unusual toys and practising on teddy or a dolly first will encourage cooperation. Eye drops may cause a brief stinging sensation in the eye and an unpleasant taste in the mouth. The drops may also blur the vision or dilate the pupil, both of which are liable to cause clumsiness in the younger child. The nurse should be aware that the younger child will not like the effect of the drops and should be encouraging. A favourite toy held above a well-supported infant to distract the child, or a toy given to hold in each hand, may secure a few seconds for the nurse to instil an eye drop as the child gazes upwards. The child's safety during the instillation of eye drops must be maintained (see 'General postoperative care' and 'Specific advice on care of the eyes at home' below).

A full preoperative checklist is also completed, including the child's weight, allergies, and the type of comforts required by the child, e.g. thumb sucker (leave favoured finger/thumb free), dummy, teddy etc. The Ametop cream is removed at the appropriate time and patient and parents are well supported as the operation time approaches.

An oral premedication may be prescribed (e.g. midazolam 0.5 mg/kg, maximum 15 mg, 30–60 minutes before procedure), though whether such sedatives should be used in paediatric day surgery remains a subject of debate among clinical staff. Parents and the child, where appropriate, should be informed of the effects of any medication given. Midazolam does not always induce sleep, but often makes the child floppy and giggly. It is fast acting and short lasting, so the timing of administering it is crucial if it is to be effective. Following administration children must stay on their beds to avoid accidents, and travel to theatre by trolley or bed.

There are often times when children may resist a certain procedure or when their courage seems to run out at a seemingly insignificant point. Much sensitivity is required and a special box of distraction toys may be reserved in each area for these difficult moments.

## GOING TO THEATRE

The nurse should escort the child and one parent (or both where this is permitted) to the anaesthetic room at the required time. If only one parent is permitted then they should be asked to decide discreetly in advance who it should be. There should be a sensitive parting on the ward to minimise the stress to the child, and the actual words 'good-bye' should not be used, as they sound too final at this emotional time. Children who have not received a premedication may walk to theatre, or even ride in a play car – something toddlers particularly enjoy. They should take a favourite toy for comfort and a dummy or snuggly blanket (the nurse can leave these personal items in the recovery area for when they awake). Colourful pictures on the theatre suite walls encourage children to come in and provide a helpful focus for chat.

Families often describe arriving at the anaesthetic room as the most stressful part of the whole day, and nurses should be aware of this (Ellerton & Merriam 1994). There should be no waiting with children in the corridor or the anaesthetic room, so timing is important, but the nurse should take a toy and book to occupy the child if there is a short wait. The anaesthetic room can be made cheerful, with pictures (on the walls and, most helpfully, on the ceiling), gentle music, toys and books. Children can sit on the parent's lap or lie on the trolley as appropriate. Quiet encouragement from the nurse helps the child and parents recall what is required of them during the anaesthetic process. The child is anaesthetised via intravenous medication or anaesthetic gas, depending on the anaesthetist and protocol. Despite having been forewarned, the parent is often shocked at the speed at which the child loses consciousness and may become distressed and cry. Parents should be encouraged to give their child a quick kiss before leaving with the nurse. They should be assured of the normality of parental tears and, if both parents are there, they can often comfort each other best, the nurse discreetly keeping back.

After regaining their composure parents should be accompanied back to the ward (though not entering upset in front of other children awaiting surgery). This is now a good time for them to take a well deserved break. They should be reminded again of the estimated length of the operation and, if they leave the ward, of the time they should return.

It is good practice for the parents to be allowed into the recovery ward when their child awakes. Where hospital protocols do not permit this, each family should be told when their child has gone into the recovery area and again before the nurse leaves to collect the child. It is an immense relief to parents to know that the actual operation is over.

## TELLING PARENTS WHAT TO EXPECT AND HOW TO COPE

After their break it is important that the nurse should discuss ways in which parents can look after their child postoperatively. Parents will often be emotional seeing their child postoperatively, so it is beneficial to empower them to look after their child effectively and confidently. They will not succeed if they feel anxious and fearful. Parents should strive to maintain calm voices and demeanour to help the child to feel secure. The nurse should offer strategies to help them cope. This should include non-pharmacological methods – soothing the face by wiping it with a cool flannel, stroking the child's forehead rhythmically, singing to them, reading or telling a story. Parents can lie on the bed and cuddle their child to sleep or hold the child snuggled up on their lap. Often a small drink, as appropriate will settle the child for sleep. Parents should be asked not to overstimulate or fuss their children at this stage with lots of talk and presents, or they will not sleep. They need to understand that age and cognitive level will affect their child's perception of what is happening, for example their understanding of pain and how their eye feels.

## IMMEDIATE POSTOPERATIVE CARE

In the immediate postoperative period, the room should be kept dim and quiet to promote rest and sleep. Many children undergoing eye surgery are photosensitive for two or three days or so afterwards and subdued lighting allows them to relax their eyes.

Children may feel quite upset if they experience difficulty in seeing properly at first and parents need to calm and reassure them. Comments such as 'There's something in my eye', 'I can't see', or 'I can't open my eye!' are common, especially from the younger child. Parents should encourage the child to sleep; most children feel better after a sleep and are able to open their eyes with little trouble. Later, gentle play in bed will normalise things and relax the child, and a favourite video often works wonders in getting children to open their eyes almost without them thinking. The bed and the ward environment must be safe for children when they start mobilising, with no objects or furniture sticking out that may cause them to trip.

Any rubbing of the affected eye is to be discouraged and distraction with stories and play should be employed. The nurse should clean the eye using an aseptic technique if required and supply clean tissues for parents to wipe the child's cheeks, and parents are encouraged to wash their hands as necessary.

# SPECIFIC POINTS IN POSTOPERATIVE CARE

## Following surgery for squint

The parent will notice changes to the child's appearance. There will be no black eye or visible bruising as many parents expect, but the white of the eye will look red and congested. The eye may also be sticky from the antibiotic cream that is often applied at the end of surgery, which may also blur the vision when children first try to open their eyes. There may also be a slight purple discoloration of the eyelids, which will quickly disappear. Parents should not panic if the affected eye does not immediately look completely 'straight', as this may take some weeks. Occasionally, the child may complain of diplopia (double vision), which should be monitored but usually passes in 1–3 days. There may be blood in the tears, but this should stop within a day or two. An eye patch is not usually used postoperatively, in order to allow the child to see as soon as possible.

## Incision and curettage

If a meibomian cyst has been removed, an eye patch will cover the eye to absorb any blood loss. A younger child, who will not tolerate the loss of vision this causes, will often remove the pad rapidly. If it remains *in situ* it will be removed later as the doctor requests. The child may be clumsy with one eye covered and safety must be ensured, in or out of bed!

## Probing of the lacrimal ducts

The infant will have no visible effects of surgery and is often awake on return to the ward. The area around the eye may be sticky due to antibiotic cream applied in theatre.

# GENERAL POSTOPERATIVE CARE

If hospital protocol allows, the parent(s) should accompany the nurse to the recovery room to return the child to the ward. Analgesia such as fentanyl, (with assisted ventilation, 1 month to 12 years initially 15 µg/kg, then 1–3 µg as required by slow IV; child 12–18 years 0.3–3.5 mg then 100–200 µg as required), diclofenac (0.3–1.0 mg/kg daily in divided doses, for a maximum of 2 days; total dose not greater than 150 mg) and paracetamol suppositories (1–5 years 125–250 mg; 6–12 years 250–500 mg every 4–6 hours) may be given intra-operatively and this ensures a comfortable child on return to the ward. It is important that the parents and children, where appropriate, have given their informed consent for rectal analgesia to be administered. An intravenous antiemetic may also have been given i.e. ondansetron, (by slow IV injection 100 µg/kg, maximum 4 mg) for children 2–12 years. This medication should have been discussed in detail at pre-assessment with the child and parents, and again with the anaesthetist. Further analgesia such as paracetamol oral elixir (4–6 hourly, maximum 4 doses in 24 hours – see above) can be used and codeine or Oramorph may also be given as necessary. All drugs for children are calculated using the *British National Formulary for Children* (2005). A pain assessment tool should always be used throughout the child's stay in hospital to monitor pain levels and the effects of analgesia and no child should be allowed to suffer pain. Parents should be informed as to which drugs the child has received.

The child should be settled in bed with the parents by his side. Observations of the child's demeanour, colour, and heart and respiratory rate are made as appropriate. The eyes are checked according to the surgery carried out. Any blood loss or discharge from the eye is monitored and eye movements are observed. Any particular swelling, discoloration around the eye, or complaints of diplopia (double vision) are noted. The last may be indicated by remarks such as 'I can see two mummies!'

The child should be allowed to sleep in this quiet environment. The call bell, tissues and vomit bowl should be to hand. Young children should be carried to the toilet to pass urine whilst older children will need help and supervision as their vision may not be clear enough to go alone.

Small amounts of tepid fluids can be offered once the child is able to drink. Blackcurrant juice seems better tolerated than the more acidic orange juice. It should be borne in mind when reintroducing fluids that the incidence of postoperative nausea and vomiting following squint surgery can be high. A dry cracker or biscuit could be offered next and, if tolerated, a snack a little later on. It is important not to rush this process and overload a small stomach too quickly, as this may increase the likelihood of vomiting which is upsetting to all the family.

Parents should be offered regular short breaks for meals, drinks, fresh air or telephone calls, as they will find the experience of sitting with their child demanding and tiring. As further recovery takes place, the child can begin gentle play and get dressed; if children have glasses, these should be worn. To preserve access for medication or fluid replacement the intravenous cannula should not be removed until the child is up and about and discharge is imminent.

Eye drops may need to be given postoperatively, using the techniques described above (see 'Preparation for theatre'). However, once children are drinking again, they can be offered a drink to relieve the nasty taste that some eye drops give. Following a squint correction, a probing of the tear ducts or removal of meibomian cysts, either antibiotics, i.e. chloramphenicol, or a mixture of antibiotic and steroid such as Predsol N may be used. This is prescribed for 3–14 days, according to the doctor's wishes. Following squint surgery, an inspection of the eye movements is undertaken by the nurse, an orthoptist or the doctor and the findings noted. All patients undergoing eye surgery have the eyes checked by the nurse and if necessary the doctor too, and children must be able to open their eyes comfortably before going home. It is deemed good practice for the surgeon to speak to the family before discharge. The nurse should be present and ensure the family understands what is said about the surgery, prognosis and further appointments. This is particularly important, of course, if the families have English as their second language.

## DISCHARGE

A child who has met the discharge criteria (see Fig. 17.9) will be ready for discharge. The exact time spent in hospital will depend on the type of surgery performed, the individual recovery rate and partly on the family's ability to continue the nursing care required at home. However, most children are admitted as day cases on the understanding that if necessary the child will remain in hospital overnight with a resident parent. It is advisable to have two adults in the car going home especially if the journey is a long one.

Children should be included in the discussion about their care at home, as appropriate to their age and stage of development, since it helps them to feel in control and can also impress on them certain aspects of this care. This is especially indicated with young people, in order that they take responsibility for themselves and understand important points.

Often they will listen to advice better from the nurse, than from their parents.

All information and advice must be written down for the family to take away with them to refer to. This is very important, as they will receive a lot of information during the day and may well not be able to recall it all. When the family go, it should be on the understanding that they can telephone at any time for advice about the eye. It is good practice to speak to the parents the day following surgery to ensure all is well at home and offer further support as necessary.

Ideally children can look back on a hospital experience as positive, and build on it should they ever need to go back into hospital.

## SPECIFIC ADVICE ON THE CARE OF EYES AT HOME

The eye should be cleaned regularly, i.e. 3–4 times a day or more, as necessary, with sterile gauze and cooled, boiled water for the first week. This may be carried out prior to the instillation of eye drops to minimise disruption to the child. The method must be thoroughly explained and demonstrated by the nurse before discharge. A single gentle wipe is made across the eye from the inner aspect of the eye outwards and the process repeated as necessary. Hands must be washed before and after with soap and hot running water and the risk of cross infection explained.

In most cases eye drops or ointment will need to be administered. The technique should be explained and practised and the child's consent obtained if at all possible. The family should understand the effects of each eye drop. At home, it is important that the parent is well prepared before starting, and help from a partner or friend sought if possible. Other children should be well occupied. The child should lie back on the sofa or bed to support the head and neck, for ease and comfort. The parent's hands must then be washed before the cleaning and drops are administered. If more than one eye drop needs administration, 2–3 minutes should be left between drops. Ideally, the child is asked to look up, fix on an object or specific point, the lower lid is gently pulled down a little and the drop or a small amount of ointment instilled. Hands are then washed again. In reality, administering the eye drops is rarely easy with younger children and infants, so having two adults to carry out the task is easier and quicker, one holding and distracting the child and one to instil the drops/ointment. If they taste unpleasant, eating a small piece of soft bread or having a drink will help. Counting to ten slowly after each drop can help too, as it gives the child something to focus on whilst the drop absorbs. In younger children who resist the drops, a simple reward scheme often proves successful, for example using a 'star chart' (see Fig. 17.10). If any situation arises whereby the nurse and family anticipate real problems in complying with the regime, an arrangement can be made for the community paediatric nurse or health visitor to visit at home. Very occasionally a child will need to be readmitted to help the family cope with this treatment.

Following the removal of a cyst an eye pad may be left on until arriving home; this prevents dust and wind from entering the eye on the way home, causing the child to rub it. Parents are instructed to remove the eye pad at a prudent time, when the child has settled in again at home. The child should be prepared and help sought.

The pad and the Jelonet gauze are gently removed and discarded and hands washed. The eye is then gently cleaned, using the method described earlier, with great care being taken not to dislodge any blood clot present. Hands should be washed before and after this procedure. The eye should be cleaned 3–4 times during the first week using the method described above. Antibiotic ointment may be prescribed and this is administered by a parent gently putting the ointment on the affected area following cleansing.

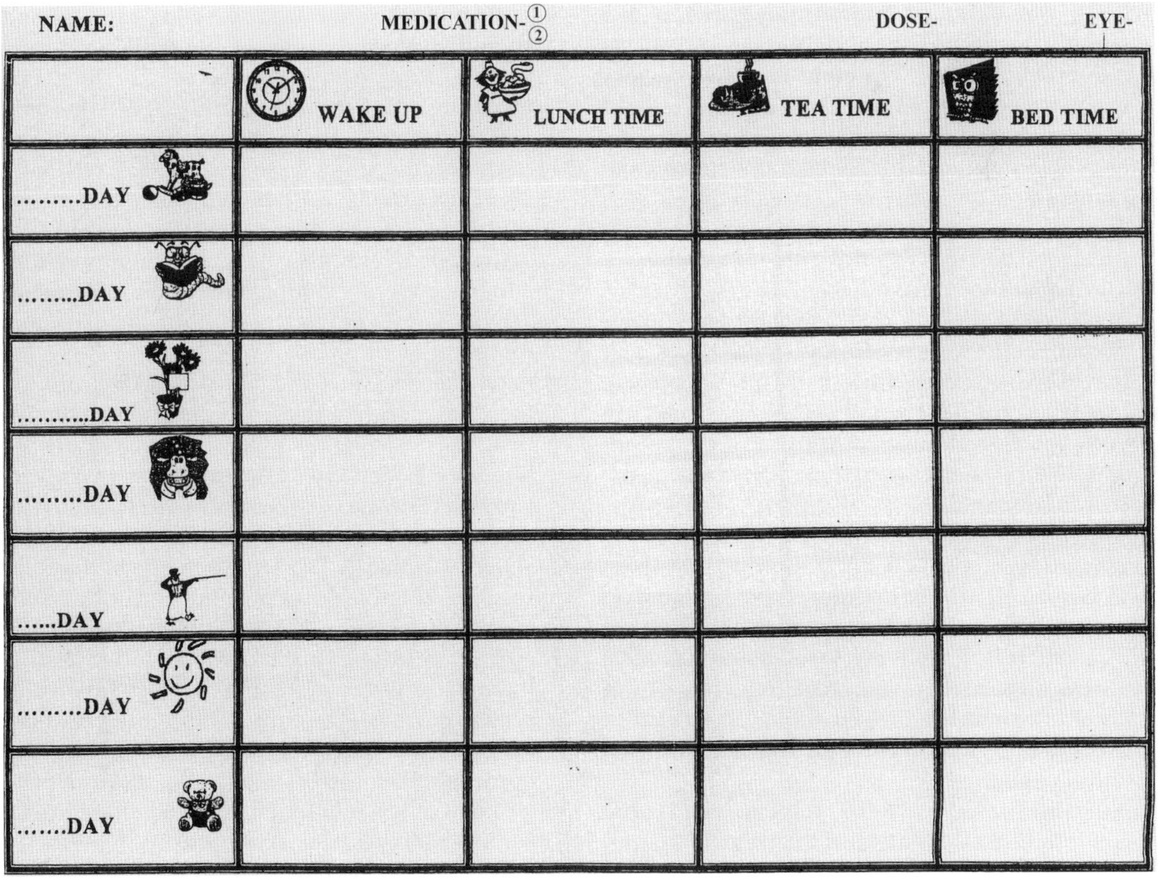

| NAME: | | MEDICATION-①② | | DOSE- | EYE- |
|---|---|---|---|---|---|
| | | WAKE UP | LUNCH TIME | TEA TIME | BED TIME |
| .........DAY | | | | | |
| .........DAY | | | | | |
| ..........DAY | | | | | |
| .........DAY | | | | | |
| ......DAY | | | | | |
| .........DAY | | | | | |
| ........DAY | | | | | |

Figure 17.10 Star chart. A 'star' or sticker is added for compliance with eye-drops and/or medication.

Whatever surgery has been undergone, the child should endeavour not to rub the eye or wipe it with used damp tissues, as this could lead to discomfort, soreness and infection.

## ADVICE ON CARE OF THE CHILD AT HOME
(see Fig. 17.9)

- The parents should be told how the eye will recover. Following squint surgery, the eye(s) will take approximately 1 month to settle down. Following cyst removal, healing should occur after approximately 1–3 weeks, depending upon the number, size and location of the cysts. If, following probing of the lacrimal ducts, the ducts are now patent, the infant should experience fewer symptoms but these may reappear if the child has an upper respiratory tract infection. Following any type of eye surgery, parents should also be aware of the signs of infection, i.e. a red, inflamed and sore eye with a discharge, the possibility of swollen eyelids or an alteration to vision. The child may also be generally unwell and have a fever. Parents should also be advised as to what to do if this situation arises, and relevant telephone numbers given to them.
- The child should be cared for by the parent/carer for at least the first 48 hours after discharge.
- The family should have 2–3 quiet days on returning home to allow the child to settle back into a regular pattern, as sleep and meal times will inevitably have been disrupted. This is especially important for babies and toddlers as they are very much creatures of routine. The parent should limit shopping trips, long journeys, visitors and so on.
- The child needs to take time off from school or playgroup. It must be borne in mind that these places can often be boisterous and hectic. Sand on the beach and sandpits are a particular hazard. As a general rule, it is advisable for children to have a week off school or playschool following squint corrections and 1–4 days off after cyst removal or other surgery, depending on individual needs and circumstances.
- No child should leave the ward in pain or discomfort. Parents are advised to give paracetamol or paediatric ibuprofen elixir regularly for at least the first 2–3 days to children recovering from squint surgery or surgery for multiple or large cysts and on an 'as required' basis to children who have undergone more minor procedures. Discomfort must be kept to a minimum to promote a quick return to normal activity and routine and help children to remain positive about their recent hospital experience. It should be remembered that young children cannot always articulate pain clearly, so pain or discomfort may manifest as altered behaviour, e.g. children may be uncooperative or tearful, hiding their face or screwing up their eyes.
- The child should have baths and not showers, to avoid splashing, and hair should not be washed for 3–4 days to avoid soap entering the eyes. Smoky, bright or windy places should be avoided to prevent the child rubbing the eye. It is advisable to wear a hat and/or sunglasses to shade the eyes, as many patients are photosensitive following eye surgery. Subdued light around the home also helps to keep the eyes and face relaxed.
- The child does not need to be kept in bed and should be able to resume gentle activities during the first few days. However, advice should be given regarding contact sports, school games, PE and swimming. The eye should be allowed to recover fully before these pastimes are resumed. As a general rule, children who have undergone squint surgery should not go swimming until the sclera look white again. This takes anything from 2 to 6 weeks, but families should be advised on activities on an individual basis, taking all factors into account.
- Parents need to realise, and research confirms the fact, that many children, especially the under 5s, demonstrate changes in behaviour on returning home, even after only 1 day in hospital (While & Crawford 1992, While & Wilcox 1994). This may manifest as 'clinginess', poor sleep patterns, anxiety or fearfulness. This will soon pass if the child receives lots of attention and encouragement from the parents. Other children in the family also need to feel particularly included at this time, in order to ensure that they feel loved and secure too. Older children and teenagers may also feel a sense of anticlimax when they get home and feel 'out of sorts' and perhaps a little irritable or tearful. They should be offered reassurance that this stage does pass.
- Girls who use cosmetics should be advised not to do so until the eye is completely healed again.

## FOLLOW-UP

Each family should receive a telephone call on the day following surgery to ensure all is well. Advice can then be given on problems that may have arisen. It is very reassuring to parents to receive this call and the assurance is given that they may telephone at any time for advice. This call and any action taken must be recorded in the case notes.

Children with squints are seen in a joint orthoptic/medical clinic within 1–2 weeks of surgery and are followed up long term, as further growth and development affect the eye. Children who have undergone surgery for cataract and glaucoma are similarly followed up on a long term basis, in order to achieve the best sight possible in both eyes. Other children may be given a follow-up appointment depending on the doctor's instructions.

## TRAUMA

A wide variety of accidents in childhood cause trauma to the eye. Trauma can also be the result of an assault with the attendant medico-legal implications (Foss 2001). Serious damage to the visual system may also occur, as a result of non-accidental injury, for example, by shaking the infant causing retinal haemorrhage (Moore 2000). Injuries to the eyes can be broadly divided into two categories, blunt and penetrating injuries, and may be minor or severe. All children with serious eye injuries should be referred to an Ophthalmic Unit, and it is these injuries that will be addressed in this section.

### Blunt injury

Common causes of a blunt injury include a fall or being hit by a tennis racquet or fast-moving ball. Children are less aware of danger than adults and are especially vulnerable and can easily be led into hazardous situations (Roper-Hall 1987).

The orbital bones offer good protection to the eye but when a blunt injury occurs the eye is flattened, and bruising occurs in the eyelid and conjunctiva (Kirton & Richardson 1987). These haemorrhages may resolve spontaneously. Bleeding into the anterior chamber (hyphaema), which can often be seen clearly, may lead to glaucoma. If a hyphaema does occur, the child needs to have complete bed rest for several days to promote healing, allow the blood to re-absorb and prevent a secondary bleed, which may occur up to 10 days after the initial event. This

serious complication can lead to raised intraocular pressure and staining of the cornea by blood (Phillips et al 1994). Various other structures, including the iris and the retina, may tear. An eye following trauma has an increased risk of retinal detachment. If torn, the retina can then also detach and injury to the optic nerve and macula may lead to permanent visual loss. A blow to the eye may also cause damage to the lens, or even a fracture of the orbital floor, which is detectable on a CT scan.

### Penetrating injury

This type of injury may occur when, for example, a pencil, scissors, glass or pellet from a gun enters the eye and the internal structures of the eye may be seriously damaged.

A traumatic cataract may occur within hours of a penetrating injury or months later. Lens matter may ooze out into the anterior chamber and cause secondary glaucoma. Trauma to the posterior part of the eye may result in retinal or optic nerve damage. Immediate surgery is often necessary following a penetrating injury (Foss 2001). An intraocular foreign body needs surgical removal in order to prevent infection and other complications, e.g. siderosis whereby a fragment of metal in the eye rusts.

Sympathetic ophthalmitis (severe uveitis in the uninjured eye) is a rare immunological response, though poorly understood, that may occur in the uninjured eye, and is a serious complication of any major eye injury. It can occur at any time. A severely injured eye with no chance of regaining useful vision may be removed to try to prevent this occurring.

There may also be trauma to the eyelids following a laceration or a burn. The lacrimal system of the eye can be damaged when a pet, often a dog, jumps up and scratches at the face, a common injury in young children.

### The specific care of trauma

The considerations described below should be taken into account by the children's nurse.

**Care of the child**    Following the incident, the child will probably be taken to a hospital Accident and Emergency department and then may have spent some hours reaching the specialised Eye Unit. This will have been frightening and distressing. The child may well be tired and disgruntled on arrival.

Pain, discomfort and other unpleasant symptoms such as watering eyes (epiphoria) and sensitivity to light (photophobia) may be experienced. The child will often appear pale and quiet and may well vomit. It is a huge psychological shock for children if their sight is affected. If a fracture of an orbital bone occurs, this will cause pain and other symptoms – double vision (diplopia), reduced eye movements and diminished facial sensation on the affected side.

If the child has sustained life threatening injuries, having been involved in a road traffic accident for example, stabilising the child's general condition will take precedence, but it is essential for the eyes to be checked if an injury is suspected. It is easy for an eye injury to be missed as deep injuries may seal themselves and not cause great pain.

If the child has sustained a head injury, regular neurological observations must be carried out to monitor consciousness levels. Pharmacological dilatation of the pupil may confuse these observations, so it should not be undertaken unless requested by the ophthalmologist in charge. If mydriatic drugs to dilate the pupil and rest the eye have been administered when a perforating injury has occurred, it may lead to the collapse of the anterior chamber.

Treatment with eye drops is prescribed on an individual basis perioperatively, but treatment is also likely to include antibiotics, steroids and a mydriatic drug e.g. homatropine 1–2%. Some drops may be required every hour to start with, which may be particularly difficult to administer to a distraught toddler or child, and this proves demanding for the parents too. If the injury was sustained in the evening or night, the child may well be exhausted and uncooperative by this stage, making it difficult to carry out an examination and other necessary tests and procedures. The child should be encouraged not to rub the affected eye and an eye shield used if there is a penetrating wound. If the shield is tolerated, it will reduce the child rubbing the eye and identifies the injured eye to other clinical staff.

It is important to give the child effective analgesia to minimise any discomfort and promote rest. Even if the child says the eye is 'not really hurting' if asked, body language often belies this – the child, looking uncomfortable, unsmiling and head down, may screw up or covers the eye and say, for example: 'It only itches' or, 'It scratches me'. In those circumstances, a simple analgesic, such as paracetamol (120 mg–1 g, 4–6 hourly, maximum 4 doses per 24 hours) or iboprufen (50–200 mg, 3–4 times daily preferably after food) will usually ease the discomfort and restore the child's appetite and desire to play. A pain tool should be used to monitor the child's pain throughout the admission.

Children should be orientated to their surroundings and careful attention paid to all aspects of their safety. Independence should be encouraged, but the nurse should be aware that the child may be relying more heavily upon non-visual senses. Gentle playing in bed if necessary, in a quiet area without bright lights and with toys, books or videos, will help the child to relax.

If the child has to undergo a CT scan or MRI scan the nurse will need to prepare the child and family for this investigation.

**Care of the parents**   The rapid admission of a child to hospital is highly traumatic for parents. They may be extremely worried and fearful at the prospect of surgery and all that it involves, the possible outcome and whether the child's sight will be lost. It is always very hard for a parent to see their own child injured and parents often feel a variety of emotions. They may be angry if the accident was caused by another adult or child, made worse if that person is a friend or a member of their own family. They can feel very guilty and remorseful if they themselves were responsible for the accident in some way, or feel that they were. Parents may have other children and domestic issues to worry about too and are usually tired and anxious on arrival. The family needs great help and support. The nurse needs to be very sensitive to all the issues involved and should support the parents to help to take care of their child at a level they feel able to, at this difficult time.

**History and examination**   A very careful history must be taken, to ascertain the full extent of injuries. This is extremely important, as a deeply penetrating wound may be relatively painless whereas a more superficial scratch, for example, can be exquisitely painful.

Children can find it hard to give an accurate account of an incident, especially if they fear punishment, are protecting their friends or siblings or are in a very distressed state, which makes them difficult to assess. They may not recall an object entering the eye or be old enough to be able to explain the incident.

The nurse may need to help the doctor examine the child and assess his or her vision, which requires great skill and ingenuity. Distraction with intriguing toys and practising the examination on the child's teddy before attempting to examine the child may help.

Large charts showing the anatomy of the eye and a model eye will help to clarify the situation for the family and improve their understanding of the injury sustained.

**Preoperative care (see 'The day of admission' and 'Preparation for theatre')**    If time is limited for the nurse to prepare the child for surgery, the priorities include administering analgesia as appropriate, obtaining parental and patient consent for surgery getting details of when the child last ate and drank, an accurate weight, the child's current medication, known allergies and the child's and family's medical history. It is essential to check the child's tetanus immunisation status with the parent (or the GP if necessary), as a tetanus booster may need to be given in some cases of perforating injury or lacerated ocular tissue.

Even if time is short, it is important that all anaesthetic procedures are explained to the child and parents. A local anaesthetic cream (e.g. Ametop) should be applied to appropriate veins prior to preoperative cannulation. A 'nurse's box' with teddies and modelling equipment will help acquaint the child with forthcoming procedures and surgery and the child's own favourite toy will provide comfort.

Nurses should support and comfort the parents in an empathetic way, give information about the predicted events over the next few hours, provide refreshments, discuss pressing domestic issues and advise on how to talk to other children at home about the incident. Worried parents often weep and may take their anger and frustration out on the nurses, who need to use tact and diplomacy when caring for them.

**Specific postoperative care (see trauma)**

- Analgesia needs to be effective postoperatively, as a child in pain or discomfort will be uncooperative, inactive and in low spirits.
- Care of the eye will include cleaning of the eye and administration of eye drops and other medication (see below, 'Preparation for theatre' and 'Specific advice on the care of eyes at home').

- The ophthalmologist will regularly check the affected eye. It is worth practising the slit-lamp examination with the child (and teddy) before the event, as the child may need to sit or kneel still for this to happen successfully. As always, parental presence is important as is distraction with toys.
- Children should be offered toys and games when they feel ready to play. This will avoid boredom and help them cope with the obvious stress of the admission.
- If visual loss has occurred it will take children time to adjust to this. They should be orientated to their environment and encouraged to be safely independent.
- Communication needs to be open and honest between clinical staff and the parents and child. Children need information about their condition, the amount of detail depending upon their age and stage of development, culture and previous life experience. This needs to be done with the greatest sensitivity, in consultation with the parents, particularly if the injury is severe.
- Some children will be afraid of what lies ahead of them and whether they will lose their vision or even the eye itself. This may then lead to fears of how their friends and peer group may react, and if bullying will ensue. Children may not even want to look in a mirror, fearing what they may look like.
- The child and parents often have a grief type of reaction to the accident over the coming days or weeks, and experience emotions similar to bereavement: shock, denial, anger and then gradual acceptance. It will take a longer period of time for the child and family to adjust emotionally to any permanent visual impairment. Help may be needed from a psychologist.
- The family must be kept accurately informed of any progress made and expected outcomes, namely the cosmetic result, the quality of vision and possible further developments. The time ahead may be very challenging for them all.
- Practical help must be given to parents whose child remains in hospital for a longer period. They must have frequent breaks and be encouraged to go home to rest and support other family members, without being made to feel guilty at leaving the injured child.

- Visits by siblings, the wider family and friends are encouraged as the family desire, as appropriate with the child's condition.
- An interpreter must be sought if the family do not speak or understand English well. It must also be remembered that some people of different cultures will respond to permanent visual loss in different ways, though not always with understanding and acceptance.

## Management of Discharge

Plans for discharge home must be made well in advance if the family are to receive seamless care and cope well at home. Parents should be fully advised about how to manage the child's return to normal life and activity.

This advice should include demonstrations by the nurse and sufficient practice by the parent, of instilling eye drops and cleaning the eye under supervision until they feel confident. A 'star chart' can be useful for encouraging younger children to comply with having eye drops (see Fig. 17.10) and helpful for parents to follow the treatment regime accurately, which may be complicated. The wearing of an eye shield will depend on the injury, but overuse may make it difficult for the child to learn how to cope without it (see 'Specific advice on the care of eyes at home' above).

The management of analgesia and safety issues must be discussed and, importantly, the emotional care of the child at home. The child's general well-being is very likely to be disrupted following such a traumatic event and parents need to know to offer much understanding and reassurance to their child. Siblings will also need extra support, particularly if they have been very upset by the accident or involved in it.

The parents will also need to know how best to integrate the child back into appropriate schooling, sports and recreation, which must be based on individual circumstances and need. All information should be discussed and repeated as often as necessary and parents should also have written information to refer to at home, including hospital telephone numbers.

The school nurse, the health visitor and GP should be contacted as appropriate, in advance, to arrange for their help in supporting the child in school and at home; the community paediatric nurses are well equipped to help children at home, but ongoing support by other agencies may also be needed. It may also be helpful for the family to meet and talk with another family who has been through a similar experience.

Parents may also need information regarding help available from agencies such as Social Services, the RNIB and local 'self help' groups.

Following discharge, regular telephone calls by the nurse to offer support to the family for the first few months are always appreciated.

## CONCLUSION

Paediatric ophthalmology is an area of paediatric nursing that is neither well known nor well researched. The needs of children attending or being admitted to an Eye Unit require identification if families are to receive the excellent paediatric care they deserve and avoid being a somewhat neglected group of patients. The impact on a family of having an infant or child with an eye disorder or injury can be very great. Vision is extremely important to growing children, who are learning rapidly about the world around them. In this speciality, paediatric nurses have a wonderful opportunity to truly be advocates of the families in their care.

## ACKNOWLEDGEMENTS

I would like to thank my husband David Bradshaw and Miss Anne Denning FRCOphth for their help in preparing this chapter.

## References

Beringer A 1991 A study to explore parents' needs for information, before their child's admission to hospital. Unpublished MSc thesis. King's College, London

Bowlby J 1953 Child care and the growth of love. Penguin, London

British National Formulary for Children (BNF) 2005 BMJ Publishing Group, London

Caress A 2003 Giving information to patients. Nursing Standard 17(43): 47–54

Charles-Edwards I 2003 Power and control over children and young people. Paediatric Nursing 15(6): 37–43

Coyne I 1996 Parent participation: a concept analysis. Journal of Advanced Nursing 23: 733–740

Dearmun A 1994 Defining differences: children's day surgery. Surgical Nurse 7(6): 7–11

Department of Health 1989 Children Act. The Stationery Office, London

Department of Health 1991 Welfare of children in hospital. HMSO, London

Department of Health 1996 The patients' charter. HMSO, London

Department of Health 2003 National service framework for children. Standard for Hospital Services. HMSO, London

Donnelly J 1995 Judy bear goes to theatre. Video. JB Productions, Garswood

Ellerton ML, Merriam C 1994 Preparing children and families psychologically for day surgery: an evaluation. Journal of Advanced Nursing 19: 1057–1062

Foss A 2001 Essential ophthalmic surgery. Butterworth/Heinemann, Oxford

Kelly M, Adkins L 2003 Ingredients for a successful paediatric pre-operative care process. AORN Journal 77(5): 1006–1011

Kirton M, Richardson M 1987 Ophthalmic nursing, 3rd edn. Baillière Tindall, London

Lambert S, Drack A 1996 Survey of ophthalmology. Major Review Infantile Cataracts 40(6): 427–458.

Mills M 1998 Perianaesthesia care of adult and paediatric strabismus surgery patients. Journal of Peri-anaesthesia Nursing 13(1): 16–23

Moore A 2000 Paediatric ophthalmology. BMJ Publishing Group, London

Nethercott S 1993 A concept for all the family. Family centred care: a concept analysis. Professional Nurse (September): 794–797

Olitsky S, Nelson L 1998 Common ophthalmologic concerns in infants and children. Paediatric Clinics of North America 45(4): 993–1013

Phillips C, Clark C, Tsukahara S 1994 Ophthalmology. Baillière Tindall, London

Roper-Hall M 1987 Eye emergencies. Churchill Livingstone, Edinburgh

Ryder A 2006 The orbit and extraocular muscles. In: Marsden J (ed) Ophthalmic care. Wiley, England

Stollery R 1997 Ophthalmic nursing, 2nd edn. Blackwell, Oxford

Thornes R 1991 Just for the day. Caring for children in the health services. NAWCH, London

While A, Crawford J 1992 Day surgery expediency or quality care. Paediatric Nursing 4: 18–20

While A, Wilcox V 1994 Paediatric day surgery: day-case unit admission compared with general paediatric ward admission. Journal of Advanced Nursing 19: 52–57

## Further reading

Department of Health 2001 The Essence of care. HMSO, London

Doverty N 1992 Therapeutic use of play in hospital. British Journal of Nursing 1(2): 77–81

Dreger V 1998 Detection and treatment of strabismus. Journal of the American Society of Ophthalmic Registered Nurses 23(3): 95

Huddleston K 1994 Strabismus repair in the paediatric patient. AORN Journal 60(5): 754–760

Khaw P, Elkington A 1999 ABC of eyes. BMJ Publishing Group, London

Knowles J 1997 Pre-assessment of the day surgery patient. British Journal of Theatre Nursing 17(4): 16–18

Smith J, Garner T 2001 Focus on children's day care – past, present and future. Journal of One Day Surgery (Spring): 10–12

# Index

Please note that page references to non-textual information such as Figure will be in *italic* print